Bipolar Disorder

Guest Editors

JEFFREY I. HUNT, MD
DANIEL P. DICKSTEIN, MD

CHILD AND ADOLESCENT PSYCHIATRIC CLINICS OF NORTH AMERICA

www.childpsych.theclinics.com

Consulting Editor
HARSH K. TRIVEDI, MD

April 2009 • Volume 18 • Number 2

SAUNDERS an imprint of ELSEVIER, Inc.

W.B. SAUNDERS COMPANY
A Division of Elsevier Inc.

Elsevier Inc. • 1600 John F. Kennedy Boulevard • Suite 1800 • Philadelphia, Pennsylvania 19103-2899
http://www.childpsych.theclinics.com

CHILD AND ADOLESCENT PSYCHIATRIC CLINICS OF NORTH AMERICA Volume 18, Number 2
April 2009 ISSN 1056–4993, ISBN-13: 978-1-4377-0459-4, ISBN-10: 1-4377-0459-X

Editor: Sarah E. Barth
Developmental Editor: Donald Mumford

Child and Adolescent Psychiatric Clinics of North America (ISSN 1056-4993) is published quarterly by Elsevier Inc., 360 Park Avenue South, New York, NY 10010-1710. Months of issue are January, April, July, and October. Business and Editorial Offices: 1600 John F. Kennedy Boulevard, Suite 1800, Philadelphia, PA 19103-2899. Customer Service Offices: 6277 Sea Harbor Drive, Orlando, FL 32887-4800. Periodicals postage paid at New York, NY and additional mailing offices. Subscription prices are $238.00 per year (US individuals), $378.00 per year (US institutions), $122.00 per year (US students), $270.00 per year (Canadian individuals), $456.00 per year (Canadian institutions), $156.00 per year (Canadian students), $321.00 per year (international individuals), $456.00 per year (international institutions), and $156.00 per year (international students). International air speed delivery is included in all *Clinics* subscription prices. All prices are subject to change without notice. **POSTMASTER:** Send address changes to *Child and Adolescent Psychiatric Clinics of North America*, Elsevier Periodicals Customer Service, 11830 Westline Industrial Drive, St. Louis, MO 63146. **Customer Service: 1-800-654-2452 (US). From outside the United States, call 1-314-453-7041. Fax: 1-314-453-5170. E-mail: JournalsCustomerService-usa@elsevier.com (for print support) or journalsonlinesupport-usa@elsevier.com (for online support).**

Reprints. For copies of 100 or more of articles in this publication, please contact the Commercial Reprints Department, Elsevier Inc., 360 Park Avenue South, New York, New York 10010-1710 Tel.: (212) 633-3812; Fax: (212) 462-1935, e-mail: reprints@elsevier.com.

Child and Adolescent Psychiatric Clinics of North America is covered in *MEDLINE/PubMed (Index Medicus), ISI, SSCI, Research Alert, Social Search, Current Contents,* and *EMBASE/Excerpta Medica.*

Printed in the United States of America.

Contributors

CONSULTING EDITOR

HARSH K. TRIVEDI, MD
Site Training Director and Director of Adolescent Services, E.P. Bradley Hospital;
Assistant Professor of Psychiatry and Human Behavior (Clinical), Brown Medical School;
President, Rhode Island Council for Child and Adolescent Psychiatry, East Providence,
Rhode Island

CONSULTING EDITOR EMERITUS

ANDRÉS MARTIN, MD, MPH

FOUNDING CONSULTING EDITOR

MELVIN LEWIS, MBBS, FRCPSYCH, DCH

GUEST EDITORS

JEFFREY I. HUNT, MD
Director of Training, Child and Adolescent Psychiatry Fellowship and Combined
Pediatrics/Psychiatry/Child Psychiatry Residency, EP Bradley Hospital, Warren Alpert
Medical School of Brown University, East Providence, Rhode Island

DANIEL P. DICKSTEIN, MD
Pediatric Mood, Imaging, & Neurodevelopment Program (PediMIND), EP Bradley Hospital,
Bradley/Hasbro Children' s Research Center, Warren Alpert Medical School of Brown
University, East Providence, Rhode Island

AUTHORS

DAVID AXELSON, MD
Department of Psychiatry, Western Psychiatric Institute and Clinic, University
of Pittsburgh Medical Center, Pittsburgh, Pennsylvania

ANDY BELDEN, PhD
Post-Doctoral-Fellow, Department of Psychiatry, Washington University School of
Medicine in St. Louis, St. Louis, Missouri

BORIS BIRMAHER, MD
Department of Psychiatry, Western Psychiatric Institute and Clinic, University
of Pittsburgh Medical Center, Pittsburgh, Pennsylvania

ALISON C. BRAZEL, BS
Pediatric Mood, Imaging, & Neurodevelopment Program (PediMIND), EP Bradley
Hospital, Bradley/Hasbro Children's Research Center, Warren Alpert Medical School
of Brown University, East Providence, Rhode Island

GABRIELLE A. CARLSON, MD
Professor of Psychiatry and Pediatrics, Director, Child and Adolescent Psychiatry, Stony
Brook University School of Medicine, Stony Brook, New York

MELISSA P. DELBELLO, MD, MS
Vice-Chair for Clinical Research, Associate Professor of Psychiatry and Pediatrics,
Department of Psychiatry, University of Cincinnati, College of Medicine, Cincinnati, Ohio

DANIEL P. DICKSTEIN, MD
Pediatric Mood, Imaging, & Neurodevelopment Program (PediMIND), EP Bradley
Hospital, Bradley/Hasbro Children's Research Center, Warren Alpert Medical School
of Brown University, East Providence, Rhode Island

STEPHEN V. FARAONE, PhD
Professor of Psychiatry, Neuroscience, and Physiology, Departments of Psychiatry,
Neuroscience and Physiology, SUNY Upstate Medical University, Syracuse, New York

JEAN A. FRAZIER, MD
Child and Adolescent Neurodevelopment Initiative, University of Massachusetts Medical
School; Department of Psychiatry, UMASS Memorial Medical Center, Worcester,
Massachusetts

ANDREW J. FREEMAN, BS
Department of Psychology, University of North Carolina, Chapel Hill, North Carolina

IRA GLOVINSKY, PhD
Adjunct Professor, Department of Education, Madonna University, Livonia, Michigan; and
Director, Mood Disorder Program, Interdisciplinary Center for the Family, West
Bloomfield, Michigan

LISA D. GOLDBERG, BA
Pediatric Mood, Imaging, & Neurodevelopment Program (PediMIND), EP Bradley
Hospital, Bradley/Hasbro Children's Research Center, Warren Alpert Medical School
of Brown University, East Providence, Rhode Island

TINA R. GOLDSTEIN, PhD
Assistant Professor, Department of Child and Adolescent Psychiatry, Western Psychiatric
Institute and Clinic, University of Pittsburgh Medical Center, Pittsburgh, Pennsylvania

ALLISON G. HARVEY, PhD
Associate Professor, Department of Psychology; and Director, Sleep and Psychological
Disorders Laboratory, University of California, Berkeley, California

JEFFREY I. HUNT, MD
Director of Training, Child and Adolescent Psychiatry Fellowship and Combined
Pediatrics/Psychiatry/Child Psychiatry Residency, EP Bradley Hospital, Warren Alpert
Medical School of Brown University, East Providence, Rhode Island

MELISSA McKEOWN JENKINS, MA
Department of Psychology, University of North Carolina, Chapel Hill, North Carolina

GAGAN JOSHI, MD
Scientific Director, Pervasive Developmental Disorders Program, Clinical and Research Programs in Pediatric Psychopharmacology, Massachusetts General Hospital; and Instructor in Psychiatry, Harvard Medical School, Boston, Massachusetts

ROBERT KOWATCH, MD, PhD
Professor, Departments of Psychiatry and Pediatrics, Cincinnati Children's Hospital Medical Center, Cincinnati, Ohio

MELISSA LOPEZ-LARSON, MD
The Brain Institute, University of Utah, Salt Lake City; Department of Psychiatry, University of Utah Medical School, Salt Lake City, Utah

JOAN L. LUBY, MD
Associate Professor, Department of Psychiatry, Washington University School of Medicine in St. Louis, St. Louis, Missouri

ERIC MICK, ScD
Assistant Professor of Psychiatry, Department of Psychiatry, Massachusetts General Hospital and Harvard Medical School, Boston, Massachusetts

ALANA MOSES, BA
Clinical Research Coordinator, Department of Pediatric Psychopharmacology, Massachusetts General Hospital, Cambridge, Massachusetts

JAYASREE J. NANDAGOPAL, MD
Assistant Professor, Department of Psychiatry, University of Cincinnati, College of Medicine, Cincinnati, Ohio

MANI N. PAVULURI, MD, PhD
Associate Professor of Psychiatry, University of Illinois at Chicago, Chicago, Illinois

MONA POTTER, MD
Child and Adolescent Psychiatry Fellow, Massachusetts General Hospital and McLean Hospital, Cambridge, Massachusetts

SUSAN RESKO, MM
Executive Director, Child and Adolescent Bipolar Foundation, Wilmette, Illinois

REGINA SALA, MD
Department of Psychiatry, Western Psychiatric Institute and Clinic, University of Pittsburgh Medical Center, Pittsburgh, Pennsylvania

MINI TANDON, DO
Post-Doctoral-Fellow, Department of Psychiatry, Washington University School of Medicine in St. Louis, St. Louis, Missouri

JANINE TERRY, BA
The Brain Institute, University of Utah, Salt Lake City, Utah

AMY E. WEST, PhD
Assistant Professor of Psychology in Psychiatry, University of Illinois at Chicago, Chicago, Illinois

TIMOTHY WILENS, MD
Director, Substance Abuse Services, Pediatric Psychopharmacology, Massachusetts General Hospital; and Associate Professor, Department of Psychiatry, Harvard Medical School, Boston, Massachusetts

JANET WOZNIAK, MD
Director, Pediatric Bipolar Disorder Clinical and Research Program, Massachusetts General Hospital, Cambridge; and Assistant Professor of Psychiatry, Harvard Medical School, Boston, Massachusetts

ERIC A. YOUNGSTROM, PhD
Associate Professor of Psychology and Psychiatry, Associate Director of the Center for Excellence in Research and Treatment of Bipolar Disorder, Department of Psychology, University of North Carolina, Chapel Hill, North Carolina

Cover artwork Courtesy of Socorro Rivera G., Mexico City, Mexico

Contents

Before the last 150 years, the use of the term mania to mean any kind of agitated state and the term childhood to include people up to their early 20s make historical identification of manic-depression in children difficult. Not long after Kraepelin's seminal work was published, similar syndromes were identified in youth, usually adolescents. Interestingly, however, the question of whether preadolescent mania should be broadly or narrowly defined–the so-called bipolar controversy–has been an issue for at least 50 years. Although the question of whether and how a disorder characterized by discrete episodes of mania and depression with periods of relative normality between episodes relates to one characterized by more fluctuating and intense mood lability/dysregulation remains unanswered, the work of researchers in the twenty-first century will be to understand not only symptoms of bipolar disorder but also how it develops and how emotion regulation relates to both the development of bipolar disorder and to other conditions that are characterized by dysregulated emotion.

Pediatric bipolar disorder (BPD) significantly affects the normal emotional, cognitive, and social development. The course of children and adolescents with BPD is manifested by frequent changes in symptoms polarity showing a dimensional continuum of bipolar symptoms severity from subsyndromal to mood syndromes meeting full DSM-IV criteria. Thus, early diagnosis and treatment of pediatric bipolar is of utmost importance.

The growing literature shows the pervasiveness and importance of comorbidity in youth with bipolar disorder (BPD). For instance, up to 90% of youth with BPD have been described to manifest comorbidity with attention-deficit hyperactivity disorder. Multiple anxiety, substance use, and disruptive behavior disorders are the other most commonly reported comorbidities with BPD. Moreover, important recent data highlight the importance of obsessive–compulsive and pervasive developmental illness in the context of BPD. Data suggest that not only special developmental relationships are operant in the context of comorbidity but also that the presence of comorbid disorders with BPD results in a more severe clinical condition. Moreover, the presence of comorbidity has therapeutic implications for the treatment response for both BPD and the associated comorbid disorder. Future longitudinal studies to address the relationship and the impact of comorbid disorders on course and therapeutic response over time are required in youth with BPD.

Bipolar disorder (BPD) is a severe and chronic disorder, ranked among the top 10 leading causes of disability worldwide. Bipolar spectrum disorders with onset in childhood and adolescence have a particularly severe course, including more suicide attempts and greater comorbidity. The evidence accrued to date indicates that sleep disturbances are common among youth with BPD. Moreover, sleep problems may be an early marker for BPD, a distinguishing feature of BPD, and a contributor to relapse. The evidence reviewed highlights that sleep problems are associated with a range of serious adverse consequences, including difficulty in regulating affect in the daytime and difficulties with cognitive functions, such as memory, learning, attention, and concentration. Evidence reviewed also points to sleep disturbance as one possible contributor to weight gain, comorbid substance use, and impulsivity. The implications for intervention are explored, and a multicomponent sleep intervention for youth with BPD is outlined.

This article describes what is known about the epidemiology of suicidal ideation and behavior in pediatric bipolar disorder. Risk factors associated with suicidality in this population are reviewed in detail. Clinical recommendations for assessment, management and treatment are provided based on the literature to date.

The overarching goal of this article is to examine the current best evidence for assessing bipolar disorder (BPD) in children and adolescents and provide a comprehensive, evidence-based approach to diagnosis. Evidence-based assessment strategies are organized around the "3 Ps" of clinical assessment: *Predict* important criteria or developmental trajectories, *Prescribe* a change in treatment choice, and inform *Process* of treating the youth and his/her family. The review characterizes BPD in youths— specifically addressing bipolar diagnoses and clinical subtypes; it then provides an actuarial approach to assessment using prevalence of disorder, risk factors, and questionnaires; discusses treatment thresholds; and identifies practical measures of process and outcomes. The clinical tools and risk factors selected for inclusion in this review represent the best empirical evidence in the literature. By the end of the article, clinicians will have a framework and set of clinically useful tools with which to effectively make evidence-based decisions regarding the diagnosis of BPD in children and adolescents.

Although some empirical work has now been added to the larger body of case material, preschool bipolar disorder (BPD) remains a highly ambiguous diagnostic area. This is notable in the context of the significant progress that has been made in many other areas of psychopathology in the preschool period. While there is a need for well controlled empirical investigations in this area, a small but growing body of empirical literature suggests that some form of the disorder may arise as early as age 3. The need for large scale and focused studies of this issue is underscored by the high and increasing rates of prescriptions of atypical antipsychotics and other mood stabilizing agents for preschool children with presumptive clinical diagnosis of BPD or a related variant. Clarifying the nosology of preschool BPD may also be important to better understand of the developmental psychopathology of the disorder during childhood. Data elucidating this developmental trajectory could then inform the design of earlier potentially preventive interventions that may have implications for the disorder across the lifespan.

Increasingly, clinicians and researchers alike are describing children presenting with emotional and behavioral problems as suffering from deficits of "affect regulation." The present article reviews the current understanding of affect regulation. The authors also discuss recent findings implicating affect dysregulation in children and adolescents with bipolar disorder.

Over the past 5–10 years, advances in neuroimaging methods and study designs have begun to appear in the literature of early-onset bipolar disorder (onset before 18 years of age). This article contains an updated review of the literature regarding neuroimaging in youths with bipolar disorder (BPD), highlighting important new study designs and techniques. Overall, structural, functional (fMRI) and magnetic resonance spectroscopy (MRS) report consistent abnormalities in regions of the frontal lobe and limbic structures. Functional MRI and MRS studies also frequently report striatal and thalamic abnormalities in early-onset BPD. Future neuroimaging studies in youths with BPD should include longitudinal studies incorporating multimodal neuroimaging techniques.

The risk of bipolar disorder (BPD) (15–42%) in first-degree relatives of children with BPD are consistently larger than the 8.7% estimate of recurrence risk of BPD in first-degree relatives of adult BPD cases. There have been no family linkage studies of pediatric BPD, but secondary analyses of adult linkage samples suggest that early-onset BPD both increases the strength of associations in linkage studies. Positive associations with pediatric BPD and the BDNF gene (Vall66), the GAD1 gene (4s2241165), and the dopamine transporter gene (rs41084) have been reported but none of these associations have been replicated in independent samples. The number of informative families examined so far is quite small and studies were vastly underpowered to detect small effects. An adequately powered sample will likely require collaborative ascertainment of cases and families from multiple sites using valid and accepted measures of pediatric BPD.

Bipolar disorder (BPD) is being diagnosed with increasing frequency in the pediatric population as the phenomenology of this disorder is becoming more clearly delineated. Early diagnosis and treatment of pediatric BPD is important to minimize psychosocial disability and improve prognosis. Traditional mood stabilizers and atypical antipsychotic agents are frequently used to treat BPD in youth, and there are emerging data to support their use in this population. This article provides a review of the literature on appropriate pharmacologic treatment strategies for BPD in children and adolescents. The complex treatment issues of comorbid BPD and attention deficit/hyperactivity disorder also are addressed.

Adjunctive psychosocial interventions are increasingly recognized as an important aspect of comprehensive treatment for bipolar disorder (BPD) in childhood and adolescence. Research in this area is relatively new, but psychosocial interventions being developed and tested include: multi-family psychoeducation groups for school-aged children with either BPD or depressive disorders; family-focused treatment, dialectical behavior therapy, and interpersonal and social rhythm therapy for adolescents with BPD; and child and family-focused cognitive-behavioral therapy for school-aged children with BPD. Preliminary evidence, where available, indicates that these interventions are feasible, well-received by families, and associated with positive outcomes. The continued study of adjunctive psychosocial interventions will help identify critical treatment ingredients that target specific areas of functioning and enhance overall treatment effectiveness for children and adolescents with BPD and their families.

There has been growing interest in the use of complementary and alternative treatments in pediatric bipolar disorder (BPD). There are limited data, however, regarding the safety and efficacy of these treatments. This article discusses select complementary and alternative treatments that have been considered for use in pediatric BPD and/or depression, including omega-3-fatty acids, inositol, St. John's wort, SAMe, melatonin, lecithin, and acupuncture. Background information, reference to available adult and pediatric data, proposed mechanisms of action, dosing, side effects, and precautions of these treatments are included. Across the board, more research is necessary and warranted regarding the long-term safety and efficacy of available complementary and alternative treatments for the management of pediatric BPD.

This article is intended to provide parents perspective on bipolar disorder in children and adolescents as is gathered from the experience of countless parents who participate in the activities of the organization known as the Child & Adolescent Bipolar Foundation (CABF; www.bpkids.org).

RELATED INTEREST

Psychiatric Clinics, June 2005 (Vol. 28, Number 2)
Bipolar Disorder
E. Sherwood Brown, MD, *Guest Editor*

THE CLINICS ARE NOW AVAILABLE ONLINE!

Access your subscription at:
www.theclinics.com

Foreword

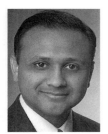

Harsh K. Trivedi, MD
Consulting Editor

"The passionate controversies of one era are viewed as sterile preoccupations by another, for knowledge alters what we seek as well as what we find."
— *Freda Adler*

I begin this foreword with the words of Freda Adler to provide perspective. If there was ever one diagnosis in child and adolescent psychiatry that could generate significant controversy, one topic that captured the collective conscience of our field, a clinical presentation that brought so many thought leaders of our field to research it, one topic to which it would be difficult to do justice within one issue of the Clinics, bipolar disorder is that diagnosis.

As debates continue across the country (and, indeed, the world) regarding how broadly to define the phenotypes of bipolar disorder; whether certain research groups are more or less restrictive in their definition of this clinical entity; whether genetic studies can validate our phenotypic interpretations; whether our treatments are effective and with acceptable side effect burdens; and, in some circles, whether this diagnosis is even valid in youth, I am reminded of the need for perspective.

Not too long ago, there was a similar belief about the presence (or rather lack) of depression in youth. Psychoanalytic theory posits that depression is the result of intrapsychic conflict between the ego and a persecutory superego. Based on a belief that the superego was formalized only after resolution of the Oedipal conflict by late adolescence, it was long held that young children could not experience intrapsychic conflict. If there is no superego and, hence, no intrapsychic conflict, then children could *not* be depressed.[1] It would be difficult to argue today that children do not experience depression. Just as importantly, the level of controversy surrounding this assertion is significantly less than when it was first made.

In selecting the guest editors for this issue, significant energies were expended in finding editors who were both highly knowledgeable about the topic and able to do justice to the multiple viewpoints that exist in the field. Jeffrey Hunt and Daniel Dickstein fit the bill—their years of clinical experience with this population, their

Child Adolesc Psychiatric Clin N Am 18 (2009) xiii–xiv
doi:10.1016/j.chc.2009.01.002
childpsych.theclinics.com
1056-4993/09/$ – see front matter © 2009 Elsevier Inc. All rights reserved.

contributions to research on this disorder, and their ability to cogently present the intricacies of this diagnosis shine through. I thank each of the excellent contributors, who are all leaders in the field, for sharing their expertise.

To paraphrase Freda Adler, may today's controversies about bipolar disorder seem like mere sterile preoccupations as we uncover knowledge and make sense of this disorder.

Harsh K. Trivedi, MD
Site Training Director and Director of Adolescent Services
E.P. Bradley Hospital
Assistant Professor of Psychiatry and Human Behavior (Clinical)
Brown Medical School
President, Rhode Island Council for Child and Adolescent Psychiatry
East Providence, RI 02915, USA

E-mail address:
harsh_trivedi@brown.edu

REFERENCE

1. Bowers RT. Child and adolescent affective disorders and their treatment. In: Klykylo WM, Kay J, editors. Clinical child psychiatry. 2nd edition. Chichester, England: Wiley & Sons, Ltd; 2005.

Preface

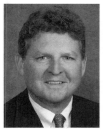 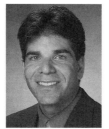

Jeffrey I. Hunt, MD   Daniel P. Dickstein, MD
Guest Editors

This issue of the *Child and Adolescent Psychiatric Clinics of North America* provides an update of our current understanding of bipolar disorder (BPD) in children and adolescents. It includes a fascinating historical perspective; an in-depth discussion of the phenomenology, outcomes, and assessment of BPD; the latest findings in neurobiology and genetics; the various treatment options available; and an important perspective from families living with children and adolescents who have BPD.

The amount of research in child and adolescent BPD has been increasing at an impressive pace. We are fortunate that many of the leaders in the field are able to contribute their expertise to this edition. Although it is no longer debated that BPD can occur in children and adolescents, many questions remain about the boundaries of the disorder, the neurobiologic underpinnings, and the optimal treatments, to name a few. We hope that this issue provides clinicians with an easily accessible and integrated source of the latest information available that may improve patient outcomes and prompt new research hypotheses.

The first article, by Carlson and Glovinsky, vibrantly describes the evolution of the conceptualization of BPD in children and adolescents. These investigators clearly define the current controversies and the pertinent historical perspectives. It is, for example, important to know that our field was debating the appropriateness of diagnosing BPD in children and adolescents in a 1950s edition of *The Nervous Child* in a way that closely parallels the main controversies of today.

The next several articles highlight the latest research on our current understanding of the phenomenology, comorbidity, and outcomes of juvenile BPD. Drs. Sala, Axelson, and Birmaher review the clinical characteristics, differential diagnosis, course, and prognosis of pediatric BPD, indicating that even though findings vary somewhat among different research groups, there are several unique features that have been consistently demonstrated in studies of the phenomenology and course of pediatric BPD. Drs. Joshi and Wilens, in their article on comorbidity, remind readers that BPD in children and adolescents seldom occurs in the absence of comorbid conditions, that the co-occurrence of additional disorders complicates the accurate

Child Adolesc Psychiatric Clin N Am 18 (2009) xv–xvii
doi:10.1016/j.chc.2009.01.001
1056-4993/09/$ – see front matter   **childpsych.theclinics.com**

diagnosis of BPD and its treatment, and that youth who have BPD and comorbid conditions are among the most impaired. Dr. Harvey extends this discussion of co-morbidity with an exploration of sleep disturbances that are common among youth who have BPD. The implications for intervention with sleep are considered, and a multicomponent sleep intervention for youth who have BPD is outlined. Dr. Gold-stein's article on suicide in pediatric BPD highlights the apparent link between early illness onset and suicidality, and discusses the appropriate assessment and manage-ment of suicidal patients who have BPD.

The best evidence for assessing BPD in children and adolescents is compre-hensively described by Drs. Youngstrom, Freeman, and Jenkins. They also define an actuarial approach to assessment—using prevalence of disorder, risk factors, and questionnaires—that many clinicians may find to be a valuable framework to effectively make evidence-based decisions regarding the diagnosis of BPD in children and adolescents. The challenge of diagnosing preschool children completes this section. Drs. Luby, Tandon, and Belden discuss the difficulty of distinguishing norma-tive extremes in mood intensity and lability that are known to characterize early child-hood from the emotions and behaviors that typically manifest in BPD. These investigators highlight the ongoing lack of clarity about the diagnostic criteria and the validity of the diagnosis in the preschool period. Although there are few studies that have systematically studied mania symptoms in preschoolers, the existing litera-ture has begun to shed some light on this area of early psychopathology. These inves-tigators also describe some important studies using novel research tools such as the Emotion Reactivity Questionnaire that have great promise in further elucidating BPD in very young children.

The neurobiologic underpinnings of mood and knowledge about the genetics of pediatric BPD are described in the next series of articles. Dr. Dickstein and colleagues amplify several aspects of affect regulation that require the interplay between many subprocesses, such as attention and processing of emotional stimuli, memory for prior events, response to rewards and punishments, and decision making. Dr. Frazier and colleagues review the advances in neuroimaging that complement the discussion of affect regulation. This article highlights important new study designs and techniques. Drs. Mick and Faraone review the current literature relevant to the genetic epidemi-ology of pediatric BPD, indicating that the risk of BPD in first-degree relatives of chil-dren who have BPD is consistently larger than the 8.7% estimate of recurrence risk of BPD in first-degree relatives of adult BPD cases. The positive candidate gene studies that have associations with pediatric BPD are reported, and future directions in the field are delineated.

It is clear that pediatric BPD is complex and not well understood, making the treat-ment of patients who have BPD even more daunting. Drs. Nandagopal, Delbello, and Kowatch summarize the extant literature of published pharmacologic studies of chil-dren and adolescents who have BPD and emphasize that some psychotropic agents have been shown to have potential neuroprotective properties in bipolar youth, indi-cating that these medications might be able to correct some of the neurobiologic alterations associated with BPD. Drs. West and Pavuluri affirm that although the devel-opment and study of psychosocial interventions for childhood BPD is in its relative infancy, several adjunctive psychosocial treatments are being developed or tested for children and adolescents who have bipolar spectrum disorders. According to Dr. Wozniak and colleagues, part of the controversy surrounding the diagnosis of BPD in youth is the concern that children given the diagnosis may be subjected to treatments fraught with potentially impairing and serious side effects. Increasingly, clinicians, researchers, and patients and their families are turning to an array of natural products considered complementary and alternative treatments. These investigators review some of the alternative agents that have the potential to be the most useful in the treatment of pediatric BPD.

This issue finishes with the perspective of Susan Resko, the Executive Director of the Child and Adolescent Bipolar Foundation, who helps to connect parents of children who have BPD using the Internet. She describes the struggles that many families with children diagnosed with BPD go through and offers resources, connection, and hope to families and teens who are struggling, often in isolation, with mood disorders.

We are honored to be guest editors of this issue and sincerely thank the *Child and Adolescent Clinics* Consulting Editor, Dr. Harsh Trivedi, for the opportunity. We thank Sarah Barth at Elsevier for her outstanding support throughout the past year and especially thank all the contributors for their dedication to excellence in this edition.

Jeffrey I. Hunt, MD

Daniel P. Dickstein, MD
Emma Pendleton Bradley Hospital
Alpert Medical School of Brown University
1011 Veteran's Memorial Pkwy
East Providence, RI 02914, USA

E-mail addresses:
Jeffrey_hunt@brown.edu (J.I. Hunt)
Daniel_dickstein@brown.edu (D.P. Dickstein)

The Concept of Bipolar Disorder in Children: A History of the Bipolar Controversy

Gabrielle A. Carlson, MD[a],*, Ira Glovinsky, PhD[b,c]

KEYWORDS

• Bipolar • Mania • Childhood • Nosology • History

Phenomenologists in child and adolescent psychiatry frequently aspire to the perceived certitude with which adult psychiatry conceptualizes bipolar disorder. However, there is a good deal of uncertainty in how this condition is operationalized, classified, and distinguished from other conditions even in adults. There are multiple issues. They include the following: (1) the degree to which mania is a spectrum that ranges from a severely psychotic, paranoid, and agitated condition that can be confused with schizophrenia to one that borders on normal behavior; (2) the degree to which depression may be punctuated by fluctuations of mood, which range from euthymia to hypomania to mania (ie, circular manic-depression, bipolar II disorder, and recurrent unipolar depression); (3) the degree to which the onset of a mood state can be distinguished from some kind of baseline state in which mood changes are part of the person's temperament or personality (eg, a hyperthymic energetic temperament or "cluster B personality disorders" in which chronic mood lability is present, exacerbations of which may or may not be related to manic-depression); (4) the degree to which the mood disorder is autonomous versus precipitated by, or associated with, another CNS condition, including drugs (prescribed or illicit) or illness, that is, the primary/secondary distinction.

To these muddy waters, child psychopathology adds two more: (1) the degree to which symptoms and behaviors thought to be basic to the definition of mania or depression mean the same thing in children of different ages and (2) the degree to

For the sake of this discussion, manic-depression will refer to a clearly episodic disorder as still described in ICD-10. Bipolar disorder refers to the post-1980 construct of people who meet symptom criteria and represent a broader spectrum.
[a] Child and Adolescent Psychiatry, Stony Brook University School of Medicine, Putnam Hall-South Campus, Stony Brook, NY 11794-8790, USA
[b] Department of Education, Madonna University, Livonia, MI 48150, USA
[c] Mood Disorder Program, Interdisciplinary Center for the Family, West Bloomfield, MI 48322, USA
* Corresponding author.
E-mail address: gabrielle.carlson@stonybrook.edu (G. A. Carlson).

Child Adolesc Psychiatric Clin N Am 18 (2009) 257–271
doi:10.1016/j.chc.2008.11.003
1056-4993/08/$ – see front matter © 2009 Elsevier Inc. All rights reserved.

which the symptoms can be distinguished from other developmental conditions in which similar symptoms might occur (eg, attention deficit hyperactivity disorder (ADHD) and other disorders in which executive function is significantly impaired, such as autism spectrum disorders).

Historically, the term mania, which identifies bipolar disorder, had different meanings, from those that are attached to the disorder now. Mania or "madness" was a term used in ancient Greece and appeared to have four different meanings:[1]

1. A reaction to an event in the meaning of rage or anger or excitation;
2. A biologically defined disease;
3. A divine state;
4. A kind of temperament, especially in mild form.

Hippocrates (460–337 BC) was probably the first to systematically describe melancholia and mania in a scientific way.[2] He formulated the first classification of mental disorders into melancholia, mania, and paranoia. In his work, he alluded to a connection between mania and melancholia using humoral theories. He stated that "black bile" could generate a variety of phenomena, depending on the temperature. He wrote,

> "Now, black bile... if it is in excessive quality in the body produces apoplexy or torpor, or despondency or fear; but if it becomes overheated, it produces cheerfulness with song, and madness... those...in whom the bile is considerable and cold become sluggish and stupid, while those with whom it is excessive and hot become mad, clever or amorous and easily moved to passion and desire, and some become more talkative... many, because this heat is near to the seat of the mind, are affected by the disease of madness or frenzy..."[3]

Aretaeus of Cappadocia has been referred to as the "father of bipolar disorder." He was perhaps the first who clearly described mania and melancholia as being two components of one disease.[4] He wrote,

> ... it appears to me that melancholia is the commencement and a part of mania... but those affected with melancholy are not every one of them affected according to one particular form; but they are either suspicious of poisoning, or flee to the desert from misanthropy, or turn superstitious, or contract a hatred of life. Or if at any time a relaxation takes place, in most cases a hilarity supervenes, but those persons go mad.

The distinguished historian of medicine, Stanley Jackson,[5] summarized the important points on the relationship between melancholia and mania from antiquity through medieval times and recognized that the conditions "appeared together among the disease of the head;" they were chronic and occurred without fever (ie, distinct from delirium), and mania referred to an excited, psychotic state.

Descriptions of children who might have had mania are virtually nonexistent, and when they did occur, it was not always clear which definition of mania was implied, whether there were other central nervous system conditions affecting the child, or indeed, what childhood included. Charles Bradley, the child and adolescent psychiatrist who observed the calming effect of Benzedrine on children with various neurological conditions, noted in 1937[6] that childhood often included people up to their early 20s and wanted to establish that it should refer only to those younger than 12 years.

Two examples from earlier centuries make this point. Greding's *Medical Aphorisms on Melancholy, etc.* described the case of a very young child that resembled mania (p 355):[7]

> On the 20th, January, 1763, was brought to bed without any assistance, a male child [age unspecified], who was raving mad. When he was brought to our

workhouse, which was on the 24th, he possessed so much strength in his legs and arms, that four women could, at times, with difficulty restrain him. These paroxysms either ended in indescribable laughter for which no evident reason could be observed, or else he tore in anger every thing near him, cloaths, linen, bed, furniture, even thread when he could get hold of it. We durst not allow him to be alone, otherwise he would get on the benches and table, and even attempt to climb up the walls.

A description of a 6-year-old girl by the nineteenth-century British alienist, Morison, (pp 317–318) noted:

When admitted to Bethelem Hospital, her conduct was violent and mischievous; striking those about her, tearing her clothes and destroying everything within her reach.[8] She was generally incoherent in her speech—repeated any words she might hear in a monotonous voice, and without appearing to understand them, such as "Poor thing, poor thing!"... She could not be induced to employ herself in any way, and was subject to violent and unaccountable outbursts of passion, in which she tore her clothes, and bit and scratched all who attempted to restrain her.

Although the descriptions are vivid, without a context in which to place the child and his behavior (it could represent delirious states secondary to infection or trauma, autism, etc), it is difficult to know what condition the child suffered. "Mania" simply was another term for "madness."

THE BIRTH OF THE MODERN CONCEPT OF MANIC-DEPRESSION (BIPOLAR DISORDER)

In the middle of the nineteenth century, two psychiatrists described manic-depression for the first time as a single entity.[9] In 1851, Jean-Pierre Falret, a pupil of Esquirol, published a 14-sentence-long statement at La Salpêtrière in the Gateaux des Hopitaux describing a mental disorder that he named "folie circulaire," which was characterized by a continuous cycle of depression, mania, and symptom-free intervals of varying length. Three years later he more formally described the sequential change from mania to melancholia and vice versa and the symptom-free interval in between as a separate disease, folie circulaire. In 1857, Jules Baillarger, a psychiatrist working at the same hospital, presented the concept of a disorder that he named "folie á double forme," in which mania and melancholia changed into one another, but the interval between was felt to have no meaning, unlike the concept of Falret in which the interval between mania and melancholia was a core component of the concept. The "battle" to gain credit for discovering the disorder continued until 1894 when Falret and Baillarger received joint credit for their work by the Académie de Médecine at a ceremony at La Salpêtrière. Shortly thereafter, in 1898, Beach[10] described a 13-year-old boy who evidenced folie circulaire and provided a vignette that more clearly reflects our current understanding of manic-depression.

He was a dull child, and had been so often punished at school, on account of his slow progress, that he became deeply melancholy and tried to kill himself. The melancholy alternated with mania, in which he whistled and sang day and night, tore his clothes, and was filthy in his habits....

In Germany, in the late 19th century, Emil Kraepelin wrote his seminal book on manic-depressive insanity in which he dichotomized the "endogeneous" psychoses into "dementia praecox" and manic-depressive insanity.[11] Kraepelin favored recurrence of depression over an emphasis on polarity. Thus, all types of affective disorders were included in a unitary concept of manic-depressive illness.

This classification was not without its opponents, for example, Carl Wernicke and Karl Kleist felt that polarity was extremely important and that single episodes of mania or melancholia, including recurrent depression or recurrent mania without cycling one into the other, were not the same as manic-depressive insanity.[9]

With respect to children, in his book on manic-depressive insanity, Kraepelin[11] described the ages of the greatest frequency of occurrence of the disorder at between 15 and 20 years and reported that only 0.4% of occurrences of the disorder were in children younger than 10 years. It is unclear if he treated those children or if his adult patients provided information about the age at onset.

To summarize, there have been several stages in the evolution of our understanding of the current thinking about the phenomenology of bipolar disorder. Clinicians over the centuries have gradually recognized the relationship between an underactive, unmotivated melancholic state and a hyperactive, hyperhedonic, elevated mood state. The next stage was separating schizophrenia from manic-depressive "insanity" and then distinguishing manic-depression from recurrent unipolar depression. Recognition of manic-depression as distinct from other forms of depression, that is, the potential importance of polarity rather than recurrence, was taken up by German (Karl Leonhard, initially), Swiss (Jules Angst), and Scandinavian (Carlo Perris) psychiatrists. Research by these psychiatrists ultimately supported the nosologic and family history differentiation between unipolar and bipolar manic-depression, and manic-depressive illness became manic-depressive illness, bipolar type. (There is no unanimity even now about the validity of these separations, however.)[9]

After the World Health Organization US/UK study of manic-depression and schizophrenia[12] revealed how two English-speaking countries can look at the same cases and make vastly different diagnoses, there was an increased interest in becoming more systematic and operational in making a diagnosis to increase the reliability of diagnosis. Structured and semistructured interviews were developed for adults, and researchers began to use operationally defined criteria for diagnosis: first the Research Diagnostic Criteria,[13] and then the American Psychiatric Association's revision of the Diagnostic and Statistical Manual of Mental Disorders, third edition, (DSM-III-R).[14] With these criteria, and even more so with the DSM-III-R,[15] in which the definition of "episodes" became less specific, the diagnosis of what has become "bipolar disorder" became symptom-driven, in contrast to the International Classification of Diseases (ICD) definitions of manic-depression, in which a template or gestalt is described.[16]

The most recent struggles in the nosology of bipolar disorder have been defining the boundaries of a bipolar spectrum, which provides "coverage" to an increasingly large population of patients with various mood states, and trying to find an endophenotype that might allow us to better understand the underpinning of whatever bipolar disorder is.

BIPOLAR DISORDER IN CHILDREN

Theodor Ziehen (1862–1950)[17] was both a physician and psychologist, which influenced his observations and many writings. With the textbook, *Mental Diseases of Childhood,* which appeared in three sections between 1902 and 1906, Ziehen created the first systematic work on child psychiatry in Germany. Ziehen apparently defined childhood as peri-puberty and older (ie, ages 11–15 years). He defined mania under the category of "composite or periodic psychoses. He wrote the following:

> "A simple, nonrecurring mania occurs only exceptionally during childhood. In most cases mania is characterized by periodic recurrences or regular alternation with melancholy, that means either by the so- called period mania or circular

insanity. The two mental diseases are clinically distinctive and therefore shall be treated separately under the heading of Composite Psychoses.

Ziehen's exquisite descriptions of manic-depressive illness bear striking similarity to classical bipolar disorder as described in contemporary literature.

Among the symptoms, pathological jocularity is the most prominent. It always shows in the facial expression of the child: the eyes shine, the face is cheerful and often the children can't keep from laughing for hours. The jocularity remains even when the children feel pain, or when they are corrected or criticized. However, it is not rare that the jocularity is associated with anger, and in severe cases there are attacks of rage.

Accelerated and associative thinking, the so-called flight-of-ideas, manifests it-self in continuous and rapid speech, so-called logorrhea. Often, parents and teachers are hardly able to speak with a manic child. During lessons at school, the child continually chatters and seems unfocused.... Closely related to flight-of-ideas is pathological distractibility or hypervigilance. Every sensory stimulus distracts the child from his occupation. Every noise, every change in the environment inspires ideas and gives rise to associative remarks.... Directly related to the increased psychomotor activity and flight-of-ideas is sleep Disturbance that almost always occurs in childhood mania, In severe cases nearly complete insomnia can be observed.... Delusions are much more frequent than disturbances of perception. They are characterized by ideas of grandeur. I many cases, however, they manifest themselves only in a change of thinking toward heightened self-assurance. These changes lead to boasting, an impertinent attitude, rebellion against the authority of parents and teachers, fantastic plans for the future, and the like (pp 214–215).

Ziehen saw this pathologic condition as being on a continuum from normal child development foreshadowing work on developmental components of bipolar patterns. He stated that the diagnosis of mania was problematic because the individual features of the disorder were similar to the behavioral features exhibited by normal children. What differentiated mania in young adolescents from the behaviors of typical young people was the fact that the symptoms reflected a *rapid change* from the child's characteristic behavior.

Interest in manic-depressive insanity among child psychiatrists increased thereafter. For example, in 1931, Kasanin[18] in studying affective psychoses in adolescents described the clinical picture of mania. He noted mild elation, overactivity, irritability, and pressured speech. In contrast, the picture of depression included withdrawal, under-talkativeness, general retardation, and occasional refusal of food. In analyzing the etiologic factors, Kasanin wrote the following:

"When it comes to the analysis of the etiologic factors it was rather striking that the immediate precipitating causes of depression or elation seemed to be quite trivial, but apparently of definite dynamic significance to the patient."[18]

Surveys of state hospitals for young people with manic-depression[19,20] revealed that cases that resembled the adult form occurred mostly postpubertally and were mostly depressive.

Kanner, in his 1935 text,[1] used Adolph Meyer's terminology to describe the different patterns of manic-depressive illness in young children. He described "thymergasic" patterns (ergasias referring to "syndrome or reaction patterns"), including hyperthymergasia, which consisted of exaggerated happiness, hilariousness, acceleration in thinking, flight of ideas, and increased psychomotor activity, and hypothymergasia, consisting of profound sadness and downheartedness, slowing of thinking processes, and depressed psychomotor activity. Kanner listed different patterns in which the disorder could start, with either a depressive phase or a manic phase that was punctuated by a period in which the child was relatively symptom free. Thus, there were 5 patterns including the following:

1. Manic phase—depressive phase—interval
2. Depressive phase—manic phase—interval
3. Manic phase—interval—depressive phase
4. Depressive phase—interval—manic phase
5. Depressive phase—interval—depressive phase

Kanner also stated that the duration of intervals could vary from very short periods to longer periods that could extend for years or even decades.

Kanner's 1935 edition of *Child Psychiatry* was the last edition to describe the disorder. The removal of a description of manic-depression from subsequent editions perhaps reflected the resistance to accepting the diagnosis in childhood and possibly the impact of psychoanalytic theory of child development on psychology (Baldessarini, personal communication, 2000).

While much of the clinical literature was based on adolescents, psychoanalysts tried to explore and explain the infancy and childhood of adults with manic-depression. Melanie Klein,[21] in describing normal child development, stated that the child in very early development goes through a transitory manic-depressive state. She added that hypomania and mania were defense mechanisms among other manic defenses, including omnipotence, identification with the superego, introjection, manic triumph, and extreme idealization. Klein maintained that manic-depressive patients had been unable to establish securely a good inner object in infancy and had not been able to work through the infantile *depressive position*, which occurred normally in the second half of the child's first year.

Abraham[22] who was also interested in early child development discussed the influence of early psychosexual stages of development as being influential on the later development of manic-depression. In dividing development into oral, anal, and phallic stages that had early and later components, he stated that mania was related to the cannibalistic (later) oral stage, and he suggested a number of etiologic factors, both constitutional and psychodynamic, that were involved in the circular insanities.

Ultimately, the diagnosis of manic-depression in children may have been dismissed because it was thought that children did not have the higher-level cognitive structures that emerge with further psychosexual development after puberty. However, influential child psychoanalytic theorists may not have been treating the population of children most expected to have manic-depression (eg, children in state hospitals), either. It did not appear that these theorists were seeing children and adolescents with mania and giving them another diagnosis.

BIRTH OF THE BIPOLAR CONTROVERSY

Although the current controversy besetting very early onset of bipolar disorder (how narrow or broad the criteria should be, whether the symptoms in young children should be given more latitude, and whether, if manic-like symptoms occur, they mean the same thing in children as adults) appears new, in fact, the controversy is quite old. In the 1950s, the question of preadolescent manic-depression was discussed in the journal, *The Nervous Child*, which had several papers with case descriptions of children as well as adolescents. Again the condition was thought to be rare

(6/1000 manic-depressive patients in Barton-Hall's private practice,[23] mostly adolescents), though there was some suggestion of an "alternate form" contained within more typical childhood behavioral psychopathology. For instance, Ernest Harms[24] looked at behaviors of children in nurseries and saw what he considered to be "reactions" that were "embryonic forms of manic-depressive behavior." He felt that many of the pre-adolescent syndromes that were classified as "primary behavior disorders" could be re-classified as "manic utterance." This is remarkably similar to the view espoused by Biederman and colleagues[25] many years later who found that almost 20% of children in their attention deficit hyperactivity disorder (ADHD) clinic could be considered manic/bipolar by their assessment.

In the opposing camp, Charles Bradley, (1902–1979), one of the most prominent and published child psychiatrists in the 1930s and 1940s, thought that when manic-depression was reported in children there was either confusion in the observations or interpretation of the child's motor activity or impulsiveness and that the diagnosis of manic-depression was inappropriate.[26] Indeed, he wrote,

Severe depressions are not seen in children. What effect puberty and the maturity of the psyche as seen in later adolescence and adult life have on the capacity of the individual to develop symptoms either of mania or depression awaits further investigation. For the present it is best to avoid the diagnosis of manic-depressive psychosis or affective psychosis in children.

In 1960, Anthony and Scott[27] quelled the controversy, such as it was at the time, by developing a set of criteria to define the manic-depression and then doing a scrupulous search of the extant literature for case reports. The criteria articulated very classic manic-depression, including premorbid cyclothymia, evidence of a recurrent or periodic and diphasic illness, minimal environmental stress associated with the phases of illness, absence of features that might indicate schizophrenia, drugs, delirium, hysteria, or infection and impairment such that "heavy sedation" or electroconvulsive therapy (ECT) treatment was needed. With this definition, manic-depression was revealed to be very rare (three cases, all peri-pubertal). On the other hand, in 1986, Weller and colleagues[28] did a similar review of case reports of severely disturbed children using a much less conservative definition (DSM-III) and found that the diagnosis of mania had been missed in 16/33 cases.

The emergence of effective treatments such as ECT, antipsychotics, and lithium added to the impetus to better define manic-depression in adults.[29] The stimulus of having a specific treatment such as lithium for mania spurred attempts to find children who would also benefit from lithium. Youngerman and Canino, in 1978,[30] reviewed the growing case report literature on the effectiveness of lithium in children and adolescents. Although these authors found 211 cases, only 46 had enough information to allow tentative conclusions about the reasons lithium was used. There were very few studies of children or even adolescents who could be considered bipolar. One concludes from their review that classic manic-depression was much less common in children than adolescents, but there had been an early interest in trying to find a symptom constellation, especially in younger children who would be lithium-responsive. It was not found.

One of the studies in the Youngerman and Canino series was another harbinger of the ADHD/bipolar controversy. Greenhill and colleagues,[31] well known for research in children with ADHD, conducted a lithium trial in children with hyperkinesis (the DSM-II term for ADHD), recognizing the similarity of this condition to mania. The study describes nine children who were poor dextroamphetamine responders and were giddy, hyperverbal, and severely disruptive (and who might have been called manic by some people today). Children were treated with lithium and placebo in a double-blind, on-off fashion. Only two children had short-term positive responses, specifically with an improvement in activity level, destructiveness, and uncooperativeness. Within a few months, however, these responses dissipated along with the idea that hyperkinesis was an alternate form of mania.

As noted earlier, the 1970s were characterized by an increased interest in precise phenomenology. Feighner, a psychiatrist at Washington University School of Medicine, published a set of criteria for mania and depression (among other disorders) that the faculty had been using in their research for the previous decade.[32] Two pediatric neurologists also at Washington University (Weinberg and Brumback)[33] adapted the Feighner criteria for both mania and depression for use in very young children in a learning disabilities clinic (Table 1). A review of these criteria reveal, however, that although the symptom descriptions are reasonable, the criteria did not specify that the symptoms had to co-occur or that episodes were important—only that each symptom represented a change in behavior. Carlson and Cantwell[34] compared Weinberg criteria for depression to DSM-III criteria and found them to be broader and include children whom DSM-III defined as behavior-disordered. There have been no tests of the mania criteria. Unfortunately, there was no way to test the validity of the modified versus unmodified criteria, and the tension between the primacy of individual symptoms versus the primacy of episodes continues to the present.

Davis, in 1979,[35] described a "manic-depressive variant syndrome of childhood" characterized by five primary features and one or more secondary features that took a tack similar to that seen currently by those who think that severe irritability and rage characterize a form of bipolar disorder. The primary features in Davis's thinking included affective storms, defined as a loss of control that was highly intense, disruptive, and transient; significant family histories of affective disturbances; mental,

Table 1
Weinberg criteria for mania and depression[31]

Childhood mania	Childhood depression
The presence of either or both symptoms 1 and 2 and 3 or more of the remaining 6:	Presence of both symptoms 1 and 2, and 2 or more of the remaining 8 symptoms
1. Euphoria: denial of problems or illness; inappropriate feelings of well-being, inappropriate cheerfulness; giddiness and silliness	1. Dysphoric mood
2. Irritability and or agitation (particularly belligerence, destructiveness, and antisocial behavior	2. Self-depreciatory ideation
3. Hyperactivity, "motor driven," intrusiveness	3. Aggressive behavior (agitation)
4. Push of speech (may become unintelligible); garrulousness	4. Sleep disturbance
5. Flight of ideas	5. Diminished socialization
6. Grandiosity (may be delusional)	6. Change in attitude toward school
7. Sleep disturbance (decreased sleep and unusual sleep pattern)	7. Somatic complaints
8. Distractibility (short attention span)	8. Change in school performance
Each symptom must be a discrete change in the individual's usual behavior and be present for longer than a month	9. Loss of usual energy
	10. Unusual change in appetite or weight
	Each symptom must be a discrete change in the individual's usual behavior and be present for longer than a month

Data from Weinberg WA, Brumback RA. Mania in childhood: case studies and a literature review. Am J Dis Child 1976;130:380–5.

verbal, and physical hyperactivity; high level of distractibility; and rapid talk or a "rapid progression of interest."

Davis pointed out that both the hyperactivity and emotional upheaval were not the same as the grandiosity of manic adults and that there were no delusions or hallucinations. These children also experienced great difficulty in social relationships. There were secondary characteristics, including sleep disturbances, possible minimal brain dysfunction, sometimes abnormal EEG patterns, possible enuresis, and associated neurological problems. No research was done to validate this proposal, either. In current parlance, this "variant" might define severe mood dysregulation[52] and again illustrates that there has been a struggle with issues of broad versus narrow definition of bipolar disorder for many decades.

The use of structured and semistructured interviews in adults spurred similar research in children, and systematic research on mood disorders in children increased dramatically. However, in children, the initial search was for depression. Pioneers like Poznanski and Mokros, who developed the Children's Depression Rating Scale,[36] Puig-Antich and Chambers, who adapted the Kiddie-Schedule for Affective Disorders and Schizophrenia for Children (K-SADS),[37] Kovacs, who used her own systematic interview and adapted Beck's Children's Depression Inventory to construct the Children's Depression Inventory,[38] and Carlson and Cantwell, who modified the Rutter Interview,[39] all explored the concept of childhood depression systematically and mania when it occurred, which was not very often. This may have been because the DSM-III criteria for mania required that symptoms be present for a week. Bipolar diagnoses did not begin to increase dramatically in adults (and then children) until DSM-III-R stopped specifying a duration requirement for episodes.

One of the reasons that manic-depression had not been diagnosed in teens after the 1950s was that schizophrenia was the most frequently diagnosed psychosis in the United States—a bias that was especially true for young people. Thus, the realization that people with mania and depression can have severe psychosis[40] was important. A number of authors came to realize that severe psychosis in adolescents can, in fact, be manic or depressive.[41] This was less of an issue in children in whom schizophrenia is rare.

By the early 1980s, there was increasing acceptance of the fact that preadolescent children could present bipolar symptomatology, though there was no attempt to establish the frequency with which this might occur. Carlson concluded based on an updated literature review[42] that younger children with mania were described as having hyperactivity, an absence of discrete episodes, greater irritability and emotional lability as opposed to euphoria, and a relative absence of grandiosity or paranoia. In contrast, children older than 9 years presented a more classical pattern marked by discrete episodes, euphoria and irritability, and grandiosity. In addition, when younger children were in a depressive phase of the disorder, they did not display specific episodes, including depressed appearance, guilt, paranoia, morbid preoccupation, or psychomotor retardation. Instead, when they were depressed they were more typically agitated or irritable in the same way as unipolar depressed children.

Almost 20 years ago (1990), before research groups were really taking hold of the question about the boundaries of mania in children, there was enough interest in the question about ADHD and mania for Carlson[43] to summarize the issues as follows:

In both ADHD/CD and mania, hyperactivity, distractibility, intrusiveness, poor judgment, volatile and irritable behavior especially when thwarted, impulsive risk taking, poor sleep habits and denial of problems prevail. Hyperactive, conduct-disordered children may brag and tell "tall stories" making them appear grandiose as well. One cannot even depend on eliciting a history of euphoria since its absence does not rule mania out and its presence is very difficult to elicit from children and their parents.[42] The major symptomatic difference is that ADHD/CD is largely chronic with an age of onset usually before age 6 or 7 whereas mania is episodic. In fact, I have made the point elsewhere that the further one gets from requiring clear-cut episodes of disorder, as part of the definition, the more muddied these waters become.[42,44]

Possible explanations for the relationship between ADHD/conduct disorder (CD) and mania/bipolar disorder are as follows:

(1) ADHD/CD is a prodrome or subsyndromal form of mania, which has been developmentally modified and will look more obvious with puberty.
(2) Children with prepubertal bipolar disorder (which is manifested by ADHD/CD) have a particularly virulent form of bipolar disorder as exemplified by its early age at onset.
(3) The ADHD/CD represents one of many nonspecific early responses to family psychopathology.
(4) Mania occurring after the onset of ADHD/CD is a condition known in the adult literature as secondary affective disorder, a concept articulated originally by Monro[45] and Woodruff and colleagues.[46] In this instance, secondary meant that another psychiatric disorder temporally preceded the affective disorder and suggested that both disorders coexist (comorbidity) without being necessarily causal.
(5) Children with ADHD/CD who develop mania have "secondary mania" as originally described by Krauthammer and Klerman,[47] that is, a manic syndrome that occurs following and is probably precipitated by such organic factors as metabolic disturbances, specific drugs, seizures, central nervous system infections, tumors, and other CNS pathology.[48]

Wozniak and colleagues, in 1995, published the first really systematic research done on a relatively large (ie, more than a few case reports) population of children[49] though other research was under way as well. By the time a specially called National Institute of Mental Health (NIMH) Roundtable on Prepubertal Bipolar Disorder in Children[50] was convened on April 27, 2000, there were at least a dozen different research groups investigating prepubertal mania. The use of one form or another of semistructured interview, usually the K-SADS,[51] was one of the areas of agreement reached at this meeting. Another was the high rate of comorbid ADHD and behavior disorders that occurred in samples of prepubertal manic children. Assessment of mood variability (and irritability) and its convergence with bipolar I disorder, versus bipolar disorder not otherwise specified, versus being an entirely separate condition, however, were left unresolved. This question prompted the intramural program at NIMH, headed by Leibenluft, to develop a line of research in which chronic, severe irritability was operationalized, combined with secondary symptoms of mania (which are indistinguishable from ADHD), and named "severe mood dysregulation."[52] In this way, the group reasoned, some headway might be made in distinguishing what some might call "bad ADHD" (and others call a bipolar subtype), from bipolar I disorder.

At present, ironically, we have a situation that did not develop purposely and that really was not recognized until recently. That is, although each research group uses usually one form or another of the K-SADS,[52] and all use DSM-IV criteria, different research groups have diverged somewhat in how the interviews are used, what kinds of questions are asked, whether criteria are modified, (and, thus, what kinds of responses are counted), and what informants are used. As Youngstrom and colleagues[53] have noted:

The concern is that the "bipolar" label often might be inappropriately applied to youths whose emotional and behavioral issues might actually not be a manifestation of the same illness connoted by that label in adults. The concern that the same label might be capturing different conditions in childhood versus adulthood has been heightened by discussions of perceived differences in the phenomenology, comorbidity, and course of bipolar disorder in pediatric versus adult samples. Adding to the complexity is the fact that different research groups have used various different diagnostic interviews, different conceptualizations of the disorder, and different ascertainment patterns and inclusion or exclusion criteria to define their samples.

Not only do these definitions often differ in potentially important respects from the DSM-IV criteria but they are also different from the definitions employed by most practicing clinicians.

The clinical implications of this observation can be seen in the results of a recent cross-national (United States and United Kingdom) study of five cases of children with mood symptoms, in whom bipolar disorder might be a diagnostic consideration.[54] In three of the five cases, there was significant disagreement about diagnosis because of different interpretations of specific manic symptoms. For example, in a preadolescent patient with classic mania, agreement was close (96.4% of US and 88.9% of UK physicians made a diagnosis of mania). However, in the prepubertal child with both ADHD and manic-like symptoms, 86.2% of US child psychiatrists diagnosed mania in contrast to only 31.1% of their UK colleagues. Indeed, the same differences emerged in a recent online American Academy of Child & Adolescent Psychiatry (e-AACAP) roundtable[55] in which two experts thought a youngster had ADHD and severe mood dysregulation, and the other two thought she had bipolar disorder.

Perhaps the heart of the matter is that the conceptualization of bipolar disorder in adults, although by no means settled, has emerged over time from the amalgamation of the clinical picture of thousands of patients observed and followed in America and Europe to form a template. Indeed, the template has been what operationalized criteria have tried to recreate. However, bipolar disorder in children has evolved from imposing adult criteria, with or without investigator imposed modifications, onto children of all ages.

SUMMARY

Although the "bipolar controversy" has become more heated as diagnostic stakes have increased, it is evident that there have been two schools of thought for many years. One is that manic-depression should be confined to a condition characterized by discrete episodes of mania and depression, during which a constellation of mood and behavioral symptoms co-occur, which are clear departures from the person's intermorbid state. The other is that bipolar disorder is a more far-reaching condition that embodies difficulty with emotion regulation, which may or may not be episodic. It is possible that for some people these conditions are related, much the same way that schizotypy and schizophrenia are related.

In children (before puberty), classic manic-depression is uncommon, though how uncommon is not clear. On the other hand, manic symptoms and severely dysregulated emotion in children are quite common and pose a significant mental health problem.[56,57] They are a heterogeneous group with manic symptoms occurring after the onset of other medical, neurological, or psychiatric disorders, or who respond to drugs (prescribed and illicit) with manic symptoms, or who may have a developmental delay or arrest in emotion regulation. In the latter instance, behavior problems and volatile emotions may continue to plague the afflicted into adulthood and underpin any number of other disorders, including manic-depression. In our view, this group of children are likely to include future manic-depressives, people on a bipolar

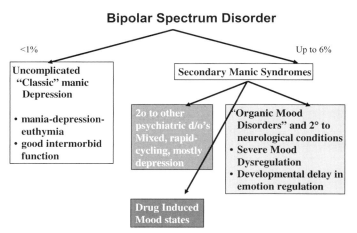

Fig. 1. A way of dividing and studying bipolar disorder.

spectrum, as well as children who have phenocopies of manic-depression and bipolar disorder (**Fig. 1**). The question is how, if at all, this group of children map onto classic manic-depression such that the same neurobiological explanations and treatment strategies can be used for both. The work of the researchers in the twenty-first century will be to understand not only symptoms of bipolar disorder but also how it develops and how emotion regulation relates to both the development of bipolar disorder and to other conditions that are characterized by dysregulated emotion.

Although the differences of opinion implicit in a "controversy" have been sometimes misinterpreted as confusion or as evidence of ineptitude in psychiatry, the questions raised have stimulated research. Work is now being done in many areas, for example, neuroscience, child development, clinical psychiatry, and psychology, which will ultimately allow us to clarify differences and to develop treatment paradigms to help children and their families who suffer from dysregulated mood and resultant behavior and dysfunction regardless of its origins.

REFERENCES

1. Kanner L. Child psychiatry. Springfield(IL): CC Thomas; 1935. p. 502–7.
2. Marneros A, Angst J. Bipolar disorders: roots and evolution. In: Marneros A, Angst J, editors. Bipolar disorders: 100 years after manic depressive insanity. AA Dordrecht (The Netherlands): Kluwer Academic Publishers; 2000. p. 1–35.
3. Pies R. The historical roots of the "bipolar spectrum": did Aristotle anticipate Kraepelin's broad concept of manic-depression? J Affect Disord 2007;100:7–11.
4. Aretaeus. The extant works of Aretaeus, The Cappadocian. (Adams F editor and translator). Sydenham Society. London: 1856. p. 301–4.
5. Jackson SW. Melancholia and depression. New Haven (CT): Yale University Press; 1986. p. 214–5.
6. Bradley C. Definition of childhood in psychiatric literature. Am J Psychiatry 1937; 94:33–6.
7. Greding J.E. Medical aphorisms on melancholy, etc. In: [Trans. in Crichton A], editor. An inquiry into mental derangement II. T Cadell, Jr W Davies, London: 1798. p. 355.

8. Morison TC. Case of mania in a child six-years old. J Psychological Med 1848;1: 317–8.
9. Goodwin FK, Jamison KR. Manic depressive illness: bipolar disorders and recurrent depression. 2nd edition. New York: Oxford University Press; 2007. p. 3.
10. Beach F. Insanity of children. J Ment Sci 1898;44:459–74.
11. Kraepelin E. Manic-depressive insanity and paranoia [Barclay M, trans.] Edinburgh (UK): Livingstone; 1921.
12. Cooper JE, Kendall RE, Gurland BJ, et al. Psychiatric diagnosis in New York and London: a comparative study of mental hospital admissions. Institute of Psychiatry, Maudsley Monographs 1972 (20).
13. Spitzer RL, Endicott J, Williams JB. Research diagnostic criteria. Arch Gen Psychiatry 1979;36(12):1381–3.
14. American Psychiatric Association. Diagnostic and statistical manual of mental disorders III. American Psychiatric Association: Washington, DC. 1980.
15. American Psychiatric Association. Diagnostic and statistical manual of mental disorders, III-R. Washington, DC: American Psychiatric Association; 1987.
16. World Health Organization. The ICD-10 Classification of mental and behavioural disorders. Clinical descriptions and diagnostic guidelines. Geneva: WHO; 1992.
17. Baethge C, Glovinsky I, Baldessarini RJ. Manic-depressive illness in children: an early twenieth-century view by Theodor Ziehen (1862–1950). Hist Psychiatry 2004;15(2):201–26.
18. Kasanin J. The affective psychoses in children. Am J Psychiatry 1931;10:897–903.
19. Strecker EA. The prognosis in manic depressive psychosis NY. J Med 1921;114: 209–16.
20. Barrett AM. Manic depressive psychosis in childhood. Nerv Child 1952;9:319–25.
21. Klein M. Mourning and its elation to manic-depressive states. London: Hogarth Press; 1952.
22. Abraham K. Notes on the psychoanalytic investigations of manic-depressive insanity and allied conditions. In: Selected papers on psychoanalysis. London: Oxford University Press; 1911. p. 137–56.
23. Barton-Hall M. Our present knowledge about manic-depressive states. Nerv Child 1952;9:319–32.
24. Harms E. Differential patterns of manic-depressive disease in childhood. Nerv Child 1952;9:326–56.
25. Biederman J, Faraone SV, Wozniak J, et al. Further evidence of unique developmental phenotypic correlates of pediatric bipolar disorder: findings from a large sample of clinically referred preadolescent children assessed over the last 7 years. J Affect Disord 2004;82:S45–58.
26. Bradley C. Psychoses in children. In: Lewis N, Pacella B, editors. Modern trends in child psychiatry. New York: International Universities Press; 1945. p. 135–54.
27. Anthony EJ, Scott P. Manic-depressive psychosis in childhood. J Child Psychol Psychiatry 1960;1:53–72.
28. Weller RA, Weller EB, Tucker SG, et al. Mania in prepubertal children: has it been underdiagnosed. J Affect Disord 1986;11(2):151–4.
29. Schou M. Lithium treatment at 52. J Affect Disord 2001;67(1):21–32.
30. Youngerman J, Canino IA. Lithium carbonate use in children and adolescents: a survey of the literature. Arch Gen Psychiatry 1978;35(2):216–24.
31. Greenhill LL, Reider RO, Wender PH, et al. Lithium carbonate treatment of hyperactive children. Arch Gen Psychiatry 1973;28:636–40.
32. Feighner JP, Robins E, Guze SB, et al. Diagnostic criteria for use in psychiatric research. Arch Gen Psychiatry 1972;26(1):57–63.

33. Weinberg WA, Brumback RA. Mania in childhood: case studies and a literature review. Am J Dis Child 1976;130:380–5.
34. Carlson GA, Cantwell DP. Diagnosis of childhood depression: a comparison of the Weinberg and DSM-III criteria. J Am Acad Child Psychiatry 1982;21(3): 247–50.
35. Davis RE. Manic-depressive variant syndrome in childhood. Am J Psychiatry 1979;136:702–6.
36. Poznanski EO, Mokros H. Children's depression rating scale. Revised (CDRS-R). Los Angeles (CA): Western Psychological Services; 1996.
37. Chambers WJ, Puig-Antich J, Hirsch M, et al. The assessment of affective disorders in children and adolescents by semistructured interview. Test-retest reliability of the schedule for affective disorders and schizophrenia for school-age children, present episode version. Arch Gen Psychiatry 1985;42(7):696–702.
38. Kovacs M. Children's depression inventory. Washington, DC: American Psychiatric Association; 1994.
39. Carlson GA, Cantwell DP. A survey of depressive symptoms in a child and adolescent psychiatric population: interview data. J Am Acad Child Psychiatry 1979;18(4):587–99.
40. Carlson GA, Goodwin FK. The stages of mania. A longitudinal analysis of the manic episode. Arch Gen Psychiatry 1973;28(2):221–8.
41. Carlson G, Strober M. Manic depressive illness in early adolescence: a study of clinical and diagnostic characteristics in six cases. J Am Acad Child Adolesc Psychiatry 1978;17:138–53.
42. Carlson GA. Bipolar affective disorder in childhood and adolescence. In: Cantwell D, Carlson G, editors. Affective disorders in childhood and adolescence. New York: Spectrum; 1983. p. 61–83.
43. Carlson G. Annotation: child and adolescent mania- diagnostic considerations. J Child Psychol Psychiatry 1990;31:331–41.
44. Carlson G. Classification issues of bipolar disorders in childhood. Psychiatr Dev 1984;4:273–85.
45. Monro A. Some familial and social factors in depressive illness. Br J Psychiatry 1966;112:429–41.
46. Woodruff RA, Murphy GE, Herjanic M. The natural history of affective disorders. I. Symptoms of 72 patients at the time of index hospital admission. J Psychiatr Res 1967;5:255–63.
47. Krauthammer C, Klerman GL. Secondary mania. Arch Gen Psychiatry 1978;35: 1333–9.
48. Stasiek C, Zetin M. Organic manic disorders. Psychosomatics 1985;26:394–402.
49. Wozniak J, Biederman J, Kiely K, et al. Mania-like symptoms suggestive of childhood-onset bipolar disorder in clinically referred children. J Am Acad Child Adolesc Psychiatry 1995;34(7):867–76.
50. NIMH Research Roundtable. Prepubertal bipolar disorder. J Am Acad Child Adolesc Psychiatry 2000;40(8):871–7.
51. Kaufman J, Birmaher B, Brent D, et al. Schedule for affective disorders and schizophrenia for school-age children-present and lifetime version (K-SADS-PL): initial reliability and validity data. J Am Acad Child Adolesc Psychiatry 1997;36(7):980–8.
52. Leibenluft E, Charney DS, Towbin KE, et al. Defining clinical phenotypes of juvenile mania. Am J Psychiatry 2003;160:430–7.
53. Youngstrom E, Meyers O, Youngstrom JK, et al. Diagnostic and measurement issues in the assessment of pediatric bipolar disorder: implications for

understanding mood disorder across the life cycle. Dev Psychopathol 2006; 18(4):989–1021.

54. Dubicka B, Carlson GA, Val A, et al. Prepubertal mania: diagnostic differences. Eur Child Adolesc Psychiatry 2007;17:153–61.

55. e-AACAP Roundtable. "What those in the know, know". Available at: www.aacap. org/cs/onlinecme#eobd. Accessed January 1, 2009.

56. Langlois JH. Emotion and emotion regulation: from another perspective. Child Dev 2004;75(2):315–6.

57. Brotman MA, Schmajuk M, Rich BA, et al. Prevalence, clinical correlates, and longitudinal course of severe mood dysregulation in children. Biol Psychiatry 2006;60(9):991–7.

Phenomenology, Longitudinal Course, and Outcome of Children and Adolescents with Bipolar Spectrum Disorders

Regina Sala, MD, David Axelson, MD*, Boris Birmaher, MD

KEYWORDS
- Mood symptomatology • Diagnosis
- Recovery and recurrence
- Rate of conversion • Consequences

It is now well established that bipolar disorder (BP) occurs in children and adolescents.[1,2] However, aspects of the phenomenology and clinical course of pediatric BP are controversial.

The goal of this article is to review the clinical characteristics, differential diagnosis, course, and prognosis of pediatric BP.

CLINICAL CHARACTERISTICS
DSM-IV Criteria

It is clear from the work of several groups that some children and adolescents meet the full Diagnostic and Statistical Manual of Mental Disorders, 4th edition (DSM-IV) criteria for BP, despite the fact that the criteria were not specifically adapted for use in the pediatric population.[1,3] When examining the DSM-IV criteria for a manic (**Box 1**) or hypomanic (**Box 2**) episode, it is obvious that normal children can exhibit many of these features to some degree, especially in certain situations or environments. Therefore, it is of utmost importance to evaluate whether the mood and symptoms are

Dr. Sala's work was supported by an Alicia Koplowitz Foundation Fellowship in Child and Adolescent Psychiatry. Dr. Birmaher's and Dr. Axelson's work was funded by the National Institute of Mental Health (MH059929).
Department of Psychiatry, Western Psychiatric Institute and Clinic, University of Pittsburgh Medical Center, Pittsburgh, PA 15213, USA
* Corresponding author.
E-mail address: axelsonda@upmc.edu (D. Axelson).

> **Box 1**
> **DSM-IV criteria for a manic episode**
>
> A. A distinct period of abnormally and persistently elevated, expansive, or irritable mood for at least 1 week (or any duration if hospitalization is necessary).
>
> B. During the period of mood disturbance, three (or more) of the following symptoms have persisted (four if the mood is only irritable) and have been present to a significant degree:
>
>   (1) Inflated self-esteem or grandiosity
>
>   (2) Decreased need for sleep (eg, feels rested after only 3 hours of sleep)
>
>   (3) More talkative than usual or pressure to keep talking
>
>   (4) Flight of ideas or subjective experience that thoughts are racing
>
>   (5) Distractibility (ie, attention too easily drawn to unimportant or irrelevant external stimuli)
>
>   (6) Increase in goal-directed activity (either socially, at work or school, or sexually) or psychomotor agitation
>
>   (7) Excessive involvement in pleasurable activities that have a high potential for painful consequences (engaging in unrestrained buying sprees, sexual indiscretions, or foolish business investments)
>
> C. The symptoms do not meet criteria for a mixed episode.
>
> D. The mood disturbance is sufficiently severe to cause marked impairment in occupational functioning or in usual social activities or relationships with others or to necessitate hospitalization to prevent harm to self or others, or there are psychotic features.
>
> E. The symptoms are not due to the direct physiological effects of a substance (eg, a drug of abuse, a medication, or other treatment) or a general medical condition (eg, hyperthyroidism).
>
> Note: Manic-like episodes that are clearly caused by somatic antidepressant treatment (eg, medication, electroconvulsive therapy, light therapy) should not count toward a diagnosis of bipolar I disorder (BP-I).

abnormal or clearly different from the child's usual mood and behavior given the context and the child's level of development.

The distinction between a manic and hypomanic episode can be difficult but must also be taken in a developmental context. Beyond the differences in minimum duration, manic episodes require marked impairment, which should be measured against what would be the expected level of functioning for a child, given his/her chronological age and intellectual capabilities, in the psychosocial domains that are relevant to youth (eg, school, family, peers). A hypomanic episode does not require impairment, although there must be an unequivocal change from usual functioning and the mood and functional changes must be observable by others. Given that lack of insight can be associated with mania or hypomania, it is imperative to obtain information from caregivers or other significant adults in the child's or adolescent's life to accurately assess symptoms and potential change in functioning.

Mood Symptomatology

Kowatch and colleagues[1] conducted a literature review and meta-analysis of seven reports describing the phenomenology of pediatric BP. The weighted average rates of irritable mood (81%) and euphoria/elated mood (70%) found in the studies were not statistically different. However, there was statistically significant heterogeneity in the rates of irritability and euphoria/elated mood among the individual studies.

Box 2
DSM-IV criteria for a hypomanic episode

A. A distinct period of persistently elevated, expansive, or irritable mood, lasting throughout at least 4 days, that is clearly different from the usual nondepressed mood.

B. Same as criterion B for manic episode.

C. The episode is associated with an unequivocal change in functioning that is uncharacteristic of the person when not symptomatic.

D. The disturbance in mood and the change in functioning are observable by others.

E. The episode is not severe enough to cause marked impairment in social or occupational functioning, or to necessitate hospitalization, and there are no psychotic features.

F. The symptoms are not due to the direct physiological effects of a substance (eg, a drug of abuse, a medication, or other treatment) or a general medical condition (eg, hyperthyroidism).

Note: Hypomanic-like episodes that are clearly caused by somatic antidepressant treatment (eg, medication, electroconvulsive therapy, light therapy) should not count toward a diagnosis of bipolar II disorder (BP-II).

For instance, the rate of euphoria/elation ranged from 14% to 89%. Grandiosity was present in an average of 78% of subjects. Increased energy was on average the most common presenting symptom of mania, occurring in an average of 89% of cases across the samples. Distractibility and pressured speech were nearly equally common. Racing thoughts, decreased need for sleep, and poor judgment were all displayed by around 70% of youths with mania. Hypersexuality was significantly less common than any other symptom or associated feature of mania, and it manifested in fewer than half of all cases in all samples with relevant data. Flight of ideas was the second rarest symptom, appearing in an average 56% of cases (**Table 1**). These patterns of symptom presentation also appear to be consistent with the 2006 analysis of a large group of children and adolescents with bipolar spectrum disorders[3] and a report in 2005 on the phenomenology of cases with early onset BP in Europe.[4]

Table 1
Symptoms of mania from meta-analysis of pediatric BP studies

Symptom	Weighted Rate (%)	95% Confidence Interval (%)
Increased energy	89	76–96
Distractibility	84	71–92
Pressured speech	82	69–90
Irritability	81	55–94
Grandiosity	78	67–85
Racing thoughts	74	51–88
Decreased need for sleep	72	53–86
Euphoria/elation	70	45–87
Poor judgment	69	38–89
Flight of ideas	56	46–66
Hypersexuality	38	31–45

Data from Kowatch RA, Youngstrom EA, Danielyan A, et al. Review and meta-analysis of the phenomenology and clinical characteristics of mania in children and adolescents. Bipolar Disord 2005;7:483–96.

Though there is less published research on the phenomenology of depression in BP youth, depressive symptoms appear to be quite common. BP youth are frequently described as having mixed states of manic and depressive symptoms or very rapid cycling between mania and depression.[5] Rates of mixed episodes vary among different studies of bipolar youth. Some groups have reported a chronic mixed state lasting years in duration and rapid cycling between mania and depression as frequently as several times per day.[6–10] The issue is complicated by the fact that there are no clear boundaries that differentiate a mixed state from an actual switch in episode polarity or from mood lability and/or transient dysphoria occurring in the midst of mania. It is not clear whether the reports of multiple mood cycles in a day represent periods in which the child switches from meeting the full criteria of the manic syndrome to a period where he or she is completely depressed or whether they are manifestations of mood lability within the manic state. However, the evidence does indicate that the majority of BP youth have symptoms of depression interspersed in some manner with manic symptoms.[11]

Bipolar children and adolescents can have clear periods of depression that meet the full criteria for a major depressive episode (MDE); more than 50% of BP youth had a prior history of an MDE in a report published in 2006.[3] An MDE may precede the onset of manic symptomatology, so that some children and adolescents who appear to have unipolar depression may actually have BP with depression as the initial presentation.

Psychotic symptoms are frequently present in youth with BP. In the Kowatch meta-analysis, hallucinations and/or delusions were present in an average of 42% of BP youth; however, there was substantial heterogeneity in the rates of psychosis across the different studies.[1] The presence of hallucinations or delusions in a youth should trigger careful evaluation for mood disorder, for even though pediatric BP is uncommon, it has a significantly higher prevalence than do early onset schizophrenia or other potential causes of psychotic features in children.

Controversies Regarding the Diagnosis of Pediatric BP

The diagnosis of children with BP may be difficult because pediatric BP usually manifests with rapid mood changes, and, therefore, many children do not have the currently required DSM-IV duration of symptoms to fulfill diagnosis for BP-I or BP-II. According to McClellan and colleagues,[5] the most common presentation among youth with BP in community settings is characterized by "outbursts of mood lability, irritability, reckless behavior, and aggression." Shifts in mood state are short-lived,[12] and irritability, rather than euphoria, tends to be the predominant and most impairing mood state.[7] Furthermore, developmental issues influencing the clinical pictures of BP in youths, the difficulties that children and adolescents have in verbalizing their emotions, and the high rates of comorbid disorders with symptoms that overlap with those of BP account for the complexity and current controversies in diagnosing children and adolescents with BP.

One factor that may contribute to the difficulty of diagnosing BP in youth is that the most common symptoms of pediatric mania from the meta-analysis by Kowatch and colleagues[1] also happen to be frequently present in other pediatric psychiatric disorders. A recent study comparing the phenomenology of BP and attention-deficit/hyperactivity disorder (ADHD) found that there were no significant differences between the BP versus the ADHD subjects in the rate of irritability (98% BP versus 72% ADHD), accelerated speech (97% versus 82%), distractibility (94% versus 96%), or unusual energy (100% versus 95%).[13] The lack of specificity makes it problematic to diagnose mania by simply counting the presence or absence of symptoms.

Symptom expressions concerning inflated self-esteem and increased goal-directed activity are best judged in the context of the child's history, because behaviors in isolation may be misleading and may be accounted for by the child's cognitive, biological, or social development.

DSM versus Cardinal Symptoms versus Irritability

The overlap of manic symptoms with features of other psychiatric illnesses emphasizes the diagnostic importance of symptoms that tend to be more specific to mania. Some authors have advocated that two of these mania-specific symptoms, elated/elevated mood and grandiosity, are core features of the manic syndrome, so they should be considered cardinal symptoms.[13–15] These two symptoms are present in most manic youth, though there was considerable heterogeneity among studies in the rates of euphoria/elation, and one of the largest studies in the analysis required the presence of either elevated mood or grandiosity as an inclusion criterion for the BP subjects. However, a subsequently published large study of BP-I youth that did not require either of these symptoms also had high rates of elated/elevated mood (86%) and grandiosity (57%).[3] Long-term longitudinal studies of youth meeting the DSM-IV criteria for mania with or without cardinal symptoms have not been completed.

Irritable mood may be a frequent presentation of manic mood disturbance, and irritability is generally accepted as one of the most impairing features of pediatric mania. Irritability can be a diagnostic feature of depression, generalized anxiety disorder, oppositional defiant disorder (ODD), post-traumatic stress disorder, or intermittent explosive disorder, and it is a clinical feature frequently associated with conduct disorder, ADHD, Asperger syndrome, autism, and a variety of other conditions. Irritability provides a sensitive marker for pediatric BP, but it is not specific to any particular condition.[1]

Some reports have prompted controversy by stating that chronic presentations of irritability alone, particularly when the irritability is severe and accompanied by aggression and volatility, is the primary mood disturbance in bipolar youth and that elevated or expansive mood is uncommon.[6–8] However, the high prevalence of elated/expansive mood in most cross-sectional pediatric BP samples stands in contrast to these reports. Prospective evaluations of the phenomenology of new manic episodes in youth have not been published, so it is difficult to assess how frequently pediatric mania presents with only irritable mood.

Children with disruptive behavior disorders (DBDs) or ADHD may also have irritability, mood lability, and episodes of anger, defined as "severe mood dysregulation."[16] These children differ from youth with BP spectrum disorders in course, response to lithium, family history, and neuroimaging.[15]

Subthreshold Presentations

Some children and adolescents present in clinical and research settings with what appears to be significant manic symptomatology, but they do not meet the DSM-IV criteria for BP-I or BP-II. Reasons for this include the following: (1) the manic symptoms are not present for sufficient time to meet the DSM-IV duration criteria for a manic, hypomanic, or mixed episode; (2) the mood disturbances and symptoms do not occur in distinct episodes; (3) the potential manic symptoms are not clearly temporally associated or do not intensify with the abnormal mood; or (4) it cannot be reliably determined whether the abnormal mood and symptoms are attributable to BP or better accounted for by another psychiatric diagnosis. The diagnosis and management of these children and adolescents are controversial, though many present for mental health treatment with significant impairment and are frequently assigned a diagnosis of BP not otherwise specified (BP-NOS). Empirical research in subthreshold presentations of bipolarity in youth is in its early stages.

A recent multicenter study examined children and adolescents who presented with a history of clinically significant subthreshold manic symptoms. Specifically, BP-NOS patients had (a) elated mood plus two "B" mania symptoms, or irritable mood plus three "B" symptoms; (b) change in level of function associated with mood symptoms; (c) at least 4 hours of symptoms within 24 hours; and (d) at least four cumulative lifetime days meeting criteria. Though the subjects could have been below the DSM-IV threshold for either the number of manic symptoms or the duration of episode, the majority of these youth fulfilled the full mood and symptom criteria for mania and/or hypomania but did not meet the 4-day duration criteria for a hypomanic episode or the 7-day duration criteria for a manic/mixed episode.[3]

These patients with BP-NOS uniformly presented with histories of significant impairment, and nearly all had some form of psychiatric treatment before assessment. There were no significant differences among the BP-I and BP-NOS groups in age of onset, duration of illness, lifetime rate of comorbid diagnoses, suicidal ideation and major depression, family history, and the types of manic symptoms that were present during the most serious lifetime episode. Compared with youth with BP-NOS, subjects with BP-I had more severe manic symptoms, greater overall functional impairment, and higher rates of hospitalization, psychosis, and suicide attempts.[3] Elevated mood was present in 82% of subjects with BP-NOS and 92% of subjects with BP-I.[3] A significant proportion (36%) of these youth with BP-NOS has converted to BP-II or BP-I diagnoses over an average 4-year follow-up period.

BP is more likely to present with hypomania or subthreshold manic symptoms in community settings. A large community study of adolescents found that the lifetime prevalence of BP (primarily BP-II and cyclothymia) was approximately 1%. An additional 5.7% of the sample reported what would be categorized in the DSM-IV as BP-NOS.[17] Lifetime prevalence for subsyndromal BP was approximately 5%. Less than 1% of adolescents with major depressive disorder (MDD) switched to BP by age 24 years. Adolescents with BP had an elevated incidence of BP from 19 to 23 years, whereas adolescents with subsyndromal BP exhibited elevated rates of MDD and anxiety disorders in young adulthood.[18]

The diagnosis of BP-NOS was addressed in the recent American Academy of Child and Adolescent Psychiatry (AACAP) practice parameter guidelines.[5] These guidelines note that irritability and emotional reactivity are nonspecific symptoms found in multiple behavioral, affective, and developmental disorders and are, therefore, not diagnostic of mania. The AACAP guidelines suggest that the BP-NOS diagnosis be given to youths with either (a) manic symptoms of insufficient duration (ie, lasting less than 4 days) or (b) youths with "chronic manic-like symptoms which constitute baseline functioning."[5] However, prominent differences between these two classifications may indicate that cases of BP-NOS, as defined by the AACAP guidelines, are clinically heterogeneous.[16]

Comorbid Disorders

Pediatric BP is usually accompanied by other psychiatric disorders. The rates of comorbid disorders vary according to the age of the child, sample selection (clinical vs community), and the methods used to ascertain the psychiatric symptomatology.[2]

Depending on the population studied, approximately 50% to 80% have ADHD, 20% to 60% DBDs, and 30% to 70% anxiety disorders.[2] Beginning in adolescence, the rates of comorbid substance abuse and conduct disorder progressively increase.[1]

To a lesser degree, other psychiatric disorders such as obsessive-compulsive disorder as well as medical conditions can accompany BP. The presence of these disorders affects the child's response to treatment and prognosis, indicating the need to identify and treat these conditions.[1]

Children with pediatric BP tend to have higher rates of ADHD than those of adolescents with BP, whereas the latter have higher rates of substance abuse.[10,17,19] Wilens and colleagues[20] found that the risk of substance abuse was 8.8 times higher in adolescent-onset BP than that in childhood-onset adolescent BP. As in adult BP, pediatric BP is specifically associated with panic disorder.[21,22] Pediatric BP can be comorbid with autistic spectrum disorders, with one report showing rates of comorbid pervasive developmental disorder to be as high as 11%.[23]

Associated Features

Psychosis appears to be associated with pediatric BP. Most research groups have found that approximately one-fifth of youths meeting diagnostic criteria for BP-I will also have hallucinations or delusions during the course of a mood episode.[1] The prevalence of psychotic features is lower in adolescent mania than that with adult mania, with lower ratings on thought disorder and delusions. It is critical to pay attention to age-specific manifestation of the symptoms.[2]

Pediatric BP significantly affects the normal psychosocial development of the child. Youth with BP have a high risk for suicidal behaviors, completed suicide, and substance abuse as well as for behavioral, academic, social, and legal problems and increase health care use rates.[2,3,24]

Differential Diagnosis

It can be difficult to diagnose pediatric BP because of the variability in clinical presentations, high comorbidity, and overlap in symptom presentation with other psychiatric disorders. Depending on their level of cognitive development, children may have problems expressing or describing their symptoms. In addition, psychotropic medications used for treatment can potentially affect a child's mood and/or behavior.[24] Use of illicit drugs or alcohol can also complicate the diagnostic picture.

In daily practice, severe DBDs and ADHD are the most frequent conditions that may be confused with BP. The DSM-IV diagnostic criteria for a manic episode overlap with those of ADHD (distractibility, motor hyperactivity, pressured speech) and ODD (irritability/anger). In addition, youth with ADHD frequently present with mood variability, difficulty falling asleep, and tendency to engage in risk-taking or thrill-seeking behavior that could be difficult to differentiate from BP. There are some symptoms that mainly occur in BP youth and may help to differentiate between BP and these disorders, such as clinically relevant euphoria, grandiosity, significant decreased need for sleep, hypersexuality (without history of sexual abuse or exposure to sex), and hallucinations.[13]

Most depressed youth seen at psychiatric clinics are experiencing their first episode of depression.[25] Some of these subjects may develop BP, but so far it is almost impossible to know at the time of first assessment who will develop BP. Thus, a careful assessment for history of manic or hypomanic symptoms is indicated. Also, the presence of psychosis, family history of BP, and pharmacologically induced mania/hypomania may indicate an increased risk to develop BP.[26–29]

Schizophrenia is rare in children, and sometimes BP may manifest with psychosis and bizarre behavior. In older adolescents, the presence of mood-incongruent delusions and hallucinations and thought disorder can lead to the misdiagnosis of BP as schizophrenia in as many as 50% of cases.[30,31] Therefore, mood disorders need to be ruled out in any child with psychosis.

Youth with pervasive developmental disorder not otherwise specified or Asperger-syndrome may have mood lability, aggression, and agitation and be misdiagnosed as having BP. Substance abuse may also induce severe mood changes that may be difficult to differentiate from BP.

The use of medications such as antidepressants, stimulants, or steroids may unmask or trigger manic symptomatology in a susceptible individual.[32] However, this does not necessarily mean that the child has BP. Family history, the severity, length, and quality of manic symptomatology, as well as the temporal association to changes in medication may help to differentiate between BP and agitation induced by these or other medications.[33]

CLINICAL COURSE
Recovery and Recurrence

There is a consensus for definitions used to characterize the longitudinal course of BP. Recovery is defined as eight consecutive weeks without meeting any of the DSM-IV criteria for mania, hypomania, depression, or mixed affective state. Remission is defined as 2 to 7 weeks without meeting any of the DSM-IV criteria for affective episodes. Relapse is defined as two consecutive weeks of DSM-IV criteria for affective episodes with clinically significant impairment (Children's Global Assessment Scale score of <60). Chronicity is defined as failure to recover from an affective episode for a period of at least 2 years. Retrospective studies[31] and naturalistic longitudinal studies of children and adolescents with BP[9,17,34–38] have reported that 40% to 100% will recover in a period of 1 to 2 years. Of those patients who recovered, however, approximately 60% to 70% showed recurrences in an average of 10 to 12 months.[2]

Birmaher and colleagues[11] reported that overall 68% of subjects recovered from their index episode a median of 78 weeks after the onset of the episode. There were no significant differences in the rates of recovery among the subjects with BP-I, BP-II, and BP-NOS, but those with BP-NOS had a significantly longer time to recovery than subjects with BP-I and BP-II (all comparisons, $P \le .05$) (**Fig. 1**). They also reported that overall 56% of subjects had at least one recurrence at a median of 61.0 weeks after recovery of the index episode. Subjects with BP-II had higher rates of recurrence than subjects with BP-NOS, and subjects with BP-NOS had significantly longer time to recurrence than those with BP-I and BP-II (all comparisons, $P \le .05$) (**Fig. 2**). In summary, subjects with BP-I and BP-II recovered from their index episode and had recurrences more frequently than those with BP-NOS. In contrast, subjects with BP-NOS had a more protracted illness; but once they recovered from their index episode, their symptoms took a longer time to recur than those with BP-I and BP-II. On average, subjects had 1.5 syndromal recurrences per year, particularly depressive episodes.

The results for BP-I subjects are similar to those of Geller and colleagues,[9] who found that 70% to 100% of children and adolescents with BP will eventually recover from their index episode over the 4-year follow-up; but of those who recover, up to 80% experience one or more recurrences in a period of 2 to 5 years. DelBello and colleagues[39] showed that 85% had syndromic recovery in an average period of 27 weeks after the onset of their index episode when evaluating the 1-year outcome after discharge from an inpatient unit of BP-I adolescents admitted for their first manic or mixed episode. However, of these subjects, about 52% had at least one syndromic recurrence 17 weeks on average after recovery.

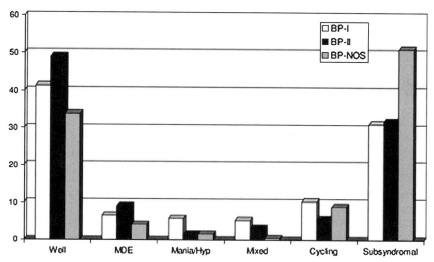

Fig.1. A comparison of the weekly symptom status of youth with bipolar I disorder, bipolar II disorder, and bipolar disorder not otherwise specified. The weekly symptoms status is the percentage of follow-up weeks that were asymptomatic or symptomatic in different mood categories. (*From* Birmaher B, Axelson D. Course and outcome of bipolar spectrum disorder in children and adolescents: a review of the existing literature. Dev Psychopathol 2006;18(4):1023–35; with permission.)

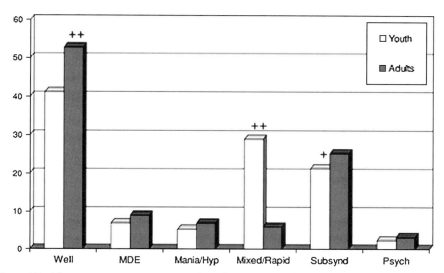

Fig. 2. Weekly symptoms status. Comparison between youth with bipolar I disorder (BP-I) versus adults with BP-I. The weekly symptom status is the percentage of follow-up weeks that were asymptomatic or symptomatic in different mood categories; $P = .05$; $P \leq .001$; $+ P = .05$; $++ P \leq .001$. (*From* Birmaher B, Axelson D. Course and outcome of bipolar spectrum disorder in children and adolescents: a review of the existing literature. Dev Psychopathol 2006;18(4):1023–35; with permission.)

Several factors have been identified that may potentially affect the course and outcome of bipolar youth. DelBello and colleagues[39] report that the comorbid presence of ADHD, anxiety disorders, low socioeconomic status, and poor adherence to pharmacological treatment was associated with longer time to recovery. Alcohol-use disorder, lack of psychotherapy treatment, and use of antidepressants were associated with shorter time to recurrence.

Preliminary analyses from the Course and Outcome of Bipolar Youth study showed that subjects with prepubertal-onset BP were approximately two times less likely to recover than those with postpubertal-onset BP.[40] In addition, subjects with prepubertal-onset BP had more chronic symptoms (defined as percentage of follow-up time with any mood symptoms), spent more follow-up time with any mood symptoms, and had more polarity changes per year than those of postpubertal-onset BP subjects. Preliminary analyses showed that mixed episodes, psychosis, low socioeconomic status, comorbid ADHD, conduct anxiety, substance abuse, and family psychopathology were associated with significantly more follow-up time with syndromal and subsyndromal symptoms.[40]

Geller and colleagues[9] found that low scores on an assessment of maternal warmth was the factor with the strongest association with worse outcome and predicted faster relapse after recovery from mania. Psychosis predicted more weeks ill with mania or hypomania.

Week-to-Week Mood Symptomatology

Recent studies have shown that BP is not only manifested by punctuated recovery and recurrences but also by ongoing fluctuating syndromal and subsyndromal symptoms.[2,9–11,24] Birmaher and colleagues[40] analyses of weekly mood symptoms showed that subjects were symptomatic approximately 60% of the follow-up time, with about 22% of the time in full syndromal episodes (manic, hypomanic, mixed, or MDEs) and 38% of the time with subsyndromal symptoms of mania and/or depression. Subjects with BP-I had more syndromal manic/hypomanic and mixed episodes than those with BP-NOS, and subjects with BP-II had more syndromal and subsyndromal depression than those with BP-I and BP-NOS. In contrast, subjects with BP-NOS showed more subsyndromal symptoms. During the follow-up, subjects with all types of BP, and particularly those with BP-NOS, with early onset or psychosis showed numerous changes in symptoms and shifts of polarity.

DelBello and colleagues[39] show that during a 1-year follow-up after hospitalization, BP adolescents spent 38% of their time meeting full syndromic criteria (mainly mixed episodes), 46% of the time with subsyndromal symptoms, and 16%, without symptoms.

Developmental Differences in Course

There are developmental differences in the course of BP between children and adults.[2,6,9,10,41,42] Youth with BP-I spent significantly more time symptomatic and had more mixed/cycling and subsyndromal episodes (see **Fig. 2**; symptomatic periods and mixed $P<.001$; subsyndromal $P = .05$), than adults with BP-I. Moreover, BP-I youth showed significantly more polarity switches than adults with BP-I (**Fig. 3**) (all comparisons $P<.001$). Thus, across the age span and especially in youth, BP usually follows an ongoing changeable course, with patient having a wide spectrum of mood symptoms ranging from mild to severe depression, mania, and/or hypomania.[40]

Early onset BP may be a particularly severe form of the illness. BP disrupts a child's developmental trajectory, limiting his or her ability to achieve critical developmental

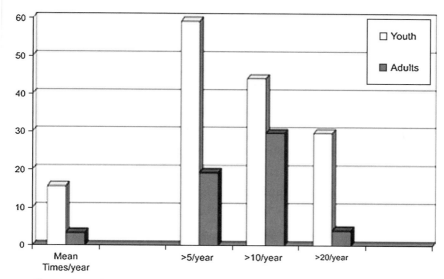

Fig. 3. Change in polarity. Comparison between youth with bipolar I disorder (BP-I) versus adults with BP-I. The change in polarity is the switch between depression and mania/hypomania or vice versa with or without intervening weeks in asymptomatic status. All comparisons are significant at *P* < .001. (*From* Birmaher B, Axelson D. Course and outcome of bipolar spectrum disorder in children and adolescents: a review of the existing literature. Dev Psychopathol 2006;18(4):1023–35; with permission.)

milestones, which has a lasting impact on his or her functioning into adulthood. Bipolar adults with onset in childhood or adolescence have higher rates of manic and depressive episodes and comorbid psychiatric disorders and spend less time in a euthymic (normal) mood state compared with those with adult onset BP.[43] Children and adolescents with BP have phenotypic features that are associated with poor prognosis in adults with BP, including high rates of mixed depressive and manic symptomatology, psychosis, and long periods of subsyndromal mood symptoms.[40] Given the severity of illness, identifying and treating BP in children is extremely important, particularly since large studies in 2004 indicate that between one-third and one-half of bipolar adults recall the onset of their symptoms during childhood or adolescence.[43,44]

Rate of Conversion Between BP-I, BP-II, and BP-NOS

Birmaher and colleagues[11] reported that approximately 20% of subjects who had an intake diagnosis of BP-II converted into BP-I. About 25% of the BP-NOS subjects converted to either BP-I or II over an average of 2 years of follow-up. Factors associated with conversion included gender (female)and longer duration of illness. The rates of conversion from BP-II to BP-I found in children[40] are higher than the cumulative rate of conversion reported in the literature on adults,[45] possibly suggesting that BP-II is less developmentally stable in the pediatric age group. However, it is currently unknown how many of the youth with BP-NOS will eventually become bipolar adults or which subthreshold presentations predict development of BP-I or BP-II versus those that are not truly bipolar.[24]

Consequences

The enduring and rapid changeability of symptoms in children and adolescents with BP occurs early in life and at crucial stages of their lives. This can deprive them of the opportunity for normal emotional, cognitive, and social develop-ment.[2,6,9,10,17,18,36,46–48] Prospective naturalistic pediatric studies as well as retro-spective reports[36,49–54] have shown a high rate of hospitalizations and health service use, psychosis, suicide attempts and completions, switch from BP-NOS to BP-I or II and from BP-II to BP-I, substance abuse, unemployment, legal problems, and poor psychosocial functioning. Ongoing BP symptoms also have a negative impact on the family and on marital and sibling relationships as well as family economics. The considerable impairment in psychosocial functioning reported in these studies is not only due to the fact that most of them were performed in clinical samples, because similar findings have been reported in BP adolescents never referred for treatment.[17,18]

Functional impairment

Pediatric BP is associated with aggressive behavior, attention problems, anxious and depressed symptoms, delinquent behavior, social problems, withdrawal, and thought problems.[55–57] Geller and colleagues[58] reported that more than half of youths diag-nosed with BP had poor social skills, had no friends, and were teased by other chil-dren. They have poor relationships with siblings and a conflictual relationship with their parents. Specifically, there was a high degree of hostility and low warmth in mother–child relationships, poor agreement between parents on child-rearing prac-tices, and minimal problem-solving skills. Parent and child reported elevated novelty-seeking traits in pediatric BP compared with those with ADHD and healthy controls.[59] Onset of bipolar illness in adolescence negatively impacts on the teen-ager's ability to function effectively in the school environment.[60] Additional studies are required to clarify whether social skill deficits are related to BP, comorbid disor-ders, family psychopathology, or demographic factors, and the interactions among these variables.

Suicidality

Longitudinal follow-up indicates that through age 18 years, 44% of patients with bipolar diagnoses (excluding BP-NOS) attempted suicide, versus 22% of patients with MDD, 18% of those with BP-NOS, and only 1% of those with no diagnosis.[61] BP was associated with the highest rates of suicidal ideation (72% of cases, versus 52% of MDD, 41% of core positive bipolar NOS, and 6% of participants with no diag-nosis), as well as younger age at first attempt (mean, 13.3 years), higher rates of multiple attempts (88% of cases), and significantly greater medical lethality of attempts.[61]

Substance abuse and behavior problems

Comorbid substance use disorders (SUDs) are common among adults with BP and are associated with markedly increased burden of illness across multiple domains. Epidemiologic and clinical studies demonstrate that youth-onset BP confers even greater risk of SUDs in comparison with adult-onset BP. Recent studies of youth with BP have not identified childhood SUDs; however, the prevalence escalates during adolescence, with estimates ranging from 16% to 39%. SUDs among adolescents with BP is associated with suicide attempts, legal problems, pregnancy, and abor-tion.[62] Several studies suggest that SUDs are more common among youth with BP than among healthy and psychiatric controls. Wilens and colleagues[20,63] found that the prevalence of SUDs was significantly higher among subjects with BP compared with those without BP. The increased prevalence of SUDs among youth with BP remained significant after controlling for conduct disorder.[20,63]

FUTURE DIRECTIONS FOR RESEARCH

Despite the growing evidence that the consequences of BP arising during childhood can be devastating, with high rates of mixed and cycling presentations, substance abuse, suicidal risk, and social, family, vocational, and academic impairment,[2,11] the long-term course of BP in youth has been insufficiently studied. Extensive follow-up time is needed to evaluate the continuity of BP symptoms from childhood to adulthood. Finally, studies should evaluate and analyze the positive or negative contributions to the child's outcome of factors such as the child's emotional and cognitive development, social and coping skills, circadian/social rhythms, and home and community environment. Regarding this last factor, important issues such as parental lifetime and current psychopathology, support, and exposure to negative life events should be considered.

SUMMARY

Though findings vary somewhat among different research groups, there are several unique features that have been consistently demonstrated in studies of the phenomenology and course of pediatric BP: (1) high rates of elevated, expansive, or elated mood; (2) prominent irritability; (3) prolonged mood episodes characterized by significant periods of subsyndromal symptomatology; (4) depressive symptoms interspersed with manic or hypomanic symptoms; (5) high rates of comorbid psychiatric disorders, especially ADHD, other DBDs, and anxiety disorders; (6) high rates of substance use disorders in older adolescents with BP; and (7) high rates of psychotic symptoms and suicide attempts and significant functional impairment. These features emphasize the need for early recognition and treatment of children and adolescents with BP to ameliorate ongoing syndromal and subsyndromal symptoms and to reduce or prevent the serious psychosocial morbidity that usually accompanies this illness.

REFERENCES

1. Kowatch RA, Youngstrom EA, Danielyan A, et al. Review and meta-analysis of the phenomenology and clinical characteristics of mania in children and adolescents. Bipolar Disord 2005;7:483–96.
2. Pavuluri MN, Birmaher B, Naylor M. Pediatric bipolar disorder: a review of the past 10 years. J Am Acad Child Adolesc Psychiatry 2005;44(9):846–71.
3. Axelson D, Birmaher B, Strober M, et al. Phenomenology of children and adolescents with bipolar spectrum disorders. Arch Gen Psychiatry 2006;63(10): 1139–48.
4. Soutullo CA, Chang KD, Diez-Suarez A, et al. Bipolar disorder in children and adolescents: international perspective on epidemiology and phenomenology. Bipolar Disord 2005;7(6):497–506.
5. McClellan J, Kowatch RA, Findling RL. Practice parameter for the assessment and treatment of children and adolescents with bipolar disorder. J Am Acad Child Adolesc Psychiatry 2007;46(1):107–25.
6. Biederman J, Faraone SV, Wozniak J, et al. Further evidence of unique developmental phenotypic correlates of pediatric bipolar disorder: findings from a large

sample of clinically referred preadolescent children assessed over the last 7 years. J Affect Disord 2004;82(Suppl 1):S45–58.

7. Mick E, Spencer T, Wozniak J, et al. Heterogeneity of irritability in attention-deficit/ hyperactivity disorder subjects with and without mood disorders. Biol Psychiatry 2005;58(7):576–82.

8. Wozniak J, Biederman J, Kiely K, et al. Mania-like symptoms suggestive of child-hood-onset bipolar disorder in clinically referred children. J Am Acad Child Ado lesc Psychiatry 1995;34(7):867–76.

9. Geller B, Tillman R, Craney JL, et al. Four-year prospective outcome and natural history of mania in children with a prepubertal and early adolescent bipolar disorder phenotype. Arch Gen Psychiatry 2004;61(5):459–67.

10. Findling RL, Gracious BL, McNamara NK, et al. Rapid, continuous cycling and psychiatric co-morbidity in pediatric bipolar I disorder. Bipolar Disord 2001; 3(4):202–10.

11. Birmaher B, Axelson D, Strober M, et al. Clinical course of children and adoles-cents with bipolar spectrum disorder. Arch Gen Psychiatry 2006;63(2):175–83.

12. Carlson GA. Who are the children with severe mood dysregulation, a.k.a. "ra-ges"? Am J Psychiatry 2007;164(8):1140–2.

13. Geller B, Zimerman B, Williams M, et al. DSM-IV mania symptoms in a prepubertal and early adolescent bipolar disorder phenotype compared to attention-deficit hyperactive and normal controls. J Child Adolesc Psychopharmacol 2002; 12(1):11–25.

14. Geller B, Zimmerman B, Williams M, et al. Phenomenology of prepubertal and early adolescent bipolar disorder: examples of elated mood, grandiose behav-iors, decreased need for sleep, racing thoughts and hypersexuality. J Child Ado-lesc Psychopharmacol 2002;12(1):3–9.

15. Leibenluft E, Charney DS, Towbin KE, et al. Defining clinical phenotypes of juve-nile mania. Am J Psychiatry 2003;160(3):430–7.

16. Leibenluft E, Rich BA. Pediatric bipolar disorder. Annu Rev Clin Psychol 2008;4: 163–87.

17. Lewinsohn PM, Klein D, Seeley JR, et al. Bipolar disorders in a community sample of older adolescents: prevalence, phenomenology, comorbidity, and course. J Am Acad Child Adolesc Psychiatry 1995;34(4):454–63.

18. Lewinsohn PM, Klein DN, Seeley JR. Bipolar disorder during adolescence and young adulthood in a community sample. Bipolar Disord 2000;2:281–93.

19. McClellan J, McCurry C, Snell J, et al. Early-onset psychotic disorders: course and outcome over a 2-year period. J Am Acad Child Adolesc Psychiatry 1999; 38(11):1380–8.

20. Wilens TE, Biederman J, Kwon A, et al. Risk of substance use disorders in adolescents with bipolar disorder. J Am Acad Child Adolesc Psychiatry 2004; 43(11):1380–6.

21. Biederman J, Faraone SV, Hatch M, et al. Conduct disorder with and without mania in a referred sample of ADHD children. J Affect Disord 1997;44(2–3): 177–88.

22. Birmaher B, Kennah A, Brent D, et al. Is bipolar disorder specifically associated with panic disorder in youths? J Clin Psychiatry 2002;63(5):414–9.

23. Wozniak J, Biederman J, Faraone SV, et al. Mania in children with pervasive developmental disorder revisited. J Am Acad Child Adolesc Psychiatry 1997; 36(11):1552–9.

24. Birmaher B, Axelson D, Pavuluri MN. Pediatric bipolar disorder. In: Martin A, Volkmar FR, editors. Lewis' child and adolescent psychiatry: a comprehensive

textbook. 4th edition. Baltimore (MD): Lippincott Williams & Wilkins; 2007. p. 513–28.

25. Birmaher B, Ryan ND, Williamson DE, et al. Childhood and adolescent depression: a review of the past 10 years. Part I. J Am Acad Child Adolesc Psychiatry 1996;35(11):1427–39.
26. Geller B, Zimerman B, Williams M, et al. Bipolar disorder at prospective follow-up of adults who had prepubertal major depressive disorder. Am J Psychiatry 2001; 158(1):125–7.
27. Kovacs M. Presentation and course of major depressive disorder during childhood and later years of the life span. J Am Acad Child Adolesc Psychiatry 1996;35(6):705–15.
28. Strober M, Carlson G. Bipolar illness in adolescents with major depression: clinical, genetic, and psychopharmacologic predictors in a three- to four-year prospective follow-up investigation. Arch Gen Psychiatry 1982;39(5):549–55.
29. Weissman MM, Wolk S, Wickramaratne P, et al. Children with prepubertal-onset major depressive disorder and anxiety grown up. Arch Gen Psychiatry 1999; 56(9):794–801.
30. Carlson GA. Child and adolescent mania-diagnostic considerations. J Child Psychol Psychiatry 1990;31(3):331–41.
31. Werry JS, McClellan JM, Chard L. Childhood and adolescent schizophrenic, bipolar, and schizoaffective disorders: a clinical and outcome study. J Am Acad Child Adolesc Psychiatry 1991;30(3):457–65.
32. Martin A, Young C, Leckman JF, et al. Age effects on antidepressant-induced manic conversion. Arch Pediatr Adolesc Med 2004;158(8):773–80.
33. Wilens TE, Wyatt D, Spencer TJ. Disentangling disinhibition. J Am Acad Child Adolesc Psychiatry 1998;37(11):1225–7.
34. Birmaher B, Williamson DE, Dahl RE, et al. Clinical presentation and course of depression in youth: does onset in childhood differ from onset in adolescence? J Am Acad Child Adolesc Psychiatry 2004;43(1):63–70.
35. Carlson GA, Bromet EJ, Sievers S. Phenomenology and outcome of subjects with early- and adult-onset psychotic mania. Am J Psychiatry 2000;157(2):213–9.
36. Carlson GA, Bromet EJ, Driessens C, et al. Age at onset, childhood psychopathology, and 2-year outcome in psychotic bipolar disorder. Am J Psychiatry 2002;159(2):307–9.
37. Jairam R, Srinath S, Girimaji SC, et al. A prospective 4–5 year follow-up of juvenile onset bipolar disorder. Bipolar Disord 2004;6(5):386–94.
38. Strober M, Schmidt-Lackner S, Freeman R, et al. Recovery and relapse in adolescents with bipolar affective illness: a five-year naturalistic, prospective follow-up. J Am Acad Child Adolesc Psychiatry 1995;34(6):724–31.
39. DelBello MP, Hanseman D, Adler CM, et al. Twelve-month outcome of adolescents with bipolar disorder following first hospitalization for a manic or mixed episode. Am J Psychiatry 2007;164(4):582–90.
40. Birmaher B, Axelson D. Course and outcome of bipolar spectrum disorder in children and adolescents: a review of the existing literature. Dev Psychopathol 2006; 18(4):1023–35.
41. Post RM, Denicoff KD, Leverich GS, et al. Morbidity in 258 bipolar outpatients followed for 1 year with daily prospective ratings on the NIMH life chart method. J Clin Psychiatry 2003;64(6):680–90.
42. Schneck CD, Miklowitz DJ, Calabrese JR, et al. Phenomenology of rapid-cycling bipolar disorder: data from the first 500 participants in the Systematic Treatment Enhancement Program. Am J Psychiatry 2004;161(10):1902–8.

43. Perlis RH, Miyahara S, Marangell LB, et al. Long-term implications of early onset in bipolar disorder: data from the first 1000 participants in the systematic treatment enhancement program for bipolar disorder (STEP-BD). Biol Psychiatry 2004; 55(9):875–81.
44. Chengappa KN, Kupfer DJ, Frank E, et al. Relationship of birth cohort and early age at onset of illness in a bipolar disorder case registry. Am J Psychiatry 2003; 160(9):1636–42.
45. Coryell W, Endicott J, Maser JD, et al. Long-term stability of polarity distinctions in the affective disorders. Am J Psychiatry 1995;152(3):385–90.
46. Weller RA, Weller EB, Tucker SG, et al. Mania in prepubertal children: has it been underdiagnosed. J Affect Disord 1986;11(2):151–4.
47. Brent DA, Perper JA, Moritz G, et al. Psychiatric risk factors for adolescent suicide: a case-control study. J Am Acad Child Adolesc Psychiatry 1993;32(3): 521–9.
48. Geller B, Bolhofner K, Craney J, et al. Psychosocial functioning in a prepubertal and early adolescent bipolar disorder phenotype. J Am Acad Child Adolesc Psychiatry 2000;39(12):1543–8.
49. Bashir M, Russell J, Johnson G. Bipolar affective disorder in adolescence: a 10-year study. Aust N Z J Psychiatry 1987;21(1):36–43.
50. Jarbin H, Ott Y, Von Knorring AL. Adult outcome of social function in adolescent-onset schizophrenia and affective psychosis. J Am Acad Child Adolesc Psychiatry 2003;42(2):176–83.
51. McGlashan TH. Adolescent versus adult onset of mania. Am J Psychiatry 1988; 145(2):221–3.
52. Rajeev J, Srinath S, Reddy YC, et al. The index manic episode in juvenile-onset bipolar disorder: the pattern of recovery. Can J Psychiatry 2003;48(1):52–5.
53. Welner A, Welner Z, Fishman R. Psychiatric adolescent inpatients: eight- to ten-year follow-up. Arch Gen Psychiatry 1979;36(6):698–700.
54. Werry JS, McClellan JM. Predicting outcome in child and adolescent (early onset) schizophrenia and bipolar disorder. J Am Acad Child Adolesc Psychiatry 1992; 31(1):147–50.
55. Youngstrom E, Youngstrom JK, Starr M. Bipolar diagnoses in community mental health: Achenbach child behavior checklist profiles and patterns of comorbidity. Biol Psychiatry 2005;58(7):569–75.
56. Kahana SY, Youngstrom EA, Findling RL, et al. Employing parent, teacher, and youth self-report checklists in identifying pediatric bipolar spectrum disorders: an examination of diagnostic accuracy and clinical utility. J Child Adolesc Psychopharmacol 2003;13(4):471–88.
57. Mick E, Biederman J, Pandina G, et al. A preliminary meta-analysis of the child behavior checklist in pediatric bipolar disorder. Biol Psychiatry 2003;53(11): 1021–7.
58. Geller B, Craney JL, Bolhofner K, et al. Two-year prospective follow-up of children with a prepubertal and early adolescent bipolar disorder phenotype. Am J Psychiatry 2002;159(6):927–33.
59. Tillman R, Geller B, Craney JL, et al. Temperament and character factors in a prepubertal and early adolescent bipolar disorder phenotype compared to attention deficit hyperactive and normal controls. J Child Adolesc Psychopharmacol 2003;13(4):531–43.
60. Quackenbush D, Kutcher S, Robertson HA, et al. Premorbid and postmorbid school functioning in bipolar adolescents: description and suggested academic interventions. Can J Psychiatry 1996;41(1):16–22.

61. Lewinsohn PM, Seeley JR, Klein DN. Bipolar disorder in adolescents: epidemiology and suicidal behavior. In: Geller B, DelBello MP, editors. Bipolar disorder in childhood and early adolescence. New York: Guilford; 2003. p. 7–24.
62. Goldstein BI, Strober MA, Birmaher B, et al. Substance use disorder among adolescents with bipolar spectrum disorder. Bipolar Disord 2008;10(4):469–78.
63. Wilens TE, Biederman J, Millstein RB, et al. Risk for substance use disorders in youths with child- and adolescent-onset bipolar disorder. J Am Acad Child Adolesc Psychiatry 1999;38(6):680–5.

Comorbidity in Pediatric Bipolar Disorder

Gagan Joshi, MD[a],*, Timothy Wilens, MD[b]

KEYWORDS

- Bipolar disorder • Comorbidity • Children and adolescents
- Clinical presentation • Treatment

Pediatric-onset BPD seldom occurs in the absence of comorbid conditions. The co-occurrence of additional disorders complicates both the accurate diagnosis of BPD and its treatment. BPD is one of the most debilitating psychiatric disorders, estimated to cost Americans $45 billion per year. It is not so infrequent as previously reported, with rates of bipolar spectrum disorder reaching an estimated 4%. Youth with BPD are among the most impaired population, and the presence of comorbidity compounds disability, complicates treatment, and appears to worsen the prognosis in this population. Comorbid disorders may have a significant impact on various indices of BPD correlates. Knowledge of their comorbid presence with BPD could be informative in determining course, prognosis, and functional and therapeutic outcomes. Early identification and appropriate management may lead to improved functioning, prevention of impending emergence of comorbid disorders (oppositional defiant disorder/conduct disorder [ODD/CD], substance use disorders [SUDs]), and attenuation of the untreated course of BPD.[1,2] On the other hand, if comorbidity is not appropriately acknowledged, then misattribution of impairing symptoms could lead to inappropriate therapeutic interventions, unnecessary exposure to neuroleptic agents, worsening of symptoms, delayed diagnosis, and misuse of mental health resources.

This work was supported by the National Institutes of Health (NIH) RO1 DA12945, K24 DA016264, the Dupont Warren Fellowship Award, the Norma Fine Pediatric Psychopharmacology Fellowship Fund, and the Pediatric Psychopharmacology Council Fund.
[a] Pervasive Developmental Disorders Program, Clinical and Research Programs in Pediatric Psychopharmacology, Massachusetts General Hospital, Harvard Medical School, 32 Fruit Street, YAW 6A, Boston, MA 02114, USA
[b] Substance Abuse Services, Pediatric Psychopharmacology Clinic, Massachusetts General Hospital, Harvard Medical School, 32 Fruit Street, YAW 6A, Boston, MA 02114, USA
* Corresponding author.
E-mail address: joshi.gagan@mgh.harvard.edu (G. Joshi).

Child Adolesc Psychiatric Clin N Am 18 (2009) 291–319
doi:10.1016/j.chc.2008.12.005   childpsych.theclinics.com

Recognition of comorbidity is important as it has therapeutic implications, such as (1) increased risk of mood destabilization, which is inherent to the therapeutic options for the comorbidity, as is the case with antianxiety, antidepressant, or anti-ADHD medications that have manicogenic potential, (2) atypical response (efficacy and tolerability) to psychotropics associated with certain disorders such as pervasive developmental disorders (PDD), or (3) less than expected antimanic response to thymoleptic agents in the presence of certain comorbid disorders (for instance ADHD, obsessive–compulsive disorder [OCD]).

Comorbid disorders may be challenging to diagnose due to overlapping symptoms and developmentally sensitive, complicated patterns of symptom development. Several methods have been applied to scientifically understand comorbidity. Structured diagnostic interviews (for instance, the Kiddie Schedule for Affective Disorders and Schizophrenia-Epidemiologic Fifth Version [K-SADS-E])[3] are helpful in clinically parsing out comorbid conditions as they comprehensively assess the spectrum of psychopathologies described in the Diagnostic and Statistical Manual of Mental Disorders (DSM), including past and present severity of symptoms. Diagnoses are considered positive only if the diagnostic criteria are met to a degree that would be considered *clinically meaningful*. "Clinically meaningful" means that the data collected from the structured interview indicate that the diagnosis should be a clinical concern due to the nature of the symptoms, the associated impairment, and the coherence of the clinical picture. For a given disorder, the overlapping nonspecific symptoms are considered for the diagnosis if the respective cardinal symptoms are present, and the disorder is cause for significant impairment. Furthermore, although DSM criteria do not permit comorbid presence of certain disorders and assign diagnoses based on hierarchy, to fully characterize the clinical picture, a nonhierarchical diagnostic approach is taken to assess for comorbid disorders. Thus, the approach taken by the structured interview objectively and comprehensively documents symptom presentation and minimizes diagnostic biases.

Perhaps the most compelling scientific method to examine comorbidity is familial risk analysis, which addresses uncertainties regarding complex phenotypes in probands by examining the transmission of comorbid disorders in families.[4,5] Therapeutic response has also provided evidence of the existence of separate conditions. For instance, in a review of clinical records in manic children, Biederman and colleagues[6] reported that whereas mood stabilizers significantly improved mania-like symptoms, antidepressants and stimulants did not, and, conversely, tricyclic antidepressants and not mood stabilizers were associated with improvement of ADHD symptoms. Finally, attributes of comorbidity can also be addressed by applying neurobiological probes to seek the existence of underlying changes commensurate with each comorbid disorder, either disorder or neither disorder indicating a unique subtype with distinct neurobiological attributes. The emerging proton magnetic resonance spectroscopic (^{1}HMRS) imaging intervention research in youth with BPD suggests a profile of cerebral metabolites in a specific region of the brain, which may facilitate the understanding of neurochemical correlates of BPD in the context of comorbidity. For instance, the ^{1}HMRS profile of cerebral metabolites in the anterior cingulate cortex region of the brain in children with ADHD appears to have a significantly higher ratio of glutamate plus glutamine to myo-inositol-containing compounds than does the profile of children with comorbid BPD and ADHD.[7]

Present studies addressing comorbidity generally rely either on cross-sectional observations or on recall of disorders over the whole life course. Both of these approaches pose limitations. Longitudinal studies that offer the best possibility for observing the developmental progression of the emergence of comorbid conditions are required.

Treatment guidelines for pediatric BPD indicate that the treatment plan must include treatment for each comorbid disorder, which may become a complex process of trial and error to find the most effective combination of medications.[8] These guidelines further recommend that in the absence of treatment trials specifically studying a population of children with BPD and specific comorbid disorders, clinicians should use psychopharmacologic and psychosocial treatments that are generally recommended for each comorbid disorder when that disorder occurs as the primary problem. Though certain comorbid disorders associated with BPD respond to antimanic agents (DBDs, PDD), there are frequently co-occurring disorders (ADHD, anxiety disorders, depression) with typical onset before the emergence of mania that require treatment with agents that have manicogenic potential. Available empiric evidence and clinical acumen dictate that treatment of comorbid conditions can be addressed only after the symptoms of BPD are stabilized.[9] Decision to treat the comorbid disorders following stabilization of mania should be guided by clinically determining the level of impairment associated with the disorder. As a rule, medications with lower manicogenic potential are preferred in this population.

Comorbid conditions frequently associated with pediatric-onset BPD include ADHD, DBDs, SUDs, anxiety disorders (including panic disorder, post-traumatic stress disorder (PTSD), OCD), and PDDs (**Fig. 1**). In the following sections, we address the characteristics and management of frequently occurring comorbid disorders in children and adolescents with BPD.

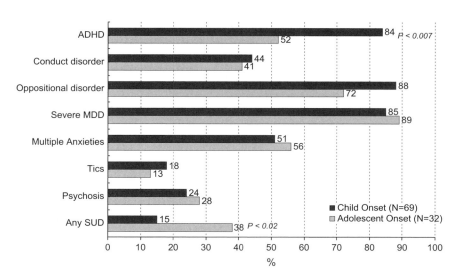

Fig. 1. Rates of psychiatric comorbidity in bipolar youth stratified by age at onset of BPD. (*Adapted from* Biederman J, Petty C, Faraone SV, et al. Moderating effects of major depression on patterns of comorbidity in referred adults with panic disorder: a controlled study. Psychiatry Res 2004;126:143.)

ATTENTION-DEFICIT HYPERACTIVITY DISORDER

Systematic studies of pediatric populations with BPD show that the rates of comorbid ADHD range from 60% to 90%.[10-12] While a high prevalence of ADHD is reported in youth with BPD, a modest rate (22%) of comorbid BPD is reported in pediatric populations with ADHD.[13] Although the rates of ADHD in youth with BPD are universally high, the age at onset modifies the risk for comorbid ADHD. ADHD comorbidity is more often associated with early onset BPD (<18 years).[14,15] Rates of ADHD in adolescents with BPD are reported to be greater in childhood-onset BPD (≤12 years) than those in adolescent-onset BPD (>13 years).[16,17] Sachs and colleagues[15] reported that, among adults with BPD, a history of comorbid ADHD was evident only in subjects with onset of BPD before the age of 19 years.

Although the literature on adult patients on the subject has been less extensive, similar findings have been documented. The National Comorbidity Survey Replication epidemiologic study documented significantly higher rates of BPD in the adult population with ADHD compared with those in adults without ADHD (19.4% versus 3.1%).[18] Consistent with the documented association of comorbid ADHD almost exclusively with early onset BPD, a relatively low lifetime prevalence (9.5%) of comorbid ADHD is reported in an adult research population with BPD.[19] Similarly, Winokur and colleagues[20] reported childhood hyperactivity in 21.3% of their adult BPD population (N = 189) and in 19% of their first-degree adult relatives with BPD. ADHD comorbidity with BPD is over-represented in males, and in its presence, BPD adults had the onset of their mood disorder approximately 5 years earlier, had shorter periods of euthymia, were more frequently depressed, and had a greater burden of additional comorbid psychiatric disorders, especially anxiety disorders and SUD.[19]

In an analysis of prepubertal children with BPD and ADHD, Wozniak and colleagues[21] demonstrated correlates of both conditions. Affected children had high rates of major depression, psychosis, multiple anxiety disorders, impaired psychosocial function, and hospitalization, consistent with BPD. Similarly, phenotypic features of ADHD and associated neuropsychiatric correlates (that is, high rates of learning disabilities and need for educational services) have striking homology to the presentation of ADHD in the context of comorbidity with BPD, suggesting that ADHD may be a bona fide disorder when comorbid with BPD.[6] As ADHD and mania diagnostically share nonspecific symptoms (distractibility, motoric hyperactivity, and talkativeness), there is a risk of unintentional overdiagnosis. Several studies have addressed this issue.[22] Biederman and colleagues[16] showed that the majority of children with the combined condition continued to meet criteria of both mania and ADHD after removing overlapping symptoms, suggesting that BPD and ADHD comorbidity is not a methodological artifact due to shared diagnostic criteria. Although limited information is available regarding the potential for different rates of comorbidity with BPD among the DSM-IV subtypes of ADHD, the rates of BPD are reported to be highest among youth with combined-type ADHD (26.5%) but also elevated among hyperactive-impulsive (14.3%) and inattentive (8.7%) youth.[23] Wilens and colleagues[12] examined a research population of adults with ADHD in which nearly half the population also met the criteria for BPD (47%); the vast majority were BPD-II (88%). Although ADHD adults with comorbid BPD shared the prototypic characteristics of both the disorders, they had higher rates of combined-type ADHD, with a greater number of DSM-IV ADHD symptoms (especially attentional symptoms), a higher prevalence of anxiety disorders, and poorer global functioning.

Although the mechanisms that mediate the association between BPD and ADHD are not entirely clear, other data suggest that subforms of these disorders share genes in common.[24] Children of bipolar parents have an elevated risk for ADHD, and relatives of ADHD children have an increased risk for BPD.[25] The transmission of these disorders has been studied in families ascertained through pediatric BPD patients, ADHD boys,[25] and ADHD girls.[26] In each of these reports, the pattern of transmission supported the hypothesis that early onset BPD may be a developmental subtype of BPD.

In BPD youth with ADHD whose mood is well stabilized, ADHD symptoms often become the second most severe presenting complaint.[9] If the symptoms of inattentiveness, distractibility, talkativeness, and impulsivity are not recognized as comorbid ADHD, then they may be inappropriately treated as residual symptoms of mania. Conversely, identification of mania in youth with ADHD has therapeutic implications, as failure to recognize comorbidity could lead to administration of anti-ADHD medications that could exacerbate the mania.

The response to lithium has been reported to be less robust in the presence of ADHD comorbidity in youth with BPD,[27,28] suggesting that this subgroup of BPD may constitute a unique genetic subform with a differential treatment response. A chart review evaluating treatment outcome of youth with BPD treated during a 4-year period showed that mood stabilizers selectively improved manic symptoms, whereas stimulants had no effect.[29] Furthermore, in youngsters with BPD, comorbid ADHD could be addressed selectively with the anti-ADHD armamentarium but only after mood stabilization.

Stimulants have been reported to be efficacious in treating comorbid ADHD without precipitating (hypo)mania in mood-stabilized BPD youth in two controlled trials. A controlled trial of stimulants as an adjunctive therapy for ADHD in BPD youth with manic symptoms stabilized on divalproex found mixed amphetamine salts to be safe and efficacious for the treatment of ADHD in the context of BPD.[30] Findling and colleagues[31] reported that in youth stabilized with a stable dose of at least one mood stabilizer, concomitant treatment with methylphenidate improved ADHD in a dose-dependent manner without destabilization of mood. Furthermore, in an open trial of the nonstimulant anti-ADHD agent bupropion in adults with predominately mood-stabilized bipolar II disorder and ADHD, we previously reported a significant improvement in ADHD without activation of mania.[32] These aggregate data suggest that treatment for BPD needs to precede ADHD treatment, and that in general, stimulants and nonstimulants may be cautiously introduced.

OPPOSITIONAL DEFIANT DISORDER

High rates with bidirectional overlap of comorbid ODD and BPD are reported by various studies. Rates of ODD in the BPD population range from 47% to 88%,[33,34] and conversely, 20% of children with ODD are reported to have comorbid BPD.[35] A meta-analysis in 2005 reported ODD as the second most common comorbidity after ADHD, with a weighted rate of 53% among samples of children and adolescents with BPD.[8]

The diagnosis of ODD in the context of BPD is challenging as nosologically ODD shares overlapping symptoms with mania without any symptom specific to ODD that could diagnostically differentiate it from mania. Because ODD is so frequently comorbid with pediatric BPD, the understanding of the relationship of ODD with BPD ranges from ODD being a secondary disorder as a consequence of bipolar illness or being a prodrome or early manifestation of BPD to ODD representing a "true independent" comorbid psychopathologic phenomenon. However, many children with DBDs do not go on to develop BPD,[13] suggesting that different forms of DBDs may exist, one that could be prodromal to BPD and another form that is not. More work is needed to further evaluate this issue.

A clinical inquiry summarized 8 reviews on ODD treatments of children and found improved behavior with a 20% to 30% decrease in disruptive or aggressive behaviors with parenting interventions and behavioral therapy including cognitive-behavioral therapy (CBT), social problem-solving skills training, and parent management training involving the child and/or parent for 12 to 25 sessions.[36]

Though treatment of ODD is primarily behavioral in nature, when comorbid with other medication-responsive psychiatric conditions (BPD, ADHD), pharmacologic treatment of the comorbid disorder often reduces overall symptoms of the ODD. Although there are currently no data available on the treatment of ODD in the context of BPD comorbidity, an emerging body of literature points to the role of thymoleptic agents in the treatment of DBD (CD, ODD, and DBD not otherwise specified), including ODD in youth with significant aggression. Evidence suggests that pharmacotherapy may be effective in youth with DBD, especially those experiencing problematic aggression, but response of the DBD per se to these thymoleptics is understudied. Multiple studies have examined the safety and efficacy of atypical antipsychotics (risperidone, olanzapine, quetiapine, and aripiprazole) in treating aggression in children with DBD. Atypical antipsychotics have generally been significantly more efficacious than placebo in treating aggression in DBD youth.

To date, risperidone is the most extensively studied atypical antipsychotic for DBD. Several trials indicate that risperidone can be useful for DBD, especially the aggressive features, in both short- and long-term use.[37–40] Short- and long-term efficacy and tolerability of risperidone as pharmacotherapy for DBDs in children with subaverage intelligence has been demonstrated in more than 1,300 children and adolescents in the literature.[37–42] In two short-term (6-week) controlled trials, Aman and colleagues (2005) studied the role of low-dose risperidone (mean dose, 1.16 and 0.98 mg/d) in borderline intellectual functioning (intelligence quotient of 36–84) DBD youth (N = 223; ages, 5–12 years) and reported an acceptable tolerability profile with significant improvement in aggression and behaviors associated with DBD.[37,42] As the five long-term (1–3 year) follow-up trials suggest, a low dose of risperidone (mean dose, 1.38–1.92 mg/d) was equally well tolerated and effective in controlling the DBD and aggressive behaviors in this population.[38–41,43] Low-dose risperidone (0.02 mg/kg/d) is also reported to be well tolerated and efficacious in treating DBD behaviors in youth with normal intelligence as suggested by short- and long-term trials.[41,44]

However, a post hoc analysis of the data from the controlled trial of risperidone in DBD conducted by Aman and colleagues[37] examined 24 candidate affective symptoms extracted from the 64-item Nisonger Child Behavior Rating Form.[45] These symptoms reflected the bipolar symptoms of explosive irritability, agitation, expansiveness, grandiosity, and depression. Risperidone was also effective in treating these putative symptoms of mania. This analysis raises the question of whether studies that examine the effects of antimanic agents on DBD may include subjects with comorbid bipolar spectrum illness, and, further, whether the improvement in DBD is a function in part of the improvement in BPD.

Quetiapine is the other most studied atypical antipsychotic for DBD in youth. In youth with DBD and ADHD who fail to respond to osmotic-release oral system methylphenidate monotherapy (dose, 54 mg/d), the addition of quetiapine (mean dose, 329 mg/d) has been shown to be effective in controlling symptoms of ODD and aggression.[46] Open-label and placebo-controlled studies suggest that divalproex is efficacious for the treatment of mood lability and explosive temper in children and adolescents with DBD.[47,48] Further prospective studies addressing the course and treatment of ODD when comorbid with BPD are warranted.

CONDUCT DISORDER

In a comprehensive literature review, Geller and Luby[49] concluded that "available data strongly suggest that prepubertal-onset BPD is a nonepisodic, chronic, rapid-cycling, mixed manic state that may be comorbid with attention-deficit hyperactivity disorder (ADHD) and conduct disorder (CD) or have features of ADHD and/or CD as initial manifestations." This observation is supported by a body of research documenting a bidirectional overlap between CD and BPD in children. As both CD and BPD are highly impairing conditions, their co-occurrence heralds a particularly severe clinical picture and raises important clinical questions. From a diagnostic standpoint, the question remains as to whether antisocial behaviors in a child with BPD, such as stealing, lying, or vandalizing, should be attributed to the disinhibition of mania with its attendant impulsivity, irritability, and grandiosity or to comorbid CD. From a treatment standpoint in such a child, the question further remains as to whether the symptoms of CD will diminish when the symptoms of BPD are adequately treated.

The association between CD and mania is consistent with the well-documented comorbidity between CD and major depression[50] and the frequently bipolar nature of juvenile depression.[51,52] Moreover, pediatric-onset BPD is frequently mixed (dysphoric) and commonly associated with "affective storms," with prolonged and aggressive temper outbursts.[53,54] These irritable outbursts often include threatening or attacking behavior toward family members, children, adults, and teachers, behaviors that overlap with CD. For example, McGlashan[55] reported that juvenile-onset BPD may be particularly explosive and disorganized and that children with mania tended to have more trouble with the law and more "psychotic assaultiveness" than that of adults with BPD. Kovacs and Pollock[56] reported that some youngsters with mania showed serious acting out behaviors including burglary, stealing, vandalism, and a history of school suspensions. Although these aberrant behaviors are consistent with the diagnosis of CD, they may be due to the behavioral disinhibition that characterizes BPD. Thus, it is not surprising that youth with BPD frequently meet diagnostic criteria for CD. High rates of CD (69%) are reported in youth with BPD,[56] and the comorbid presence of BPD and CD in youth heralds a more complicated course with high rates of hospitalization (42%).[57] Furthermore, CD is reported to be severe in the presence of comorbid BPD.[58]

Epidemiologic studies report high rates of comorbidity between BPD and DBD.[59,60] There seems to be an increase in the risk for BPD with a higher number of CD symptoms[60] and a nearly seven-fold increase in the risk for BPD in individuals with antisocial personality disorder.[61] The risk of CD is 3-fold higher in younger bipolar individuals (<30 years) with comorbid SUD than that in those without SUD (52% versus 14.8%).[62]

Comorbid CD in BPD youth might confuse the clinical presentation of childhood BPD and possibly account for some of the documented failure to detect bipolarity in children. Isaac[63] examined a group of adolescents found to be the most problematic, crisis prone, and treatment resistant in a special educational day school and treatment program. These authors found that two-thirds of these youngsters satisfied DSM-III-R criteria for BPD, which had often been misdiagnosed as ADHD and CD. Most of the remaining youngsters showed significant bipolar features but did not fully satisfy DSM-III-R criteria for BPD. Considering the heterogeneity of BPD and that of CD, these findings may have important implications in helping to identify a subtype of BPD with early onset characterized by high levels of comorbid CD[56] and a subtype of CD with high levels of dysphoria and explosiveness.

In a large, well-characterized, prospective sample of children referred with ADHD,[64] ADHD children with comorbid BPD and CD reported higher familial and personal risk for mood disorders than youth with ADHD and CD alone, who were found to have higher personal risk for antisocial personality disorder. This suggests that the presence of BPD in some CD children could be clinically meaningful, at least in the context of ADHD. Further analysis of structured interview-derived data from a large sample of consecutive, clinic-referred children and adolescents showed again a large and symmetric overlap between BPD and CD.[27] Examination of the clinical features, patterns of psychiatric comorbidity, and functioning in multiple domains showed that children with CD and BPD had similar features of each disorder irrespective of comorbidity with the other disorder. These findings further supported the hypothesis that children satisfying diagnostic criteria for BPD and CD suffer from both disorders, rather than one being misdiagnosed as the other, even outside the context of comorbid ADHD. These authors also documented that psychiatric hospitalizations among CD probands were almost entirely accounted for by those with comorbid BPD. This finding is consistent with the notion that CD plus BPD probands, along with other symptoms of CD, engage in a disorganized type of aggression associated with BPD. Since many children in psychiatric hospitals with the diagnosis of CD commonly have a profile of severe aggressiveness, it is likely that these children required psychiatric hospitalizations because of the manic picture and not necessarily due to the CD.

Further evidence that a subtype of CD linked to BPD could be identified derives from pilot familial risk analyses.[65,66] These results suggest that relatives of BPD probands were at an increased risk for BPD but not CD. On the other hand, relatives of CD probands had an increased risk for CD but not for BPD, whereas relatives of CD plus BPD probands had an elevated risk for both disorders.[66] Among relatives in this latter group, BPD and antisocial disorders showed significant cosegregation, that is, relatives with one disorder were highly likely to have the other. As a result of this cosegregation, CD plus BPD was significantly elevated among relatives of CD plus BPD probands but was rare among the relatives of the other proband groups. Probands with the combined condition of CD and BPD also had high rates of non-BPD conduct/antisocial disorders among the relatives, suggesting a genetic loading with two subtypes of CD: with and without BPD. These results provide compelling evidence that subtypes of CD and of BPD can be identified based on patterns of comorbidity with the other disorder, suggesting that their co-occurrence may correspond to a distinct familial syndrome.[21,23,24,65,66]

The delineation of a subgroup of manic CD children would have important clinical implications. It could lead to improvement in our efforts to ameliorate the guarded outcome of some CD youth. Since BPD may respond to specific pharmacologic treatments, correctly identifying CD children with BPD may afford the opportunity to introduce these medications in the treatment of antisocial and aggressive youth.

There is limited evidence from various trials of atypical antipsychotics in youth with BPD on the possible role of thymoleptics in managing CD when comorbid with BPD. In our open-label, short-term (8-week) trials of risperidone (N = 30) and ziprasidone (N = 21) in children and adolescents aged 6 to 17 years with BPD, these atypical antipsychotics were associated not only with significant improvement in symptoms of pediatric BPD but also with improvement in the severity of comorbid CD (a Clinical Global Impression rating of much or very much improved) in the subset of BPD youth with comorbid CD.[67,68] Likewise, a similar response of comorbid CD to an open-label, short-term trial (8-week) of risperidone (N = 16) and olanzapine (N = 15) is recorded in a younger population of preschool-age children (4–6 years) with BPD.[68] The promising role of atypical antipsychotics in treating comorbid CD in youth with BPD as suggested by these open trials requires further validation by conducting controlled studies that apply specific measures to assess the response of CD.

As discussed earlier under the role of thymoleptic agents in the DBD population, potential pharmacotherapy for CD with marked aggression includes mood stabilizers, typical and atypical antipsychotics—the very medications most commonly recommended for the treatment of BPD. The antimanic agent lithium has been found to be an effective antiaggressive agent in youth with CD as reported by various studies conducted in ambulatory and hospitalized youth with CD.[1,69] A small proportion of the literature suggests that typical antipsychotic medications such as haloperidol and molindone are helpful in decreasing aggression in youth with CD.[70–72] However, typical antipsychotic treatment was associated with a range of problematic adverse effects. This led to the use of the atypical antipsychotic agents in treating CD with aggressive features.

In an open-label, short-term (8-week; N = 17) followed by long-term (18-week; N = 9) trial of quetiapine (at median dose 150 mg/d) in children aged 6 to 12 years with the primary diagnosis of CD, quetiapine was found to be effective in treating aggression and conduct problems by week 8; the benefit was sustained during long-term treatment with quetiapine in children who responded to an acute therapeutic trial of quetiapine.[73,74] In this trial, no subject developed extrapyramidal symptoms or discontinued the trial due to adverse events, suggesting that short- and long-term treatment with quetiapine was safe and well tolerated. In a controlled trial in 2008, quetiapine 294 (±78) mg/d was reported to be superior to placebo in treating adolescents with CD (N = 9/10) on clinician-assessed measures of global severity but failed to separate from placebo on parent-assessed specific measures of aggression and conduct behaviors; this discrepancy could be attributed to small sample size, leading to diminished statistical power to detect differences.[75]

There is preliminary evidence on the role of olanzapine in treating aggression with CD from a retrospective chart review of adolescents with CD (N = 23) who were treated with olanzapine (mean dose, 8±3.2 mg/d) for an extended period of time (6–12 months).[76] Treatment with olanzapine resulted in improvement of aggression but was also associated with a modest weight gain (4.6±3 Kg). The aforementioned empiric evidence from clinical trials exclusively conducted in CD populations in addition to the previous discussion of trials conducted in DBD populations strongly suggests the role of atypical antipsychotics in managing behaviors related to CD and aggression (**Fig. 2**).

SUBSTANCE USE DISORDERS

In recent years, a focus on mood disorders in SUD youth has emerged as a major clinical and public health concern, particularly given the implications for reduction of SUD, delinquency, and mood symptoms with treatment.[77] In epidemiologic and clinically based studies, SUD is one of the most common comorbidities found in BPD in adolescents and adults.[20,78,79] McElroy and colleagues[77] reported that drug and alcohol use disorders were found in 39% and 32% of BPD adults, respectively. In terms of linking SUD to early onset adult BPD, Dunner and Feiman[79] showed that BPD onset before adulthood was strongly and specifically related to SUD development in young adults. Similarly, McElroy and colleagues[77] showed a retrospective association between early onset BPD, mixed symptoms and comorbidity, and SUD.

The literature increasingly shows that juvenile-onset BPD is a risk factor for SUD.[80] An excess of SUD has been reported in the literature in adolescents with BPD or prominent mood lability and dyscontrol, and BPD is over-represented in youth with SUD.[81–83] A high prevalence of SUD (40%) is reported in an inpatient adolescent population with BPD.[82] In a 5-year follow-up study of 54 inpatient adolescents with BPD, Strober and

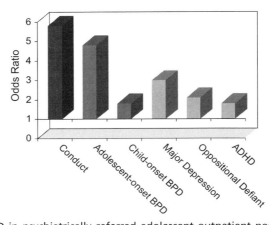

Fig. 2. Risk of SUD in psychiatrically referred adolescent outpatient population. (*Adapted from* Wilens TE, Biederman J, Millstein R, et al. Risk for substance use disorders in youth with child- and adolescent-onset bipolar disorder. J Am Acad Child Adolesc Psychiatry 1999; 38:680–5; with permission.)

colleagues[84] reported an increase in the rates of SUD from 10% at baseline (mean age, 16 yrs) to 22% at follow-up and described a mixed presentation with a highly relapsing course in the presence of comorbidity with SUD.

We previously documented that adolescents with SUD referred to a psychiatric ambulatory care clinic were more likely than those without SUD to have comorbid BPD.[83] Preliminary prospective findings from our longitudinal study of ADHD youth signaled that youth with earlyonset BPD, independent of ADHD, were reported to be at risk for SUD[81] and were also found to be at higher risk for early initiation and higher rates of cigarette smoking.[85] Similarly, clinically referred adolescents with BPD are at heightened risk for the development of SUD, independent of the status of CD, compared with that of non-BPD psychiatric adolescents.[86]

In 2008, Wilens and colleagues reported the baseline findings of an ongoing, controlled, longitudinal, family-based study of SUD in BPD adolescents[87] where the relationship between SUD and the age at onset of BPD (child versus adolescent onset) and the presence of comorbid CD was specifically evaluated. Participating youth (N = 105 BPD and 98 non–mood-disordered controls; mean age of 13.6 ± 2.5 years) did not differ by group (BPD versus controls) for any clinical characteristics or demographics. Nicotine dependence was found in 23% of BPD and 4% of controls, whereas full SUD was found in 34% of BPD youth compared with 4% of controls. BPD youth with SUD had higher rates of additional comorbidities and poorer overall functioning than those of youth with BPD without SUD and controls. Comorbidity with ADHD, conduct, or anxiety disorders did not account for the high risk of SUD in BPD.[87]

We previously reported that the onset of BPD in adolescence was more pernicious in terms of SUD onset than if the BPD began prepubertally[86] (**Fig. 3**). We further evaluated the relationship between the developmental effect of BPD onset and the onset of SUD. Interestingly, we replicated our previous findings in that youth with the onset of BPD in adolescence were at higher risk for cigarette smoking and SUD compared with that of those with the onset prepubertally.[87]

Because CD is an important comorbidity of BPD and predictor of SUD, we very recently examined the contribution of CD on later development of SUD. We found that while CD increases the risk for SUD in BPD, the risk of SUD in BPD was not

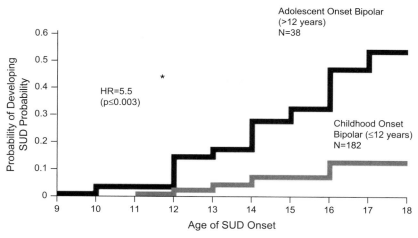

*This trend is not due to comorbidity with conduct disorder

Fig. 3. Development of SUDs in child and adolescent-onset BPD. (*Adapted from* Wilens TE, Biederman J, Millstein R, et al. Risk for substance use disorders in youth with child- and adolescent-onset bipolar disorder. J Am Acad Child Adolesc Psychiatry 1999;38:680–5; with permission.)

substantially changed with or without CD.[88] Thus, we can conclude that juvenile BPD is a risk factor for SUD irrespective of the status of CD, ADHD, or other comorbid psychopathology. Youth with the onset of BPD during adolescence were at particularly high risk for SUD, and the severity and course of both the disorders are worse when comorbid.

Mechanism of SUD Risk in BPD

The reasons for juvenile BPD being a risk factor for SUD in particular and why adolescent- versus child-onset BPD confers a differential risk for SUD remain unclear. Given the prominent genetic influences in both BPD and ADHD (as individual disorders and perhaps cosegregating), it remains unclear if SUD in BPD youth represents a subtype of BPD and/or SUD or if a vulnerability to SUD development exists in these youth. For instance, we previously speculated that the development of BPD may be particularly predictive of the development of SUD during adolescence, considering that adolescence is a time of vulnerability for the development of SUD.[86,89]

Among disturbances reported in BPD youth, severe affective and self-regulation problems may predispose them to seek drugs of abuse.[76] By nature of their intrapsychic distress and behavioral disinhibition, these youth may try to modulate their irritable and labile mood with substances of abuse; this has been described in adults.[90] Recently, Lorberg and colleagues examined this issue and found evidence that youth with BPD tended to initiate substances of abuse to attenuate mood relative to non–mood-disordered adolescents who reported using substance more often to get high.[91]

Genes and Adolescent SUD

Child- and adolescent-onset BPD may be etiologically distinct with a variable course and outcome, including the risk for SUD. It may also be that adolescent-onset BPD and adolescent-onset SUD may represent variable expressivity of a shared risk factor.[92,93] To better understand these competing influences, family studies are necessary. To this end, we examined the parents of our adolescents with and without BPD (and/or SUD) as part of our NIH-funded longitudinal study. We found that the parents of proband youth with BPD (without SUD) and BPD with SUD were more likely to develop BPD than the parents of controls (omnibus test $\chi^2 = 10.18$, $P = .006$); we also found no differences between the two bipolar groups. Parents of proband youth with BPD and with BPD with SUD were more likely than relatives of controls to develop SUD (omnibus test $\chi^2 = 14.69$, $P<.001$); however, we found no differences between the parents of the 2 proband bipolar groups. Among the parents of proband youth with BPD along with SUD, we found higher risk of SUD in parents with BPD than that in those without BPD ($\chi^2 = 8.39$, $P = .004$), leading us to speculate that BPD and SUD are prevalent in the first-degree relatives of adolescents with BPD, adults with BPD were more likely to manifest SUD, and that BPD and SUD cosegregated. Interestingly, work from our group (2008) with a candidate gene for BPD—namely the dopamine transporter protein[94]—has also been found to be associated with the development of early onset SUD.

Diagnostic and Treatment Considerations

The first consideration that clinicians should have in mind in the establishment of a specific treatment plan for adolescents with co-occurring mental and substance-related disorders is the determination of the level of care needed. When treating dually diagnosed disorders such as BPD and SUD, clinicians should consider a simultaneous approach. Given limited, albeit important, data on the effects of medication treatment reducing SUD in BPD, both psychosocial and medication strategies should be considered simultaneously in these comorbid adolescents. There is evidence that pharmacologic interventions are effective for youth with SUD and BPD. Two studies, including one randomized controlled study, have reported that mood stabilizers, specifically lithium and valproic acid, significantly reduced substance use in bipolar youth.[95,96] In a controlled, 6-week study of treatment with lithium in youth with affective dysregulation and substance dependence, Geller and colleagues[96] reported a clinically significant decrease in the number of positive urines as well as a significant increase in overall global functioning.

In a 5-week, open trial of valproic acid in adolescent outpatients with marijuana abuse/dependence and "explosive mood disorder" (mood symptoms were not classified using the DSM IV), Donovan and colleagues[95] reported significant improvement in their marijuana use and their affective symptoms. The use of atypical neuroleptics as mood-stabilizing agents in comorbid SUD-BPD remains understudied, albeit compelling, and further work in this area is needed.

ANXIETY DISORDERS

The presence of anxiety disorders in individuals who suffer from BPD has been under-recognized and understudied. One reason for this lack of recognition could be the notion that it is counterintuitive to suggest that BPD, which is characterized by high levels of disinhibition, could coexist with anxiety, which is characterized by fear and inhibition. However, in the first article to demonstrate the high frequency of BPD in an outpatient pediatric psychopharmacology clinic (16%), 56% of the children with BPD suffered from two or more lifetime anxiety disorders (multiple anxiety disorders) comorbidly. Furthermore, a recent detailed analysis of the comorbidity between pediatric BPD and anxiety disorders in a clinically referred population revealed that 76% of youth with BPD have one or more anxiety disorders comorbid with their BPD.[97] In a community sample, Lewinsohn and colleagues[56] reported that a third of nonreferred BPD adolescents had comorbid anxiety disorders, a significantly higher rate than that found in those without a history of BPD. Because the anxiety disorders are heterogeneous (eight are included in the DSM-IV)[98] and as most studies lump them, uncertainties remain as to which anxiety disorders are associated with BPD. Various clinical and epidemiologic studies in adult and pediatric populations have identified a wide range of anxiety disorders associated with BPD, with rates ranging between 12.5% and 76% (**Fig. 4**).[17,25,59,87,97,99–107]

Among various anxiety disorders, a specific association of certain anxiety disorders more than others has been suggested in youth with BPD.[106,108] A number of of investigators have suggested that a particular link exists between panic disorder and BPD in adults[109,110] and children.[108] Data from adult studies report a lifetime prevalence of panic disorder in 21% to 33% of individuals with BPD,[109–111] and, conversely, lifetime BPD in 6% to 23% of individuals with panic disorder.[105,112] MacKinnon and colleagues[113,114] use family genetic methodology in 57 families to argue that panic disorder with BPD is a genetic subtype of BPD. Savino and colleagues[115] systematically explored the intraepisodic and longitudinal comorbidity of 140 adults with panic disorder and reported comorbidity with BPD in 13.5% of the patients with panic disorder. They also note that an additional 34.3% met features of "hyperthymic temperament," a possible bipolar spectrum condition. Biederman and colleagues[99] reported high rates of panic disorder (52%) among youth with BPD consistent with the observation by Birmaher and colleagues,[108] suggesting that the association between BPD and panic disorder in children and adolescents might be unique and specific. However, emerging literature indicates high prevalence of various anxiety disorders—including but not limited to panic disorder—in pediatric[97,101,103] and adult[104,116,117] populations with BPD, which challenges the notion of a specific link between BPD and panic disorder. Thus, more information is needed as to whether the association between BPD and anxiety disorders in youth is limited to a single anxiety disorder or is more extensive and includes other anxiety disorders as well.

In the presence of high levels of anxiety, adults with BPD experience greater symptom severity, increased risk for suicide and alcohol abuse, higher frequency of

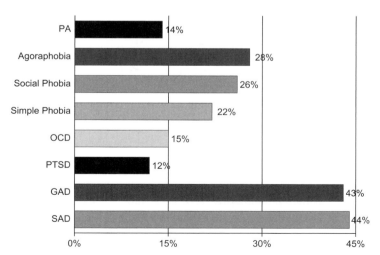

Fig. 4. Anxiety disorders in clinically referred youth with BPD. (*Adapted from* Harpold T, Biederman J, Kwon A, et al. Examining the association between pediatric bipolar disorder and anxiety disorders in psychiatrically referred children and adolescents. Journal of Affective Disorders 2005;88(1):19–26.)

a polypharmacy regimen, more severe adverse effects, poor treatment response, and higher rates of nonremission with poor course and functioning.[100,118–120] Olvera and colleagues[121] found that children with BPD and multiple anxiety disorders displayed manic symptoms at an earlier age and were more likely to have been hospitalized for their illness.

Improving the understanding of the relationship between anxiety disorders and BPD in youth has important treatment implications. Masi and colleagues[103] reported high rates of pharmacologic hypo/mania in youth with anxiety disorders, with the mean age at onset for anxiety disorders preceding that for BPD. This finding suggests caution when considering antidepressant pharmacotherapy in a pediatric population with multiple anxiety disorders.

Considering that treatments for BPD with traditional mood stabilizers do not generally treat anxiety disorders and that treatment of anxiety disorders with selective serotonin reuptake inhibitors (SSRIs) can aggravate BPD, the pharmacologic approach to bipolar children with comorbid anxiety disorders needs to be defined. As BPD and anxiety disorders respond to different treatments, identification of the comorbid state is essential for proper treatment and for achieving optimal functioning.

No systematic data are available that examine treatment of anxiety disorders in the context of bipolar comorbidity. Trials of pediatric anxiety disorders exclude children with BPD by protocol design, and, similarly, children with a BPD diagnosis are typically excluded from the trials of treatment for both depression and anxiety.

To-date, only one open-label trial has assessed response of co-occurring panic attacks and generalized anxiety disorder in adults with BPD, reporting significant decrease in or remission of anxiety symptoms with divalproex therapy.[122] Corroborative evidence for antianxiety effect of mood stabilizers comes from various open-label and controlled trials in adult population with anxiety disorders that suggest valproate to be effective in treating panic disorder and PTSD.[123–129] Antianxiety response of certain mood stabilizers could be specific to certain anxiety disorder(s). For instance, carbamazepine, though effective in treating certain symptoms of PTSD, is found to be ineffective in treating other anxiety disorders in adults, namely panic disorder and OCD.[130–134]

Obsessive–Compulsive Disorder

Descriptions of OCD symptoms in bipolar patients date back to the nineteenth century.[135] Most data on comorbid OCD and BPD are not based on systematic studies[136,137] but are documentation from naturalistic studies. In adults, evidence of a higher-than-expected overlap between OCD and BPD first came from the epidemiologic catchment area study, in which 23% of patients with BPD also met criteria for OCD.[60] Subsequent studies have consistently found the overlap between OCD and BPD at rates as high as 15% to 35%.[87,109,138] When comorbid with BPD, OCD in adults has a more episodic course, often featuring higher rates of sexual and religious obsessions, lower rates of checking rituals, and greater frequency of concurrent major depressive episodes and panic disorder. They also exhibit increased rates of suicidality, more frequent hospitalizations, and more complex pharmacologic interventions than those of patients without BPD.[109,138–140] A recent survey conducted among the French Association of OCD patients provides corroborating evidence for this comorbidity in subjects giving retrospective childhood reports. Although reporting a high prevalence of comorbid lifetime bipolarity, they also noted that many of these subjects had a juvenile onset of OCD.[141,142]

Although the available literature suggests substantial impact on clinical presentation, global functioning, and treatment decisions when BPD and OCD co-occur in young patients,[102] the nature of this relationship is not clearly delineated. For example, the agitation, racing thoughts, and feelings of distress, which can be associated with severe OCD, could mimic a bipolar picture; conversely, the manic symptom of increase in goal-directed activity ("mission mode" behavior) or repetitive, unwanted hypersexual thoughts in a child or adolescent with BPD could mimic an OCD presentation. In one of the two studies that addresses this comorbid presentation, Masi and colleagues[102] reported that in comparison with OCD, comorbid OCD and BPD youth were significantly more impaired, had earlier age at onset of OCD, and had more frequent existential, philosophical, odd, and/or superstitious obsessions, indicating that comorbidity with BPD may have a clinically relevant influence on the symptom expression of the OCD. Half of the comorbid population in this study had type II BPD, and one-third experienced pharmacologic hypomania. This high risk of (hypo) manic switches reported with antidepressant treatment in pediatric OCD is suggestive of a bipolar diathesis.[143,144]

In another study of youth ascertained for family genetic study of BPD and OCD, we[145] documented a significant and symmetric bidirectional overlap between BPD and OCD (21% of the BPD cohort and 15% of the OCD cohort satisfied criteria for both BPD and OCD). In the presence of comorbid BPD, youth with OCD more often presented with the symptom of hoarding/saving, experienced a higher prevalence of other comorbid disorders, especially ODD, major depressive disorder, and psychosis, suffered from poorer psychosocial functioning, and required hospitalization at a greater frequency. Higher prevalence of comorbidity with multiple anxiety disorders, especially general anxiety disorder (GAD) and social phobia, was observed in youth with comorbid OCD and BPD than when either disorder occurred in youth without reciprocal comorbidity. Limited family genetic data suggest a genetic linkage between OCD and BPD. Coryell[146] reported an equal incidence (2.3%) of BPD in families of probands with OCD and in families with BPD. Similarly, an increased incidence of obsessional traits has been reported in the offspring of bipolar probands.[147]

Though no systematic data to date are available that address the therapeutic response of BPD in the presence of comorbid anxiety disorder, Joshi and colleagues[148] conducted a secondary data analysis to examine the antimanic response of BPD youth to olanzapine in the context of comorbidity status with OCD and GAD and concluded that in children and adolescents with BPD the comorbid presence of lifetime OCD, but not GAD, is associated with poor antimanic response (**Fig. 5**). This suggests that certain anxiety disorders when comorbid with BPD may have a larger mediating effect on BPD treatment outcome than others.

Conversely, the presence of BPD with anxiety disorders may have a negative effect on the treatment outcome of the anxiety disorder. For instance, compared with OCD youth without comorbid BPD, children and adolescents with comorbid OCD and BPD have been reported to show poor response to psychotropic medications and are more frequently on a combined pharmacy regimen.[149] Nonpharmacologic treatments such as CBT have been found to be useful and should be instituted when possible, along with any of the pharmacologic alternatives to SSRIs.

Post-Traumatic Stress Disorder

Individuals who work with trauma victims make the clinical observation that mood swings are common in this group. Although considerable literature implicates psychosocial stresses in the onset and recurrence of BPD,[150–152] there is paucity of research on the association of PTSD with BPD. While Breslau and colleagues and Giaconia and colleagues[153,154] reported that 40% to 76% of children had been exposed to a traumatic event by 17 years, the estimated lifetime prevalence of the full syndromic PTSD

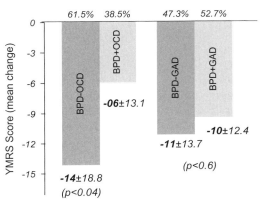

Fig. 5. Endpoint YMRS score mean change BPD+OCD vs BPD+GAD. BPD–OCD, bipolar disorder without comorbid OCD; BPD+OCD, bipolar disorder with comorbid OCD; BPD–GAD, bipolar disorder without comorbid GAD; BPD+GAD, bipolar disorder with co-morbid GAD. (*Adapted from* Joshi G, Mick E, Wozniak J, et al. Impact of obsessive-compulsive disorder on antimanic response of pediatric bipolar disorder to second generation atypical antipsychotics. In 53rd Annual Meeting of the American Academy of Child and Adolescent Psychiatry, San Diego (CA); October 24–29, 2006.)

in the general population is between 1% and 14%, and its prevalence in children is around 6%.[154] By contrast, reported rates of PTSD comorbidity in patients with BPD have varied widely from 7% to 50%.

Rates of SUD are substantially higher in youths who had a lifetime diagnosis of PTSD before 18 years compared with those in youth who had never experienced a trauma.[57] Given the increasing recognition of SUD in BPD and PTSD, we further examined the relationship of BPD, SUD, and PTSD in an older group of adolescents with BPD. We found significantly more PTSD in adolescents with BPD compared with that in non–mood-disordered controls. Sixteen percent of youth with BPD had broad PTSD compared with that in 4% of controls. Moreover, a higher risk of SUD was found in BPD adolescents with PTSD. Although exploratory in nature, interesting temporal patterns emerged suggesting a pattern of onset of BPD first, followed by substance use, trauma, PTSD, and then the onset of full SUD. These data highlight the high risk of PTSD in BPD adolescents that appears to be related to SUD in these youth.[155]

Although many studies have looked at possible links between early traumatic events and development of psychopathology during the life span,[156–158] few studies have examined the potential role of early traumatic life stresses on the development of BPD and PTSD. Emerging evidence suggests that trauma significantly compromises the course of BPD. Leverich and colleagues[159] evaluated 631 outpatients with BPD and reported that nearly half of the females (49%) and one-third of the males (36%) reported early sexual and physical abuse. Those who endorsed a history of child or adolescent physical or sexual abuse, compared with those who did not, had significantly higher rates of comorbid PTSD, a history of an earlier onset of bipolar illness, and a higher rate of suicide attempts. On the other hand, Geller and colleagues[31] reported high rates (43%) of the symptom of hypersexuality (higher in pubertal vs prepubertal BPD population) and low rates (< 1%) of history of sexual abuse in their prepubertal and early adolescent BPD cohort, suggesting that the symptom of hypersexuality in pediatric BPD is etiologically unrelated to sexual abuse and more reflective of mania and puberty. Similarly, Garno and colleagues[160] studied 100 adult patients with BPD, and half (51%) reported a history of abuse, whereas a quarter suffered from comorbid PTSD (24%).

A report by Wozniak and colleagues[161] raises the question as to whether a diagnosis of BPD may pose a risk factor for trauma. Using data from a large longitudinal sample of well-characterized boys with and without ADHD, these authors failed to find meaningful associations between ADHD, trauma, and PTSD. Instead, they identified early BPD as an important antecedent for later trauma. When traumatized children present with severe irritability and mood lability, there may be a tendency to associate these symptoms to the trauma. On the contrary, these longitudinal results suggest that rather than a consequence, BPD may be an antecedent risk factor for later trauma (possibly because of the attendant reckless, disinhibited state). If confirmed, these results could help dispel the commonly held notion that mania-like symptoms in youths represent a reaction to trauma and would further suggest that children with BPD should be adequately treated and monitored closely to avoid trauma.

Though no empiric evidence is available for the treatment of comorbid BPD and PTSD, corroborative evidence comes from trials of mood stabilizers in adult population, suggesting valproate to be effective in treating certain combat-related (but not noncombat-related) PTSD symptoms.[123–125,128,129] Certain mood stabilizers have shown promise in treating specific symptoms of PTSD. Several open trials report that carbamazepine may be useful for treating PTSD symptoms of flashbacks, nightmares, and intrusive thoughts.[131,132,134] In a preliminary controlled trial lamotrigine exhibited potential efficacy in the treatment of PTSD symptoms of re-experiencing, avoidance, and numbing in adults.[162]

PERVASIVE DEVELOPMENTAL DISORDERS

Recently, there has been immense interest in the overlap of BPD and autistic spectrum disorders. A limited literature exists on the diagnosis and treatment of comorbid BPD and PDD in children and adolescents. In the absence of systematic research on comorbid BPD and PDD, indirect evidence suggestive of comorbid BPD in pediatric populations with PDD comes from high rates of aggressive behaviors documented in children with PDD, a high incidence of BPD in family members of children with PDD, and from a small body of literature documenting the presence of BPD comorbidity in PDD populations.

High rates of aggressive behaviors and severe mood disturbances are documented in children with PDD.[163–166] There is considerable evidence suggesting that a subset of PDD youth with extreme disturbance of mood suffer from a symptom cluster that is phenomenologically consistent with the syndrome of BPD. In a study of a group of patients with Asperger's disorder who were followed into adolescence, Wing[167] found that nearly half of the patients developed affective disorders. Conversely, high rates of PDD or PDD traits are reported in children and adolescents with BPD. The presence of significant PDD traits is reported to be as high as 62% in pediatric mood and anxiety disorder research populations.[168]

In the first study using accepted operationalized criteria, our group assessed clinically referred children and adolescents (N = 727) using a comprehensive diagnostic battery, including structured diagnostic interview. We reported a bidirectional overlap: BPD occurred in 21% of PDD, and PDD occurred in 11% of BPD youth.[169] There was striking homology in the clinical characteristics of PDD and BPD when clinical features were compared based on the presence or absence of reciprocal comorbidity. BPD and

PDD irrespective of the reciprocal comorbidity were similar in phenotypic features, including symptom profile, pattern of comorbidity, and measures of functioning. This work suggests that BPD and PDD are bona fide disorders when they co-occur in youth.

Recently, we replicated our earlier findings and reported that one-third of our clinically referred population of children and adolescents with PDD also received the diagnosis of BPD on structured diagnostic interviews.[170] Similarly, we found consistently high rates of comorbid PDD (15%) in our research populations of children and adolescents with BPD irrespective of the aims for ascertainment—family genetic study or treatment trials of BPD.[171,172] In the presence of comorbid PDD, youth with BPD experience an earlier age at onset and increased severity of BPD with a poorer level of functioning.[170–172] Furthermore, PDD youth with a family history of BPD are more often high functioning, and their mood disturbance is characterized by a severe cycling pattern, agitation, and aggression along with neurovegetative disturbances.[173] There is an accumulating body of literature from family genetic studies suggesting higher than expected incidence of BPD in first-degree relatives of about one-third of the population with PDD.[173–175]

Treatment response to psychotropics in youth with PDD is noted to be less robust with higher rates of adverse effects to both medication and placebo.[176–178] Thus, due to an atypical response and higher susceptibility to adverse effects, it is advisable to initiate and titrate psychotropics at a lower dose and titrate upward in smaller increments in this population.

Though there is substantial evidence documenting the role of pharmacotherapy for the management of extreme mood difficulties, there is minimal published literature and no systematic data on the treatment of comorbid BPD in this population. Limited literature on the treatment of comorbid BPD in children with PDD suggests that first-generation antipsychotics (haloperidol, chlorpromazine, thioridazine) and traditional mood stabilizers (lithium, carbamazepine) are minimally effective for the treatment of mania.[179] On the contrary, in a recent secondary analysis of acute atypical antipsychotic monotherapy trials in BPD youth, we reported acceptable tolerability and robust antimanic response to atypical antipsychotics (risperidone, olanzapine, quetiapine, ziprasidone, or aripiprazole) in the presence of PDD comorbidity.[171] No difference was observed in the rate of antimanic response and tolerability, with the exception that PDD youth were more susceptible to the adverse effect of slurred speech and teary eyes. Furthermore, compared with other atypical antipsychotics, risperidone had a superior antimanic response in BPD youth with comorbid PDD. However, this study is limited by the retrospective nature of post hoc analysis and lack of direct measures of PDD symptomatology.

There is evidence from the treatment trials of risperidone, aripiprazole, and ziprasidone that second-generation neuroleptics are well tolerated and efficacious in treating symptoms of irritability and aggression in youth with PDD, a spectrum of symptoms suggestive of BPD. Controlled trials of risperidone consistently report favorable safety, tolerability, and efficacy profiles for treating symptoms of irritability and aggression in youth with PDD.[180–182] Although risperidone is the only atypical antipsychotic that is Food and Drug Administration approved for the treatment of irritability and aggression in autistic children, weight gain associated with risperidone is a significant adverse effect that often limits continuation of treatment in this population. In contrast, results from recent short-term open trials with newer atypical antipsychotics—aripiprazole and ziprasidone—show promise as a treatment for irritability in children with PDD and are associated with negligible weight gain.[183,184] Contrary to the encouraging response observed with the aforementioned atypical antipsychotics, the atypical antipsychotics quetiapine and olanzapine are noted to be ineffective in treating symptoms of irritability and aggression in this population.[185–187]

Thus, in choosing a thymoleptic agent for the treatment of BPD in youth with comorbid PDD, consideration should be given to those antimanic agents that are also shown to be efficacious in treating associated and core features of PDD. Furthermore, in this population due to higher susceptibility to adverse effects, it is advisable to initiate and titrate psychotropics at a lower dose. As the afore-mentioned empiric evidence suggests, risperidone appears to be efficacious in treating both core and associated features of PDD and may be superior to other atypical antipsychotics as an antimanic agent in youth with PDD. Youth should be closely monitored for adverse effects, especially weight gain, as it remains a concern in short- and long-term therapy with risperidone.

SUMMARY

The diagnosis and treatment of BPD needs to address psychiatric comorbidity given its ubiquitous nature. ADHD comorbidity is particularly associated with very early onset BPD, whereas the risk of SUD comorbidity is much higher for adolescent-onset versus child-onset BPD. Onset of pediatric BPD is generally either before or simultaneous to the onset of SUD, and severity of both the disorders is worse in the comorbid state. A higher than expected prevalence of anxiety disorders is documented in individuals with BPD. In the presence of an anxiety disorder, individuals with BPD experience greater symptom severity, poorer treatment response, and poorer course and functioning. Hypersexuality in pediatric BPD is etiologically unrelated to sexual abuse and more reflective of dysregulation related to mania and puberty. BPD may be an antecedent risk factor for later trauma and subsequent PTSD and not merely represent a reaction to the trauma. There is an accumulating body of literature that suggests that a subset of PDD youth with extreme disturbance of mood suffer from a symptom cluster that is phenomenologically consistent with the syndrome of BPD, and this is equally substantiated by family genetic studies that document a higher than expected incidence of BPD in first-degree relatives of youth with PDD.

In general, the presence of comorbid disorders with BPD results in a more severe clinical condition. Earlier onset BPD seems to be related to additional comorbidity and more severe episodes and cycle acceleration. Identifying and treating these co-occurring psychiatric conditions may help alleviate the severity of impairment and shorten the duration of mood episodes in BPD.

Knowledge of the impact of comorbid disorders on the therapeutic response in youth with BPD is growing rapidly. BPD response to lithium is less robust in the presence of ADHD comorbidity. Stimulants are safe and efficacious for the treatment of comorbid ADHD once mania is stabilized in youth with BPD. Treatment of BPD with lithium or valproic acid results in attenuation of active SUD. In youth with BPD, the comorbid presence of lifetime OCD, but not GAD, is associated with poor antimanic response. Response to psychotropics in PDD youth with mood dysregulation is noted to be less robust with higher susceptibility to adverse effects.

The scientific interface between BPD and comorbidities remains unclear. Comorbidity may represent an important genetic and clinical subtype with distinct psychopathology, familiality, and cognitive, neural, and genetic underpinnings. Future longitudinal studies addressing the impact of comorbidity on the clinical presentation, course, and response to treatment along with studies examining the cognitive correlates, genetic-candidate genes, and neurobiological overlap would assist in further clarifying the relationship of BPD with its comorbidities.

REFERENCES

1. Campbell M, Cueva JE. Psychopharmacology in child and adolescent psychiatry: a review of the past seven years. Part II. J Am Acad Child Adolesc Psychiatry 1995;34:1262–72.
2. Tarter RE. Evaluation and treatment of adolescent substance abuse: A decision tree method. Am J Drug Alcohol Abuse 1990;16:1–46.
3. Ambrosini PJ. Historical development and present status of the schedule for affective disorders and schizophrenia for school-age children (K-SADS). J Am Acad Child Adolesc Psychiatry 2000;39:49–58.
4. Faraone SV, Tsuang MT. Methods in psychiatric genetics. In: Tohen M, Tsuang MT, Zahner GEP (editors). Textbook in psychiatric epidemiology. New York: John Wiley; 1995. p. 81–134.
5. Faraone SV, Tsuang MT, Tsuang D. Genetics and mental disorders: a guide for students, clinicians, and researchers. New York: The Guilford Press; 1999.
6. Biederman J, Mick E, Bostic J, et al. The naturalistic course of pharmacologic treatment of children with manic-like symptoms: a systematic chart review. J Clin Psychiatry 1998;59:628–37.
7. Moore CM, Biederman J, Wozniak J, et al. Differences in brain chemistry in children and adolescents with attention deficit hyperactivity disorder with and without comorbid bipolar disorder: a proton magnetic resonance spectroscopy study. Am J Psychiatry 2006;163:316–8.
8. Kowatch RA, Fristad M, Birmaher B, et al. Treatment guidelines for children and adolescents with bipolar disorder. J Am Acad Child Adolesc Psychiatry 2005;44: 213–35.
9. Wozniak J, Biederman J. A pharmacological approach to the quagmire of comorbidity in juvenile mania. J Am Acad Child Adolesc Psychiatry 1996;35:826–8.
10. Geller B, Sun K, Zimmerman B, et al. Complex and rapid-cycling in bipolar children and adolescents: a preliminary study. J Affect Disord 1995;34:259–68.
11. West S, McElroy S, Strakowski S, et al. Attention deficit hyperactivity disorder in adolescent mania. Am J Psychiatry 1995;152:271–3.
12. Wilens T, Biederman J, Forkner P, et al. Patterns of comorbidity and dysfunction in clinically referred preschoolers with bipolar disorder. J Child Adolesc Psychopharmacol 2003;13:495–505.
13. Biederman J, Faraone SV, Mick E, et al. Attention deficit hyperactivity disorder and juvenile mania: an overlooked comorbidity? J Am Acad Child Adolesc Psychiatry 1996;35:997–1008.
14. Chang KD, Steiner H, Ketter TA. Psychiatric phenomenology of child and adolescent bipolar offspring. J Am Acad Child Adolesc Psychiatry 2000;39: 453–60.
15. Sachs GS, Baldassano CF, Truman CJ, et al. Comorbidity of attention deficit hyperactivity disorder with early- and late-onset bipolar disorder. Am J Psychiatry 2000;157:466–8.
16. Biederman J, Petty C, Faraone SV, et al. Moderating effects of major depression on patterns of comorbidity in referred adults with panic disorder: a controlled study. Psychiatry Res 2004;126:143–9.
17. Faraone SV, Biederman J, Wozniak J, et al. Is comorbidity with ADHD a marker for juvenile onset mania? J Am Acad Child Adolesc Psychiatry 1997;36:1046–55.
18. Kessler RC, Adler L, Barkley R, et al. The prevalence and correlates of adult ADHD in the United States: results from the national comorbidity survey replication. Am J Psychiatry 2006;163:716–23.

19. Nierenberg AA, Miyahara S, Spencer T, et al. Clinical and diagnostic implications of lifetime attention-deficit/hyperactivity disorder comorbidity in adults with bipolar disorder: data from the first 1000 STEP-BD participants. Biol Psychiatry 2005;57:1467.

20. Winokur G, Coryell W, Akiskal HS, et al. Alcoholism in manic-depressive (bipolar) illness: Familial illness, course of illness, and the primary-secondary distinction. American Journal of Psychiatry 1995;152:365–72.

21. Wozniak J, Biederman J, et al. Mania-like symptoms suggestive of childhood onset bipolar disorder in clinically referred children. J Am Acad Child Adolesc Psychiatry 1995;34:867–76.

22. Milberger S, Biederman J, Faraone SV, et al. Attention deficit hyperactivity disorder and comorbid disorders: issues of overlapping symptoms. Am J Psychiatry 1995;152:1793–9.

23. Faraone SV, Biederman J, Mennin D, et al. Bipolar and antisocial disorders among relatives of ADHD children: parsing familial subtypes of illness. Am J Med Genet 1998;81:108–16.

24. Faraone S, Glatt S, Tsuang M. The genetics of pediatric onset bipolar disorder. Biol Psychiatry 2003;53:970–7.

25. Faraone SV, Biederman J, Mennin D, et al. Attention-deficit hyperactivity disorder with bipolar disorder: a familial subtype? J Am Acad Child Adolesc Psychiatry 1997;36:1387–90.

26. Faraone SV, Biederman J, Monuteaux MC. Attention deficit hyperactivity disorder with bipolar disorder in girls: further evidence for a familial subtype? J Affect Disord 2001;64:19–26.

27. State RC, Frye MA, Altshuler LL, et al. Chart review of the impact of attention-deficit/hyperactivity disorder comorbidity on response to lithium or divalproex sodium in adolescent mania. J Clin Psychiatry 2004;65:1057–63.

28. Strober M, DeAntonio M, Schmidt-Lackner S, et al. Early childhood attention deficit hyperactivity disorder predicts poorer response to acute lithium therapy in adolescent mania. J Affect Disord 1998;51:145–51.

29. Biederman J, Faraone SV, Chu MP, et al. Further evidence of a bidirectional overlap between juvenile mania and conduct disorder in children. J Am Acad Child Adolesc Psychiatry 1999;38:468–76.

30. Scheffer RE, Kowatch RA, Carmody T, et al. Randomized, placebo-controlled trial of mixed amphetamine salts for symptoms of comorbid ADHD in pediatric bipolar disorder after mood stabilization with divalproex sodium. Am J Psychiatry 2005;162:58–64.

31. Findling RL, Short EJ, McNamara NK, et al. Methylphenidate in the Treatment of Children and Adolescents With Bipolar Disorder and Attention-Deficit/Hyperactivity Disorder. J Am Acad Child Adoles Psychiatry 2007;46:1445–53.

32. Wilens T, Prince J, Spencer T, et al. An open trial of bupropion for the treatment of adults with attention deficit hyperactivity disorder and bipolar disorder. Biol Psychiatry 2003;54:9–16.

33. Findling RL, Gracious BL, McNamara NK, et al. Rapid, continuous cycling and psychiatric co-morbidity in pediatric bipolar I disorder. Bipolar Disord 2001;3:202–10.

34. Geller B, Zimerman B, Williams M, et al. Diagnostic characteristics of 93 cases of a prepubertal and early adolescent bipolar disorder phenotype by gender, puberty and comorbid attention deficit hyperactivity disorder. J Child Adolesc Psychopharmacol 2000;10:157–64.

35. Greene RW, Doyle AE. Toward a transactional conceptualization of oppositional defiant disorder: implications for assessment and treatment. Clin Child Fam Psychol Rev 1999;2:129–48.

36. Farley SE, Adams JS, Lutton ME, et al. Clinical inquiries. What are effective treatments for oppositional and defiant behaviors in preadolescents? J Fam Pract 2005;54:162, 164–5.

37. Aman MG, De Smedt G, Derivan A, et al. Double-blind, placebo-controlled study of risperidone for the treatment of disruptive behaviors in children with subaverage intelligence. Am J Psychiatry 2002;159:1337–46.

38. Croonenberghs J, Fegert JM, Findling RL, et al. Risperidone in children with disruptive behavior disorders and subaverage intelligence: a 1-year, open-label study of 504 patients. J Am Acad Child Adolesc Psychiatry 2005;44:64–72.

39. Findling RL, Aman MG, Eerdekens M, et al. Long-term, open-label study of risperidone in children with severe disruptive behaviors and below-average IQ. Am J Psychiatry 2004;161:677–84.

40. Turgay A, Binder C, Snyder R, et al. Long-term safety and efficacy of risperidone for the treatment of disruptive behavior disorders in children with subaverage IQs. Pediatrics 2002;110:e34.

41. Reyes M, Buitelaar J, Toren P, et al. A randomized, double-blind, placebo-controlled study of risperidone maintenance treatment in children and adolescents with disruptive behavior disorders. Am J Psychiatry 2006;163:402–10.

42. Snyder SH. Forty years of neurotransmitters: a personal account. Arch Gen Psychiatry 2002;59:983–94.

43. Reyes M, Croonenberghs J, Augustyns I, et al. Long-term use of risperidone in children with disruptive behavior disorders and subaverage intelligence: efficacy, safety, and tolerability. J Child Adolesc Psychopharmacol 2006;16:260–72.

44. Haas M, Karcher K, Pandina GJ. Treating disruptive behavior disorders with risperidone: a 1-year, open-label safety study in children and adolescents. J Child Adolesc Psychopharmacol 2008;18:337–45.

45. Biederman J, Mick E, Faraone SV, et al. Risperidone in the treatment of affective symptoms: a secondary analysis of a randomized clinical trial in children with disruptive behavior disorder. Clin Ther 2006;28:794–800.

46. Kronenberger WG, Giauque AL, Lafata DE, et al. Quetiapine addition in methylphenidate treatment-resistant adolescents with comorbid ADHD, conduct/oppositional-defiant disorder, and aggression: a prospective, open-label study. J Child Adolesc Psychopharmacol 2007;17:334–47.

47. Donovan S, Susser E, Nunes E, et al. Divalproex treatment of disruptive adolescents: a report of 10 cases. J Clin Psychiatry 1997;58:12–5.

48. Donovan SJ, Stewart JW, Nunes EV, et al. Divalproex treatment for youth with explosive temper and mood lability: a double-blind, placebo-controlled crossover design. Am J Psychiatry 2000;157:818–20.

49. Geller B, Luby J. Child and adolescent bipolar disorder: a review of the past 10 years. J Am Acad Child Adolesc Psychiatry 1997;36:1168–76.

50. Angold A, Costello EJ. Depressive comorbidity in children and adolescents: Empirical, theoretical and methodological issues. Am J Psychiatry 1993;150:1779.

51. Geller B, Fox L, Clark K. Rate and predictors of prepubertal bipolarity during follow-up of 6- to 12-year-old depressed children. J Am Acad Child Adolesc Psychiatry 1994;33:461–8.

52. Strober M, Carlson G. Bipolar illness in adolescents with major depression: clinical, genetic, and psychopharmacologic predictors in a three- to four-year prospective follow-up investigation. Arch Gen Psychiatry 1982;39:549–55.
53. Carlson GA. Classification issues of bipolar disorders in childhood. Psychiatr Dev 1984;2:273–85.
54. Davis RE. Manic-depressive variant syndrome of childhood: a preliminary report. Am J Psychiatry 1979;136:702–6.
55. McGlashan T. Adolescent versus adult onset of mania. Am J Psychiatry 1988; 145:221–3.
56. Kovacs M, Pollock M. Bipolar disorder and comorbid conduct disorder in childhood and adolescence. J Am Acad Child Adolesc Psychiatry 1995;34:715–23.
57. Kutcher SP, Marton P, Korenblum M. Relationship between psychiatric illness and conduct disorder in adolescents. Can J Psychiatry 1989;34:526–9.
58. Moore JM Jr, Thompson-Pope SK, Whited RM. MMPI-A profiles of adolescent boys with a history of firesetting. J Pers Assess 1996;67:116–26.
59. Lewinsohn P, Klein D, Seeley J. Bipolar disorders in a community sample of older adolescents: prevalence, phenomenology, comorbidity, and course. J Am Acad Child Adolesc Psychiatry 1995;34:454–63.
60. Robins L, Price R. Adult disorders predicted by childhood conduct problems: results from the NIMH epidemiologic catchment area project. Psychiatry 1991; 54:116–32.
61. Boyd JH, Burke JD, Gruenberg E, et al. Exclusion criteria of DSM-III: A study of co-occurrence of hierarchy-free syndromes. Arch Gen Psychiatry 1984;41:983–9.
62. Carlson G, Kelly K. Manic symptoms in psychiatrically hospitalized children-what do they mean? J Affect Disord 1998;51:123–35.
63. Isaac G. Misdiagnosed bipolar disorder in adolescents in a special educational school and treatment program. J Clin Psychiatry 1992;53:133–6.
64. Biederman J, Faraone S, Hatch M, et al. Conduct disorder with and without mania in a referred sample of ADHD children. J Affect Disord 1997;44:177–88.
65. Biederman J, Faraone SV, Wozniak J, et al. Parsing the association between bipolar, conduct, and substance use disorders: a familial risk analysis. Biol Psychiatry 2000;48:1037–44.
66. Wozniak J, Biederman J, Faraone SV, et al. Heterogeneity of childhood conduct disorder: further evidence of a subtype of conduct disorder linked to bipolar disorder. J Affect Disord 2001;64:121–31.
67. Biederman J, Mick E, Spencer TJ, et al. A prospective open-label treatment trial of ziprasidone monotherapy in children and adolescents with bipolar disorder. Bipolar Disorders 2004;9:888–94.
68. Biederman J, Mick E, Wozniak J, et al. An open-label trial of risperidone in children and adolescents with bipolar disorder. J Child Adolesc Psychopharmacol 2005;15:311–7.
69. Sheard MH. Lithium in the treatment of aggression. J Nerv Ment Dis 1975;160: 108–18.
70. Campbell M, Anderson LT, Green WH. Behavior-disordered and aggressive children: new advances in pharmacotherapy. J Dev Behav Pediatr 1983;4:265–71.
71. Campbell M, Small AM, Green WH, et al. Behavioral efficacy of haloperidol and lithium carbonate: a comparison in hospitalized aggressive children with conduct disorder. Arch Gen Psychiatry 1984;41:650–6.
72. Greenhill LL, Solomon M, Pleak R, et al. Molindone hydrochloride treatment of hospitalized children with conduct disorder. J Clin Psychiatry 1985;46:20–5.

73. Findling RL, Reed MD, O'Riordan MA, et al. Effectiveness, safety, and pharma-cokinetics of quetiapine in aggressive children with conduct disorder. J Am Acad Child Adolesc Psychiatry 2006;45:792–800.
74. Connor DF, McLaughlin TJ, Jeffers-Terry M. Randomized controlled pilot study of quetiapine in the treatment of adolescent conduct disorder. J Child Adolesc Psychopharmacol 2008;18:140–56.
75. Masi G, Milone A, Canepa G, et al. Olanzapine treatment in adolescents with severe conduct disorder. Eur Psychiatry 2006;21:51–7.
76. Riggs P, Mikulich S, Coffman L, et al. Fluoxetine in drug-dependent delinquents with major depression: an open trial. J Child Adolesc Psychopharmacol 1997;7: 87–95.
77. McElroy SL, Strakowski SM, Keck PE, et al. Differences and similarities in mixed and pure mania. Compr Psychiatry 1995;36:187–94.
78. Strakowski S, Sax K, McElroy S, et al. Course of psychiatric and substance abuse syndromes co-occurring with bipolar disorder after a first psychiatric hospitalization. J Clin Psychiatry 1998;59:465–71.
79. Dunner DL, Feinman J, The effect of substance abuse on the course of bipolar disorder. In 34th Annual Meeting of the American College of Neuropsychophar-macology, San Juan, Puerto Rico; December 11–15, 1995. p. 171.
80. Wilens TE, Gignac M. Treatment of bipolar disorder in children and adolescents. In: Geller B, DelBello MP (editors). Pediatric bipolar disorder and substance use disorders: 2008.
81. Biederman J, Wilens T, Mick E, et al. Is ADHD a risk for psychoactive substance use disorder? Findings from a four year follow-up study. J Am Acad Child Adolesc Psychiatry 1997;36:21–9.
82. West SA, Strakowski SM, Sax KW, et al. Phenomenology and comorbidity of adolescents hospitalized for the treatment of acute mania. Biol Psychiatry 1996;39:458–60.
83. Wilens T, Biederman J, Abrantes A, et al. Clinical characteristics of psychiatri-cally referred adolescent outpatients with substance use disorders. J Am Acad Child Adolesc Psychiatry 1997;36:941–7.
84. Strober M, Schmidt-Lackner S, Freeman R, et al. Recovery and relapse in adolescents with bipolar affective illness: a five-year naturalistic, prospective follow-up. J Am Acad Child Adolesc Psychiatry 1995;34:724–31.
85. Wilens T, Biederman J, Milberger S, et al. Is bipolar disorder a risk for cigarette smoking in ADHD youth? Am J Addict 2000;9:187–95.
86. Wilens TE, Biederman J, Millstein R, et al. Risk for substance use disorders in youth with child- and adolescent-onset bipolar disorder. J Am Acad Child Adolesc Psychiatry 1999;38:680–5.
87. Wilens TE, Biederman J, Adamson JJ, et al. Further evidence of an association between adolescent bipolar disorder with smoking and substance use disor-ders: a controlled study. Drug Alcohol Depend 2008;95:188–98.
88. Wilens T, Martelon M, Kruesi M. Does conduct disorder mediate the develop-ment of substance use disorders in adolescents with bipolar disorder? A controlled study. J Clin Psychiatry, in press.
89. Chambers RA, Taylor JR, Potenza MN. Developmental neurocircuitry of motiva-tion in adolescence: a critical period of addiction vulnerability. Am J Psychiatry 2003;160:1041–52.
90. Khantzian EJ. The self-medication hypothesis of substance use disorders: a reconsideration and recent applications. Harv Rev Psychiatry 1997;4:231–44.

91. Lorberg B, Martelon M, Parcell T, et al. Self medication in BPD adolescents. In AACAP, Chicago; 2008.
92. Comings D, Comings B, Muhleman D, et al. The dopamine D2 receptor locus as a modifying gene in neuropsychiatric disorders. JAMA 1991;266:1793–800.
93. Ebstein R, Novick O, Umansky r, et al. Dopamine D4 receptor exon III polymorphism associated with the human personality trait of novelty seeking. Nat Genet 1996;12:78–80.
94. Mick E, Kim JW, Biederman J, et al. Family based association study of pediatric bipolar disorder and the dopamine transporter gene (SLC6A3). Am J Med Genet B Neuropsychiatr Genet 2008;147B:1182–5.
95. Donovan S, Nunes E. Treatment of comorbid affective and substance use disorders therapeutic potential of anticonvulsants. Am J Addict 1998;7:210–20.
96. Geller B, Cooper T, Sun K, et al. Double-blind and placebo controlled study of lithium for adolescent bipolar disorders with secondary substance dependency. J Am Acad Child Adolesc Psychiatry 1998;37:171–8.
97. Harpold T, Biederman J, Kwon A, et al. Examining the association between pediatric bipolar disorder and anxiety disorders in psychiatrically referred children and adolescents. Journal of Affective Disorders 2005;88(1):19–26.
98. Diagnostic and Statistical Manual of Mental Disorders. 4th edition. Washington, DC: American Psychiatric Association; 1994.
99. Biederman J, Faraone SV, Marrs A, et al. Panic disorder and agoraphobia in consecutively referred children and adolescents. J Am Acad Child Adolesc Psychiatry 1997;36:214–23.
100. Feske U, Frank E, Mallinger AG, et al. Anxiety as a correlate of response to the acute treatment of bipolar I disorder. Am J Psychiatry 2000;157:956–62.
101. Johnson JG, Cohen P, Brook JS. Associations between bipolar disorder and other psychiatric disorders during adolescence and early adulthood: a community-based longitudinal investigation. Am J Psychiatry 2000;157:1679–81.
102. Masi G, Perugi G, Toni C, et al. Obsessive-compulsive bipolar comorbidity: focus on children and adolescents. J Affect Disord 2004;78:175–83.
103. Masi G, Toni C, Perugi G, et al. Anxiety disorders in children and adolescents with bipolar disorder: a neglected comorbidity. Can J Psychiatry 2001;46: 797–802.
104. McElroy SL, Altshuler LL, Suppes T, et al. Axis I psychiatric comorbidity and its relationship to historical illness variables in 288 patients with bipolar disorder. Am J Psychiatry 2001;158:420–6.
105. Perugi G. Depressive comorbidity of panic, social phobic, and obsessive compulsive disorders re-examined: is there a bipolar II connection? J Psychiatr Res 1999;33:53–61.
106. Tillman R, Geller B, Bolhofner K, et al. Ages of onset and rates of syndromal and subsyndromal comorbid DSM-IV diagnoses in a prepubertal and early adolescent bipolar disorder phenotype. J Am Acad Child Adolesc Psychiatry 2003;42: 1486–93.
107. Wozniak J, Biederman J, Monuteaux MC, et al. Parsing the comorbidity between bipolar disorder and anxiety disorders: a familial risk analysis. J Child Adolesc Psychopharmacol 2002;12:101–11.
108. Birmaher B, Kennah A, Brent D, et al. Is bipolar disorder specifically associated with panic disorder in youths? J Clin Psychiatry 2002;63:414–9.
109. Chen Y, Dilsaver S. Comorbidity of panic disorder in bipolar illness: Evidence from the epidemiologic catchment area survey. Am J Psychiatry 1995;152:280–3.

110. Goodwin RD, Hoven CW. Bipolar-panic comorbidity in the general population: prevalence and associated morbidity. J Affect Disord 2002;70:27–33.

111. Kessler RC, Stang PE, Wittchen HV, et al. Lifetime panic-depression comorbidity in the National Comorbidity Survey. Arch Gen Psychiatry 1998;55:801–8.

112. Bowen R, South M, Hawkes J. Mood swings in patients with panic disorder. Can J Psychiatry 1994;39:91–4.

113. MacKinnon D, Xu J, McMahon F, et al. Bipolar disorder and panic disorder in families: an analysis of chromosome 18 data. Am J Psychiatry 1998;155:829–31.

114. MacKinnon DF, Zandi PP, Cooper J, et al. Comorbid bipolar disorder and panic disorder in families with a high prevalence of bipolar disorder. Am J Psychiatry 2002;159:30–5.

115. Savino M, Perugi G, Simonini E, et al. Affective comorbidity in panic disorder: is there a bipolar connection? J Affect Disord 1993;28:155–63.

116. Cassano GB, Pini S, Saettoni M, et al. Multiple anxiety disorder comorbidity in patients with mood spectrum disorders with psychotic features. Am J Psychiatry 1999;156:474–6.

117. Freeman MP. The comorbidity of bipolar and anxiety disorders: prevalence, psychobiology, and treatment issues. J Affect Disord 2002;68:1–23.

118. Gaudiano BA, Miller IW. Anxiety disorder comorbidity in bipolar I disorder: relationship to depression severity and treatment outcome. Depress Anxiety 2005;21:71–7.

119. Otto MW, Simon NM, Wisniewski SR, et al. Prospective 12-month course of bipolar disorder in out-patients with and without comorbid anxiety disorders. Br J Psychiatry 2006;189:20–5.

120. Young L, Cooke R, Robb J, et al. Anxious and non-anxious bipolar disorder. J Affect Disord 1993;29:49–52.

121. Olvera RL, Hunter K, Fonseca M, et al. Juvenile onset bipolar disorder and co-morbid anxiety. In The 52nd Annual Meeting of American Academy of Child and Adolescent Psychiatry, Toronto; October 18–23, 2006.

122. Calabrese J, Delucchi G. Spectrum of efficacy of valproate in 55 patients with rapid-cycling bipolar disorder. Am J Psychiatry 1990;147:431–4.

123. Baetz M, Bowen RC. Efficacy of divalproex sodium in patients with panic disorder and mood instability who have not responded to conventional therapy. Can J Psychiatry 1998;43:73–7.

124. Clark RD, Canive JM, Calais LA, et al. Divalproex in posttraumatic stress disorder: an open-label clinical trial. J Trauma Stress 1999;12:395–401.

125. Fesler FA. Valproate in combat-related posttraumatic stress disorder. J Clin Psychiatry 1991;52:361–4.

126. Lum M, Fontaine R, Elie R, et al. Divalproex sodium's anti-panic effect in panic disorder: a placebo-controlled study. Biol Psychiatry 1990;27:164A–5A.

127. McElroy SL, Keck PE Jr, Lawrence JM. Treatment of panic disorder and benzodiazepine withdrawal with valproate. J Neuropsychiatry Clin Neurosci 1991;3:232–3.

128. Otte C, Wiedemann K, Yassouridis A, et al. Valproate monotherapy in the treatment of civilian patients with non-combat-related posttraumatic stress disorder: an open-label study. J Clin Psychopharmacol 2004;24:106–8.

129. Petty F, Davis LL, Nugent AL, et al. Valproate therapy for chronic, combat-induced posttraumatic stress disorder. J Clin Psychopharmacol 2002;22:100–1.

130. Joffe RT, Swinson RP. Carbamazepine in obsessive-compulsive disorder. Biol Psychiatry 1987;22:1169–71.

131. Looff D, Grimley P, Kuller F, et al. Carbamazepine for PTSD. J Am Acad Child Adolesc Psychiatry 1995;34:703–4.
132. Stewart JT, Bartucci RJ. Posttraumatic stress disorder and partial complex seizures. Am J Psychiatry 1986;143:113–4.
133. Tondo L, Burrai C, Scamonatti L, et al. Carbamazepine in panic disorder. Am J Psychiatry 1989;146:558–9.
134. Wolf ME, Alavi A, Mosnaim AD. Posttraumatic stress disorder in Vietnam veterans clinical and EEG findings; possible therapeutic effects of carbamazepine. Biol Psychiatry 1988;23:642–4.
135. Morel BA. Traite de maladies metales. Paris: Libairie Victor Masson; 1860.
136. Goodwin F, Jamison K. Manic-depressive illness. New York: Oxford University Press; 1990.
137. Rasmussen S, Eisen J. The epidemiology and differential diagnosis of obsessive compulsive disorder. J Clin Psychiatry 1992;53:4–10.
138. Perugi G, Akiskal HS, Pfanner C, et al. The clinical impact of bipolar and unipolar affective comorbidity on obsessive-compulsive disorder. J Affect Disord 1997;46:15–23.
139. Centorrino F, Hennen J, Mallya G, et al. Clinical outcome in patients with bipolar I disorder, obsessive compulsive disorder or both. Hum Psychopharmacol 2006; 21:189–93.
140. Perugi G, Toni C, Frare F, et al. Obsessive-compulsive-bipolar comorbidity: a systematic exploration of clinical features and treatment outcome. J Clin Psychiatry 2002;63:1129–34.
141. Hantouche EG, Demonfaucon C, Angst J, et al. Cyclothymic obsessive-compulsive disorder. Clinical characteristics of a neglected and under-recognized entity. Presse Med 2002;31:644–8 [French].
142. Kochman FJ, Hantouche EG, Millet B, et al. Trouble obsessionnel compulsif et bipolarite attenuee chez l'enfant et l'adolescent: re sultants de l'enquete 'ABC-TOC'. Neuropsychiatr Enface Adolesc 2002;50:1–7.
143. Diler RS, Avci A. SSRI-induced mania in obsessive-compulsive disorder. J Am Acad Child Adolesc Psychiatry 1999;38:6–7.
144. King RA, Riddle MA, Chappel PB, et al. Case study: emergence of self-destructive phenomena in children and adolescents during fluoxetine treatment. J Am Acad Child Adolesc Psychiatry 1991;30:179–86.
145. Joshi G, Wozniak J, Geller D, et al. Clinical characteristics of comorbid obsessive-compulsive disorder and bipolar disorder in children and adolescents. In The 52nd Annual Meeting of American Academy of Child and Adolescent Psychiatry, Toronto; October 18–23, 2005.
146. Coryell W. Obsessive-compulsive disorder and primary unipolar depression. Comparisons of background, family history, course, and mortality. J Nerv Ment Dis 1981;169:220–4.
147. Klein D, Depue R, Slater J. Cyclothymia in the adolescent offspring of parents with bipolar affective disorder. J Abnorm Psychol 1985;94:115–27.
148. Joshi G, Mick E, Wozniak J, et al. Impact of obsessive-compulsive disorder on antimanic response of pediatric bipolar disorder to second generation atypical antipsychotics. In 53rd Annual Meeting of the American Academy of Child and Adolescent Psychiatry, San Diego (CA); October 24–29, 2006.
149. Masi G, Millepiedi S, Mucci M, et al. A naturalistic study of referred children and adolescents with obsessive-compulsive disorder. J Am Acad Child Adolesc Psychiatry 2005;44:673–81.

150. Brown GW, Harris T. Disease, distress and depression. A comment. J Affect Disord 1982;4:1–8.
151. Hlastala SA, Frank E, Kowalski J, et al. Stressful life events, bipolar disorder, and the "kindling model." J Abnorm Psychol 2000;109:777–86.
152. Kraepelin E. Manic-depressive insanity and paranoia. Edinburgh (MN): E. and S. Livingstone; 1921.
153. Breslau N, Lucia VC, Alvarado GF. Intelligence and other predisposing factors in exposure to trauma and posttraumatic stress disorder: a follow-up study at age 17 years. Arch Gen Psychiatry 2006;63:1238–45.
154. Giaconia RM, Reinherz HZ, Silverman AB, et al. Traumas and posttraumatic stress disorder in a community population of older adolescents. J Am Acad Child Adolesc Psychiatry 1995;34:1369–80.
155. Steinbuchel P, Wilens TE, Adamson J, et al. Posttraumatic stress disorder and substance use disorder in adolescent bipolar disorder. 2008; in press.
156. Grilo CM, Sanislow C, Fehon DC, et al. Psychological and behavioral functioning in adolescent psychiatric inpatients who report histories of childhood abuse. Am J Psychiatry 1999;156:538–43.
157. Kaplan SJ, Pelcovitz D, Salzinger S, et al. Adolescent physical abuse: risk for adolescent psychiatric disorders. Am J Psychiatry 1998;155:954–9.
158. Kessler RC, Davis CG, Kendler KS. Childhood adversity and adult psychiatric disorder in the US National Comorbidity Survey. Psychol Med 1997;27:1101–19.
159. Leverich GS, Altshuler LL, Frye MA, et al. Risk of switch in mood polarity to hypomania or mania in patients with bipolar depression during acute and continuation trials of venlafaxine, sertraline, and bupropion as adjuncts to mood stabilizers. Am J Psychiatry 2006;163:232–9.
160. Garno JL, Goldberg JF, Ramirez PM, et al. Impact of childhood abuse on the clinical course of bipolar disorder. Br J Psychiatry 2005;186:121–5.
161. Wozniak J, Crawford MH, Biederman J, et al. Antecedents and complications of trauma in boys with ADHD: findings from a longitudinal study. Journal of the American Academy of Child and Adolescent Psychiatry 1999;38:48.
162. Hertzberg MA, Butterfield MI, Feldman ME, et al. A preliminary study of lamotrigine for the treatment of posttraumatic stress disorder. Biol Psychiatry 1999;45:1226–9.
163. Kerbeshian J, Burd L. Case study: comorbidity among tourette's syndrome, autistic disorder, and bipolar disorder. J Am Acad Child Adolesc Psychiatry 1996;35:681–5.
164. Komoto J, Seigo U, Hirata J. Infantile autism and affective disorder. J Autism Dev Disord 1984;14:81–4.
165. Sovner R, Hurley AD. Do the mentally retarded suffer from affective illness? Arch Gen Psychiatry 1983;40:61–7.
166. Steingard R, Biederman J. Lithium responsive manic-like symptoms in two individuals with autism and mental retardation. J Am Acad Child Adolesc Psychiatry 1987;26:932–5.
167. Wing L. Asperger's syndrome: a clinical account. Psychol Med 1981;11:115–29.
168. Towbin KE, Pradella A, Gorrindo T, et al. Autism spectrum traits in children with mood and anxiety disorders. J Child Adolesc Psychopharmacol 2005;15:452–64.
169. Wozniak J, Biederman J, Faraone S, et al. Mania in children with pervasive developmental disorder revisited. J Am Acad Child Adolesc Psychiatry 1997;36:1552–60.
170. Joshi G, Morrow EM, Wozniak J, et al. Prevalence and clinical correlates of pervasive developmental disorders in clinically referred population of children

and adolescents. In 6th International Meeting for Autism Research, Seattle; May 2007.

171. Joshi G, Biederman J, Wozniak J, et al. Response to second generation neuroleptics in youth with comorbid bipolar disorder and pervasive developmental disorders. In 161st American Psychiatric Association Annual Meeting, Washington; May 2008.

172. Joshi G, Wozniak J, Wilens T, et al. Clinical characteristics of youth with comorbid bipolar disorder and autism spectrum disorders. In NIMH sponsored Annual Pediatric Bipolar Disorder Conference, Boston; March 2008.

173. DeLong GR, Nohria C. Psychiatric family history and neurological disease in autistic spectrum disorders. Dev Med Child Neurol 1994;36:441–8.

174. DeLong GR, Dwyer JT. Correlation of family history with specific autistic subgroups: Asperger's syndrome and bipolar affective disease. J Autism Dev Disord 1988;18:593–600.

175. Herzberg B. The families of autistic children. In: Coleman M, editor. The autistic syndromes. Amsterdam: North Holland; 1976. p. 151–72.

176. Research Units on Pediatric Psychopharmacology Autism Network. Randomized, controlled, crossover trial of methylphenidate in pervasive developmental disorders with hyperactivity. Arch Gen Psychiatry 2005;62:1266–74.

177. Aman MG, Arnold MDL, McDougle CJ, et al. Acute and long-term safety and tolerability of risperidone in children with autism. J Child Adolesc Psychopharmacol 2005;15:869–84.

178. Posey DJ, Wiegand RE, Wilkerson J, et al. Open-label atomoxetine for attention-deficit/hyperactivity disorder symptoms associated with high-functioning pervasive developmental disorders. J Child Adolesc Psychopharmacol 2006; 16:599–610.

179. Lainhart JE, Folstein SE. Affective disorders in people with autism: a review of published cases. J Autism Dev Disord 1994;24:587–601.

180. Research Units on Pediatric Psychopharmacology Autism Network. Risperidone in children with autism and serious behavioral problems. N Engl J Med 2002; 347:314–21.

181. Nagaraj R, Singhi P, Malhi P. Risperidone in children with autism: randomized, placebo controlled, double-blind study. J Child Neurol 2006;21:450–5.

182. Shea S, Turgay A, Carroll A, et al. Risperidone in the treatment of disruptive behavioral symptoms in children with autistic and other pervasive developmental disorders. Pediatrics 2004;114:e634–41.

183. Malone RP, Delaney MA, Hyman SB, et al. Ziprasidone in adolescents with autism: an open-label pilot study. J Child Adolesc Psychopharmacol 2007;17: 779–90.

184. Stigler KA, Diener JT, Kohn AE, et al. A prospective, open-label study of aripiprazole in youth with Asperger's disorder and pervasive development disorder not otherwise specified. Neuropscyhopharmacology 2006;31:S194.

185. Findling RL, McNamara NK, Gracious BL, et al. Quetiapine in nine youths with autistic disorder. J Child Adolesc Psychopharmacol 2004;14:287–94.

186. Hollander E, Wasserman S, Swanson EN, et al. A double-blind placebo-controlled pilot study of olanzapine in childhood/adolescent pervasive developmental disorder. J Child Adolesc Psychopharmacol 2006;16:541–8.

187. Martin A, Koenig K, Scahill L, et al. Open-label quetiapine in the treatment of children and adolescents with autistic disorder. J Child Adolesc Psychopharmacol 1999;9:99–107.

The Adverse Consequences of Sleep Disturbance in Pediatric Bipolar Disorder: Implications for Intervention

Allison G. Harvey, PhD

KEYWORDS

- Bipolar disorder • Sleep • Insomnia • Hypersomnia
- Mood • Obesity • Substance use • Impulsivity

The emergence of bipolar disorder during childhood and adolescence is of particular concern, because it may predict a more severe presentation and course,[1–6] including more suicide attempts,[7,8] greater comorbidity,[9] more psychotic features, and worse response to treatment with lithium.[10] Prevalence rates of early onset bipolar disorder are similar to those in adults.[11] However, a minority of bipolar adolescents meet full criteria for bipolar I disorder (BP-I), with the remainder meeting diagnostic criteria on the bipolar spectrum (bipolar II disorder [BP-II], cyclothymia, or bipolar disorder not otherwise specified [BP-NOS]). Even with the inclusion of those who did not meet full criteria for BP-I, youth with bipolar spectrum disorders had twice the rate of suicide attempts and significantly worse levels of overall functioning compared with adolescents with major depressive disorder. Moreover, recent findings have shown that youth meeting criteria for BP-NOS are similar to those with BP-I on many factors, including age of onset, duration of illness, rates of comorbid diagnoses, suicidal ideation, prior major depressive episodes, family history, and the types of manic symptoms that were present during the most serious lifetime episode.[12]

Important advances in treatments for early onset bipolar disorder include pharmacological treatment,[13,14] individual psychotherapy,[15] and family intervention.[16,17] However, a high proportion of individuals continue to remain symptomatic; the risk of recurrence over 2 years is as high as 50%;[1] and the probability of recovery from

Department of Psychology, University of California, 3210 Tolman Hall #1650, Berkeley, CA 94720-1650, USA
E-mail address: aharvey@berkeley.edu

Child Adolesc Psychiatric Clin N Am 18 (2009) 321–338
doi:10.1016/j.chc.2008.11.006
1056-4993/08/$ – see front matter. Published by Elsevier Inc.
childpsych.theclinics.com

episodes is lower,[18] relative to adults with bipolar disorder. Thus, bipolar spectrum disorder represents a common and serious disorder in youth with poor outcomes extending into adulthood.

SLEEP IN YOUTH WITH BIPOLAR DISORDER

Table 1 presents an overview of the studies that have reported the nature and extent of sleep disturbance in children and teenagers with bipolar disorder. Overall, the data suggest that sleep disturbance is a prominent feature of bipolar disorder in youth, although it is notable that only a handful of these studies were explicitly conducted to investigate sleep. Hence, much of our existing knowledge is derived from studies examining other aspects of the disorder in which sleep also happened to be assessed.

As evident in **Table 1**, reduced need for sleep was commonly observed, along with high rates of insomnia. Objective estimates of sleep (ie, polysomnography, actigraphy) were included in only a few studies. These indicate that compared with healthy controls, youth with bipolar disorder exhibit lower sleep efficiency, longer slow-wave sleep, and reduced rapid eye movement (REM) sleep.

A number of methodological issues emerge from this review (see also Harvey and colleagues[19] for more detail). First, there is a need to develop and use psychometrically validated self-report and/or observational methods for assessing sleep disturbance. In addition, there is a need for more studies to include objective estimates of sleep, such as polysomnography and actigraphy. Other limitations in existing studies include absence of a control group and limited assessments of psychiatric comorbidity. Given the high comorbidity rates in bipolar disorder, it will be important for future studies to track comorbidity so as to determine interactions with sleep disturbance. Finally, the strategies for dealing with medication confounders varied across the studies, with several studies not reporting the details. The impact of medications on sleep is an important methodological issue that has been discussed in detail elsewhere.[20]

CONSEQUENCES OF SLEEP DISTURBANCE FOR YOUTH WITH BIPOLAR DISORDER

There are several lines of evidence indicating that sleep disturbances represent a critical issue for the functioning of youth with bipolar disorder. Moreover, data are beginning to emerge in support of the hypothesis that sleep disturbances may contribute mechanistically to the core pathophysiology of pediatric bipolar disorder—a little-studied but potentially very important line of investigation, which could inform early treatment approaches. Several aspects of the relationship between sleep disturbance and pediatric bipolar disorder are briefly reviewed below.

Sleep Disturbance as an Early Marker for Bipolar Disorder

There is evidence that sleep disturbance may be an early marker for bipolar disorder in youth. Compared with children of control parents, children of parents with bipolar disorder exhibited shorter sleep latency and lower Pittsburgh Sleep Quality Index score as well as a trend toward less variable sleep and greater sleep duration.[21] In a study of early onset bipolar disorder (n = 82), sleep disturbance was reported by about half of the parents as one of the earliest symptoms observed.[22] In another study, sleep disturbances (and anxiety disorders) were identified as an antecedent to the onset of bipolar disorder in a subset of high-risk youth.[23] Further evidence is provided by findings reported by Shaw and colleagues[24] who studied a group of 100 at-risk children with a parent with BP-I disorder as well as a control group of 112 children with well parents. Decreased sleep was one of the distinguishing features of the high-risk group.

Table 1
Summary of studies documenting the nature of sleep disturbance in youth with bipolar disorder

Authors	Sleep Disturbance
Ballenger et al[105]	67% reduced need for sleep in child group (n = 6) vs 100% in adult group (n = 12)
Faedda et al[22]	95.1% exhibited some form of sleep disturbance (n = 82; including insomnia and parasomnias)
Faedda & Teicher[106]	Compared with normative data, children with bipolar disorder exhibited: decreased sleep efficiency and sleep duration increased sleep onset latency increased nocturnal activity
Ferreira et al[107]	87.5% decreased need for sleep (n = 7)
Findling et al[108]	Children = 69.6% (n = 56); teens = 76.5% (n = 34)
Geller et al[25]	39.8% decreased need for sleep (versus 6.2% reduced need in attention deficit hyperactivity disorder versus 1.1% in controls
Holtmann et al[26]	The BP profile group reported 66.7% reduced need for sleep compared to both clinical control (39.3%) and healthy control (10.2%) groups
Jerrell & Shugart[109]	Symptoms of mania. 21% hardly slept but not tired
Lofthouse et al[110]	96.2% had moderate to severe sleep problems. Initial insomnia was the most pervasive problem
Lofthouse et al[111]	Large sample collected over the internet (n = 494). 98.6% reported mood-related sleep problems. Also, 96.9% had psychosocial impairment (home, school, or with peers) and nearly two-thirds (64.0%) had problems across all three spheres. Phase shifts were also associated with sleep difficulties (eg, 3-d weekends, daylight savings)
Mehl et al[112]	PSG: Compared to control group, BP group exhibited sleep continuity disturbance, lower SE, less REM sleep, longer SWS, and a trend towards more awakenings. Subjective measures: Compared to control group, BP group reported more difficulty initiating sleep, more restless sleep, nightmares, and morning headaches
Papolos et al[113]	Strongest concordance coefficients between probands and siblings and widest contrasts between BP sibling pairs and comparison sibling pairs included sleep—wake cycle disturbances

Specific Types of Sleep Disturbance May Be a Distinguishing Feature of Bipolar Disorder

Several studies raise the possibility that sleep disturbances may help to distinguish manifestations of bipolar illness from the early development of other psychopathology. First, compared with children with attention deficit hyperactivity disorder (ADHD) and healthy controls, children diagnosed with bipolar disorder have significantly higher rates of sleep difficulties.[25] Second, a decreased need for sleep is more common among children with bipolar profile symptoms than in children with comparable levels of psychopathology, excluding bipolar disorder symptoms.[26] Finally, Dahl and colleagues[27] prospectively followed youth with unipolar depression who had undergone polysomnographic studies as adolescents for the following 7 years (into their early 20s). A clinical interview was administered to determine their disease course.[28] Five of the 26 patients who were diagnosed with unipolar depression at the first assessment had switched to bipolar disorder by the time of the follow-up. Based on these new categorizations, the original polysomnography data were reanalyzed. The results indicated that depressed participants who followed a unipolar course showed reduced REM latency, higher REM density, and increased overall REM sleep, whereas those who moved to a bipolar course demonstrated increased stage one sleep and decreased stage four sleep. These findings raise the possibility that sleep abnormalities may distinguish bipolar from unipolar trajectories in adolescence.

Sleep Disturbance Contributes to Relapse

There are several lines of evidence, based on adults with bipolar disorder, suggesting that sleep disturbance contributes to relapse in bipolar disorder. First, in a systematic review of 73 reports of prodromal symptoms in bipolar disorder and unipolar depression, Jackson and colleagues[29] reported that the majority of patients (more than 80%) were able to identify early symptoms. Among patients with bipolar disorder, sleep disturbance was the most common prodrome of mania and the sixth most common prodrome of depression. Second, a handful of experimental studies and case studies have reported that induced sleep deprivation is associated with the onset of hypomania or mania in a proportion of patients.[30–32] Finally, several prospective studies (which were reviewed by the author in a 2008 review)[33] indicate an association between sleep disturbance and mood. There is an urgent need for research programs to test the presumed generalizability of these findings to youth with bipolar disorder.

Sleep is Critical for Affect Regulation (and Thus, Sleep Disturbances May Exacerbate Bipolar Symptoms)

There is robust evidence that sleep deprivation undermines emotional regulation the following day.[34,35] A study by Zohar and colleagues[36] suggests that the context in which the emotion is experienced is important for determining the direction of the effect of sleep disturbance on affective functioning. These researchers examined the relationship between sleep loss and emotional reactivity in 78 medical residents who were monitored for 5 to 7 days every 6 months over a 2-year period. The results indicated that sleep loss not only intensified negative emotions following a goal-thwarting event but also diminished positive emotions following a goal-enhancing event. Although this evidence is based on adults, it seems safe to presume that it is highly relevant to youth, who may even be substantially more vulnerable to these effects given their increased sleep need.[37]

Sleep Is Important for Cognitive Functioning (and Thus, Sleep Disturbances May Exacerbate Performance Deficits Noted on Neuropsychological Testing)

Deficits in neuropsychological performance have been demonstrated in pediatric bipolar samples.[38,39] Although such findings point to disrupted brain networks that may elucidate underlying neural mechanisms as well as functional impairments suffered by patients, the extent to which sleep disturbance contributes to, or partially accounts for, these findings has not, to the author's knowledge, been examined. It seems plausible that sleep disturbance may contribute given that adverse and severe effects of sleep deprivation on cognitive functioning have been clearly demonstrated.[40,41] Adverse effects in this domain are likely to be particularly critical for bipolar youth, whose educational achievements (so reliant on cognitive function) will have far-reaching and long-term consequences.

Sleep Impacts Obesity (and Thus, Sleep Disturbance May Exacerbate Critical Medication Side Effects)

In adults, it is well established that bipolar disorder is associated with a wide range of medical problems, with the most common being cardiovascular disease, diabetes mellitus, and thyroid disease.[42] The physical health of youth with bipolar disorder has been less studied, although there is evidence of weight problems and obesity and indications that obesity is associated with worse outcome.[43] There is no doubt that many of the medications used to treat bipolar disorder are associated with weight gain.[44,45] It also seems likely that depressive symptoms may be associated with physical inactivity, which is a likely contributor to obesity. Another possible explanation, given that sleep deprivation increases appetite, weight gain, and insulin tolerance,[46] is that sleep disturbance may be an additional contributor. Indeed, in a recent meta-analysis involving 30 studies (12 in children) and 634,511 participants, an association between short sleep and obesity was observed across the age range. Specifically, there was a 60% to 80% increase in the odds of being a short sleeper among children who were obese.[47]

Sleep Deprivation Is Associated with Substance Use (and Thus, Sleep Disturbances May Be One Contributor to Substance Use Comorbidity in Bipolar Youth)

Several studies indicate that the presence of bipolar disorder in adolescence is associated with elevated risk for alcohol abuse, drug abuse, and cigarette smoking. This finding could not be attributed to comorbid conduct disorder,[48] ADHD, or multiple anxiety disorders.[49] Again, the contributors to these high rates of comorbidity with substance use problems are going to be complex and multifactorial. One possibility is that the sleep disturbance that is characteristic of bipolar disorder may be one contributor. Indeed, among a Finnish sample of adolescents, irregular sleep schedules and daytime sleepiness accounted for 26% of the variance in substance use in 15-year-old boys and 12% in 15-year-old girls.[50] Another large study of 4,500 12- to 17-year-olds found that adolescents who had trouble sleeping reported greater use of alcohol (odds ratio, 2.6), marijuana (odds ratio, 2.4), and cigarettes (odds ratio, 2.2).[51] It is possible that the effects of drugs and alcohol may be sought out for the sedation and/or emotional regulatory effects or for rewarding and/or stimulating effects.

Sleep Deprivation Contributes to Suicidality, Impulsivity, and Risk Taking (and Thus, May Exacerbate These Problems in Youth with Bipolar Disorder)

Youth with bipolar disorder have particularly high rates of suicide attempts,[7,8] and impulsivity and risk taking are core symptoms. Sleep disturbance may be relevant to both. First, there is accruing evidence that sleep disturbance[52] and sleep loss[53,54] signal increased risk for suicidality. Second, the single largest source of mortality in adolescents is deaths due to accidents—particularly lethal automobile crashes. There is compelling evidence that sleep deprivation contributes to nighttime accidents in youth.[55,56] Third, a study by Haynes and colleagues[57] found that improvements in sleep time were associated with significant decreases in aggressive thoughts and actions among adolescents with substance dependence difficulties. Again, these data raise the possibility that sleep disturbance may be an important but understudied contributor to particularly dangerous aspects of bipolar disorder.

Taken together, these lines of evidence indicate that sleep disturbance may contribute in several direct and indirect ways to core problems and symptoms of bipolar disorders in youth. Accordingly, treatment targeting sleep may represent unique opportunities for intervention.

CURRENT OPTIONS AND PRACTICES FOR TREATMENT OF SLEEP DISTURBANCE IN CHILDREN AND ADOLESCENTS (BROADLY, NOT FOCUSING ON BIPOLAR DISORDER)

There is robust evidence for the use of a psychological intervention, cognitive behavior therapy (CBT), for *treating adults* with sleep disturbance.[58] The research literature on the treatment of sleep disturbance with psychological interventions in *children and adolescents* is small but promising as are the data on the behavioral and/or emotional improvements after the treatment of sleep problems in children and adolescents.[59–62] For example, Bootzin and colleagues[63] developed a six-session (90 minutes per session) group treatment for sleep disturbance in adolescents with substance-related problems (ages, 12–19). The intervention was based on the CBT intervention for adults with sleep disturbance but was carefully developmentally adapted to enhance the motivation, commitment, and compliance of the youth. Participants who completed four or more sessions showed improved sleep, and improving sleep led to a reduction in substance abuse problems at the 12-month follow-up. In a separate report, improvements in sleep were associated with significant decreases in aggressive thoughts and actions.[64] These data show the feasibility of improving sleep through a short-term psychological intervention in adolescents and provide promising preliminary results suggesting that improved sleep in youth can contribute to improvements in behavioral and emotional functioning.

One of the most contentious issues in the domain of treating sleep problems in children and adolescents with difficulty going to sleep is the use of medications to promote sleep onset.[65] Indeed, there are large numbers of medications prescribed by pediatricians, child psychiatrists, and family practitioners for children of all ages in attempts to hasten sleep onset. Adult sleep pharmacology has seen numerous advances, including new generation agents with a much better specificity for sleep, duration of action, and relatively low risk and side effects *in adults*. Therefore, one might logically argue that some of these medications might represent better treatment options for insomnia in children and adolescents. However, until there are empirical data and controlled trials using these medications in youth (including dosing, side effects, and efficacy), it seems wise to be reluctant to advocate any specific medication at this time. There are currently some studies underway that may provide these needed data soon.

CURRENT OPTIONS AND PRACTICES FOR TREATMENT OF SLEEP DISTURBANCE IN ADULTS WITH BIPOLAR DISORDER

To the best of the author's knowledge, there are no clinical trials of interventions for sleep disturbance in adults with bipolar disorder (or in youth with bipolar disorder). However, several of the psychological adjunctive interventions for bipolar disorder include one or more components targeting sleep. Interpersonal and social rhythm therapy includes instruction in behavioral techniques designed to regularize routines and reduce social rhythm disruption.[66] CBT provides education about the importance of a regular social routine and sleep–wake cycle via the monitoring of mood and sleep as well as the use of activity scheduling. It also involves identifying prodromes, which typically include sleep disturbance, and to develop effective coping strategies for such prodromes.[67,68] Family interventions[69] group psychoeducation, and individual psychoeducation[17] also include content that encourages sleep–wake stabilization. Although these approaches have been shown to reduce relapse in adults and youth,[70–73] there are not yet data on sleep-specific outcomes. In addition, these approaches have yet to draw from advances in knowledge on the psychological treatment of sleep disturbance in adults with insomnia.[58]

For medication interventions, there have been a handful of case reports and case series. Weilburg and colleagues[74] reported that triazolam induced brief episodes of mania in an elderly woman, and Sattar and colleagues[75] reported a case in which the interaction between valproic acid and zolpidem induced somnambulism (sleepwalking) in a 47-year-old man with bipolar disorder. In a retrospective case series of 96 patients with bipolar disorder, treating insomnia during an episode of depression with sedative antidepressants was associated with worse prognosis.[76] Hence, to date, data on the effects of sleep medication for bipolar patients are not encouraging.

Although under-researched, medications targeting the circadian system appear to be promising *in adults* with bipolar disorder. A response to 3 mg of melatonin at night has been reported in an open trial of 11 patients with insomnia during mania.[77] A case series of 5 individuals with rapid-cycling bipolar disorder treated using melatonin was negative.[78] The melatonin agonists such as agomelatine and ramelteon are also potentially of interest, although they have yet to be adequately studied for efficacy in bipolar disorder. Calabrese and colleagues[79] studied adjunctive open-label agomelatine at 25 mg/d with some positive results.

In addition, modafinil, an alertness-promoting agent, is being trialed for the treatment of fatigue and perhaps also hypersomnia in adults with bipolar disorder. For example, Frye and colleagues[80] recently published the first double-blind placebo-controlled study of adjunctive modafinil. The sample included depressed bipolar patients (n = 86) who had not adequately responded to a mood stabilizer with or without antidepressant therapy. Compared with the placebo group, those receiving modafinil treatment improved significantly on the clinician-rated Inventory of Depressive Symptoms (particularly on a four-item fatigue/energy subset) by week 2, and these gains remained throughout the 6 weeks of administration. However, the response and remission rates were only 44% and 39%, respectively (relative to 23% and 18% in the placebo group). Moreover, post-treatment follow-up was not conducted to evaluate long-term outcomes. Adverse side effects included headache, nausea, insomnia, and rapid heart rate. The author emphasizes that all of this research has been conducted in adults with bipolar disorder. In the absence of data demonstrating the safety and efficacy of these approaches in youth, their use is not advocated.

TOWARD A PSYCHOLOGICAL INTERVENTION FOR SLEEP DISTURBANCE IN YOUTH WITH BIPOLAR DISORDER

Given the prevalence of sleep disturbance among youth with bipolar disorder, the associated adverse consequences, and the lack of empirically tested treatments, a high priority for future research is to develop an intervention for the sleep disturbance experienced by youth with bipolar disorder. An intervention for sleep may be particularly acceptable to youth as the payoffs of improving sleep are immediate, and sleep is often perceived by patients to be an aspect of health that is free of the strong association with mental health (and the associated stigma). It is hypothesized that delivering such an intervention to youth with bipolar disorder may help protect this high-risk group against the potential negative vicious cycles of escalating sleep disturbance and emotion dysregulation, leading to school failure, unemployment, and withdrawal of social supports, along with reducing the other hypothesized adverse outcomes described earlier.

The advantages of developing a psychological intervention to improve sleep, as compared with a pharmacological intervention, are (1) A psychological intervention will improve sleep without causing adverse side effects. (2) Youth with bipolar disorder are often already taking more than 1 psychotropic medication, so adding an additional medication to target sleep has the potential to lead to drug interactions and result in youth having very complicated medication regimens. (3) There is evidence from the adult literature that a psychological intervention for sleep disturbance is more likely to produce durable effects, relative to pharmacotherapy. (4) There is evidence from the adult literature that psychological interventions for sleep disturbance are more acceptable to patients than medication treatments.[81,82] (5) While there is evidence of the efficacy and feasibility of a psychological intervention for treating sleep disturbance in youth,[63] there is not yet equivalent evidence for sleep medication.

In the section that follows several treatment components are offered as important building blocks of a treatment for sleep disturbance in youth with bipolar disorder. This section draws on treatment development work by a team of clinical researchers (the author and Ron Dahl, Erica Forbes, Laura Trubnick, Greg Clarke, Dick Bootzin, and Rachel Manber) who are currently developing sleep-focused interventions for youth with anxiety disorders and depression, but it extends this work to target the specific needs of youth with bipolar disorder. *It is emphasized that there is an urgent need for a focused treatment development process and then formal testing of the resultant intervention*. In particular, sleep interventions need to be adapted and/or designed to address the normal and substantial maturational changes in sleep and circadian functioning across childhood and adolescence.[83] Also varying over development is the extent of parent involvement in bedtimes and choice of evening activities and bedtimes. Sleep disturbance is often amplified by increasing levels of independence from parental and adult influences on sleep-relevant decisions. Clinical decision making about the extent of involvement in the intervention should be on the basis of the youth's age and level of maturity, although an emphasis must be placed on the young person taking responsibility and initiative and inviting the parent or caregiver for support when needed.

Functional Analysis and Case Formulation

This involves a detailed clinical interview in which the clinician probes the frequency, intensity, and duration of the sleep disturbance as well as its antecedents, behaviors, and consequences. For homework, the patient is asked to complete a daily sleep diary, supplementing standard sleep diary questions with additional probes to enable the collection of information on the psychological and contextual variables that might be contributing. If available, actigraphy can be a useful adjunct and, in younger children, it can be helpful to enlist a parent's help in sleep diary completion.

Motivational Interviewing

This involves a straightforward review with the young person to explore how he or she sees the pros and cons of working toward managing the sleep disturbance.[84] By using motivational interviewing techniques, the patient's motivation can be clarified and enhanced. Many sleep-incompatible/interfering behaviors used by youth are rewarding (such as text messaging with friends into the night and freely surfing the Internet once parents have gone to bed). Moreover, as children move into adolescence, parental influence over bedtime and bedroom activities wanes. Hence, following other treatments for youth with sleep disturbance,[85] it is likely to be necessary to begin treatment with a motivational component designed to assist young persons to find their internal motivation for enhancing sleep.

Sleep and Circadian Education

This module aims to target specific factors and behaviors that interfere with good sleep.[86] Erratic sleep–wake schedules including large discrepancies between wake time on school days (typically 6—7 AM) versus weekends and holidays (typically 11 AM–2 PM) constitute a weekly experience of severe "jetlag" and contribute to high rates of insufficient sleep in adolescents in general and may represent a particularly important target for youth with bipolar disorder. This module has three core aims: to correct unhelpful sleep habits (eg, surfing the Internet until late), to develop new healthy sleep habits (eg, on waking up being active and, if possible during the day, having bright light exposure, such as walking outdoors), and to maintain these new healthier habits. After an initial education session, two steps are followed to correct habits: behavioral contracting and monitoring healthy sleep behaviors and sleep-interfering behaviors on a daily basis. The maintenance of healthy habits will be achieved by regular check-ins on progress throughout the remaining sessions and by including the targets of change in the relapse prevention plan.

There are two additional core parts to this module for bipolar youth. These are added in recognition of two sets of empirical findings on sleep in bipolar disorder. First, based on the finding that sleep disturbance is the most common prodrome of mania and the sixth most common prodrome of depression,[29] we discuss sleep disturbance as a possible early warning of an episode. The therapist then collaborates with the young person to establish and practice effective coping strategies for such prodromes.[87] This needs to be individualized to each patient, because some youth with bipolar disorder appear to be characterized by less "classic" cycles of mania and depression and more by chronic displays of irritable, explosive, and "mixed" mood states.[88] Second, on the basis that bipolar disorder is a disorder of emotional regulation,[89] along with the evidence suggesting that sleep has a key mood regulatory function,[90,91] a link is drawn between sleep disturbance and daytime mood dysfunction. In the patients treated thus far, these 2 aspects have been addressed by education and appear to serve to increase the internal motivation for working to enhance sleep.

For those with hypersomnia (addressed in more detail below) it can also be helpful to educate the young person about two additional domains.[92] The first involves education about the operation of the circadian system, the environmental influences acting on it (eg, light), the tendency if left unchecked to move toward a delayed phase, and the difficulty achieving fast shifts in circadian patterns. The second involves education about sleep inertia. This includes the fact that among both adults and youth, most mornings, there is a period between 5 minutes and 20 minutes when we feel dazed and sleepy and that this is a normal transitional state between a state of sleep and a state of wakefulness. Acknowledging that these feelings are not pleasant and that the feelings are not necessarily indicative of having had a poor night of sleep can be helpful.

Regularizing the Sleep–Wake Schedule

Delayed phase is common in teenagers, particularly those with bipolar disorder. Indeed, a significant delay in the circadian sleep–wake cycle has been hypothesized to be a core deficit of pediatric bipolar disorder.[93] It often begins with a tendency to stay up late at night, sleeping in late, and/or taking a late afternoon nap. This process often starts on weekends, holidays, or summer vacations. Problems become apparent when school schedules result in morning wake-up battles and difficulties in getting to school. Often, these adolescents cope by taking afternoon naps and getting catch-up sleep on the weekends. Although some of these behaviors occur in many healthy adolescents, in extreme cases, the circadian system can become set to such a late time that even highly motivated adolescents can have difficulty shifting their sleep back to an earlier time.

An adapted version of Bootzin's stimulus control intervention,[94] which was a core component of the sleep intervention administered to youth with substance-related difficulties,[63] is an important component for regularizing the sleep–wake cycle and strengthening the association between the bed and sleeping by limiting sleep-incompatible behaviors within the bedroom environment, while developing a consistent sleep–wake schedule.[94] The traditional components of this intervention involve the therapist providing a detailed rationale for, and assisting the patient to achieve, the following: (a) use the bed only for sleep (ie, no television watching or talking on cell phones); (b) go to bed only when sleepy; (c) get out of bed and go to another room when unable to fall asleep or return to sleep within approximately 15–20 minutes and return to bed only when sleepy again; and (d) arise in the morning at the same time each day (no later than plus 2 hours on weekends).[63] The goal is to gradually move toward a regular schedule 7 days a week. In the bipolar youth we have treated thus far, we have retained (a) and (d) but omitted (b) and (c). Point (b) was omitted because patients with bipolar disorder often need to get into bed, even though not yet sleepy, to begin the process of downregulating sufficiently to fall off to sleep. Point (c) was omitted to avoid sleep deprivation during the early phase of treatment; getting out of bed risks getting caught up in rewarding and arousing activities that reduce the potential for sleep. The latter is key for patients with bipolar disorder in whom hypomania and mania are often related to elevated achievement motivation, ambitious goal setting, and excessive goal pursuit.[95] To achieve (a) and (d) we use the standard CBT manualized methods[96] that include providing a rationale, setting goals for bedtime and wake time, keeping a daily sleep diary to monitor progress toward goals, and reviewing the diary on a weekly basis. For difficulty falling asleep, we replace the traditional stimulus control instruction (get up out of bed) with training in imagery following[97] and relaxation techniques following[96] with the goal of reducing arousal and promoting sleep onset.

Hypersomnia

In our experience, daytime sleepiness is common among youth, especially youth with a bipolar spectrum disorder. In addition, during phases of depression, patients commonly suffer from periods of hypersomnia.[98] Hypersomnia has adverse consequences for school attendance and performance, relationships, mood, and sense of self-worth. There is very little existing literature on either the mechanisms that contribute to hypersomnia in bipolar disorder or the methods to treat it.[92] In the author's clinical experience, treating hypersomnia is likely to begin with goal setting, which involves reducing nightly sleep as well as setting goals for life. The latter is based on the author's clinical experience that "having nothing to get up for" can be a key contributor to hypersomnia in patients with mood disorders. Often the combination of the mood disorder and the sleep disorder has led to unemployment and disrupted social networks. After setting the "sleep" and "life" goals for the treatment, the young person is asked to identify one small step toward these goals for the coming week. After a detailed discussion of how to achieve those goals, possible obstacles are identified. We engage in problem solving to limit the impact of these obstacles on reaching the goal, and a method is developed for monitoring the extent to which the goal is achieved (see Kaplan and Harvey[92] for further details).

Wind-Down, Wake-Up, and Regularity

Often youth need assistance to devise a "wind-down" period of 30–60 minutes before sleep in which relaxing, sleep enhancing activities are engaged in. A central issue influencing bedtime is the use of electronic media (Internet, cell phones, MP3 players) for entertainment and social interaction at night. A crucial aspect of achieving earlier sleep onset requires a behavioral contract by each individual wherein he or she voluntarily *chooses* a time for turning off all access to these devices. Equally important is the "wake-up protocol" (eg, not hitting snooze on the alarm; making the bed so the incentive to get back in is reduced; head for the shower; take a quick brisk walk; get sunlight). Finally, we emphasize the importance of minimal fluctuation in the sleep–wake schedule across weekday and weekend nights.

Behavioral Experiments

Educational approaches are often very helpful, but there is evidence that arranging situations that allow clients to experience the issue being discussed can bring about more profound change.[99] To give an example, hypersomnia patients typically believe that the only way they can feel less tired is to try to sleep more. *Telling* them that being active can generate energy is less effective than setting up an experience that allows them to *experience* the energy-generating effects of activity. Here is a brief description of a behavioral experiment recently conducted with a hypersomnia patient to provide him with *experience*. Over 2 days the patient tested his belief that the only way to get energy is to keep sleeping or go back to sleep. On the first day he spent one 3-hour block *conserving* energy (eg, sleeping in each morning, going back to bed, and when out of bed attempting only mundane tasks) and then a 3-hour block *using* energy (eg, taking a 10-minute walk, arranging to see a friend). The following day he did this in the reverse order. Contrary to his beliefs, his mood and energy were *improved* by "using" energy. As a result of this experiment, "using" energy became synonymous with "generating" energy, and this became one strategy for managing daytime tiredness.

Unhelpful Beliefs about Sleep

Holding dysfunctional beliefs about sleep is an important maintainer of insomnia in adults. There are preliminary data in adults with bipolar disorder showing that they also hold a number of unhelpful beliefs about sleep.[100] In the author's clinical work with bipolar youth, it has become clear that altering beliefs about the sleep–wake cycle is important for reducing sleep disturbance. Typical unhelpful beliefs about sleep held by youth include "there is no point going to bed earlier because I won't be able to fall asleep," "sleep is a waste of time," "sleep is boring," and "getting more sleep doesn't help me." Hence, we suggest that including a module to target such beliefs will be important. The intervention for dysfunctional beliefs typically involves a four-step process: (a) identification of dysfunctional beliefs; (b) use of guided discovery and Socratic questioning to challenge the beliefs; (c) individualized experiments to test the validity and utility of dysfunctional beliefs and to collect data on new beliefs; and (d) the identification and dropping of safety behaviors that prevent disconfirmation of dysfunctional beliefs. The foundation of this module is manualized.[101,102]

Bedtime Worry, Rumination, and Vigilance

Our research on adults with bipolar disorder and our clinical experience with bipolar youth suggest that they attribute difficulty getting to sleep to excessive negative (worry/rumination) and positive cognitive activity.[100] As anxiety[103] and negative or positive worry/rumination[104] are antithetical to sleep onset, it will be important to include a module to help the young person manage bedtime worry, rumination, and anxiety. The intervention will likely include Beckian cognitive therapy to teach methods to assist the patient to evaluate worry and rumination, diary writing or scheduling a "worry period" to encourage the processing of worries several hours before bedtime, creating a "to do" list before getting into bed to reduce worry about future plans/events, training to disengage from pre-sleep worry and redirect attention to pleasant (distracting) imagery, demonstrating the adverse consequences of thought suppression while in bed, and scheduling a pre-sleep "wind-down" period before bedtime to promote disengagement from daytime concerns. The foundation of this module is already manualized.[96,101]

Relapse Prevention

The goal is to consolidate and maximize maintenance of gains and to set the child and parent on a trajectory for continued improvement. It is guided by an individualized summary of learning and achievements. Areas needing further intervention are addressed by setting specific goals and creating a specific plan for achieving each goal.

SUMMARY

Sleep disturbance in youth with bipolar disorder is critically important, yet surprisingly understudied. We have reviewed evidence on the prevalence and nature of sleep disturbance in youth with bipolar disorder. Evidence pointing to the importance of sleep includes that sleep disturbance appears to be an early marker for bipolar disorder; is a distinguishing feature of pediatric bipolar disorder; contributes to relapse, affect dysregulation, and deficits in cognitive functioning; and may also contribute to weight problems, comorbid substance use problems, and impulsivity. The implications for intervention are explained and a multicomponent sleep intervention is outlined. At a simple pragmatic level, one can make a compelling argument for the advantages of implementing cognitive and behavioral interventions to improve sleep and regularize sleep–wake schedules in ways that are likely to have a positive impact on mental and physical health (and affect regulation) in youth with bipolar disorder. At a scientific level, there is an equally compelling case regarding the potential advances for mechanistic understanding of the interactions between sleep and affect regulation in bipolar disorder. Clearly, there is an urgent need for research to delineate the specific genetic, neurobiological, and psychosocial contributors to sleep disturbance in youth. In addition, there is a critical need for a focused treatment development process and then formal testing of the resultant intervention.

ACKNOWLEDGMENTS

The author gratefully acknowledges David Axelson, Natasha Dagys, Ron Dahl, Anda Gershon, Tina Goldstein, Steve Hinshaw, and Ben Mullin for helpful discussions relating to the content covered in this article.

REFERENCES

1. Birmaher B, Axelson D, Strober M, et al. Clinical course of children and adolescents with bipolar spectrum disorders. Arch Gen Psychiatry 2006;63:175.
2. Cate Carter TD, Mundo E, Parikh SV, et al. Early age at onset as a risk factor for poor outcome of bipolar disorder. J Psychiatr Res 2003;37:297.
3. Geller B, Craney JL, Bolhofner K, et al. Two-year prospective follow-up of children with a prepubertal and early adolescent bipolar disorder phenotype. Am J Psychiatry 2002;159:927.
4. Geller B, DelBello MP. Bipolar disorder in childhood and early adolescence. New York: Guilford; 2003.

5. Perlis R, Miyahara S, Marangell L, et al. Long-term implications of early onset in bipolar disorder: data from the first 1000 participants in the systematic treatment enhancement program for bipolar disorder (STEP-BD). Biol Psychiatry 2004;55: 875.
6. Tohen M, Angst J. Epidemiology of bipolar disorder. In: Tsuang MT, Tohen M, editors. Textbook in psychiatric epidemiology. 2nd edition. New York: Wiley-Liss; 2002. p. 427.
7. Bellivier F, Golmard J-L, Henry C, et al. Admixture analysis of age at onset in bipolar I affective disorder. Arch Gen Psychiatry 2001;58:510.
8. Tsai S-Y, Lee J-C, Chen C-C. Characteristics and psychosocial problems of patients with bipolar disorder at high risk for suicide attempt. J Affect Disord 1999;52:145.
9. Bashir MR, Russell J, Johnson G. Bipolar affective disorder in adolescence: a 10-year study. Aust N Z J Psychiatry 1987;21:36.
10. Schurhoff F, Bellivier F, Jouvent R, et al. Early and late onset bipolar disorders: two different forms of manic-depressive illness? J Affect Disord 2000;58:215.
11. Lewinsohn PM, Klein DN, Seeley JR. Bipolar disorders in a community sample of older adolescents: prevalence, phenomenology, comorbidity, and course. J Am Acad Child Adolesc Psychiatry 1995;34:454.
12. Axelson D, Birmaher B, Strober M, et al. Phenomenology of children and adolescents with bipolar spectrum disorders. Arch Gen Psychiatry 2006;63:1139.
13. Kowatch RA, DelBello MP. Pharmacotherapy of children and adolescents with bipolar disorder. Psychiatr Clin North Am 2005;28:385.
14. Ryan ND. The pharmacological treatment of child and adolescent bipolar disorder. In: Geller B, DelBello MP, editors. Bipolar disorder in childhood and early adolescence. New York: Guilford Press; 2003.
15. Pavuluri MN, Birmaher B, Naylor MW. Pediatric bipolar disorder: a review of the past 10 years. J Am Acad Child Adolesc Psychiatry 2005;44:846.
16. Fristad MA, Goldberg-Arnold JS, Gavazzi SM. Multifamily psychoeducation groups (MFPG) in the treatment of children with mood disorders. J Marital Fam Ther 2003;29:491.
17. Miklowitz DJ, Johnson SL. The psychopathology and treatment of bipolar disorder. Annual Review of Clinical Psychology 2006;2:199.
18. Strober M, Schmidt-Lackner S, Freeman R, et al. Recovery and relapse in adolescents with bipolar affective illness: a five-year naturalistic, prospective follow-up. J Am Acad Child Adolesc Psychiatry 1995;34:724.
19. Harvey AG, Mullin BC, Hinshaw SP. Sleep and circadian rhythms in children and adolescents with bipolar disorder. Dev Psychopathol 2006;18:1147.
20. Harvey AG, Talbot LS, Gershon A. Sleep disturbance in bipolar disorder across the lifespan. Clinical Psychology, in press.
21. Jones SH, Tai S, Evershed K, et al. Early detection of bipolar disorder: a pilot familial high-risk study of parents with bipolar disorder and their adolescent children. Bipolar Disord 2006;8:362.
22. Faedda GL, Baldessarini RJ, Glovinsky IP, et al. Pediatric bipolar disorder: phenomenology and course of illness. Bipolar Disord 2004;6:305.
23. Duffy A, Alda M, Crawford L, et al. The early manifestations of bipolar disorder: a longitudinal prospective study of the offspring of bipolar parents. Bipolar Disord 2007;9:828.
24. Shaw JA, Egeland JA, Endicott J, et al. A 10-year prospective study of prodromal patterns for bipolar disorder among Amish youth. J Am Acad Child Adolesc Psychiatry 2005;44:1104.

25. Geller B, Zimerman B, Williams M, et al. DSM-IV mania symptoms in a prepubertal and early adolescent bipolar disorder phenotype compared to attention-deficit hyperactive and normal controls. J Child Adolesc Psychopharmacol 2002;12:11.

26. Holtmann M, Bolte S, Goth K, et al. Prevalence of the child behavior checklist-pediatric bipolar disorder phenotype in a German general population sample. Bipolar Disord 2007;9:895.

27. Dahl RE, Puig-Antich J, Ryan ND, et al. EEG sleep in adolescents with major depression: the role of suicidality and inpatient status. J Affect Disord 1990;19:63.

28. Rao U, Dahl RE, Ryan ND, et al. Heterogeneity in EEG sleep findings in adolescent depression: unipolar versus bipolar clinical course. J Affect Disord 2002;70:273.

29. Jackson A, Cavanagh J, Scott J. A systematic review of manic and depressive prodromes. J Affect Disord 2003;74:209.

30. Colombo C, Benedetti F, Barbini B, et al. Rate of switch from depression into mania after therapeutic sleep deprivation in bipolar depression. Psychiatry Res 1999;86:267.

31. Wehr TA, Goodwin FK, Wirz-Justice A, et al. 48-hour sleep-wake cycles in manic-depressive illness: naturalistic observations and sleep deprivation experiments. Arch Gen Psychiatry 1982;39:559.

32. Wehr TA, Sack DA, Rosenthal NE. Sleep reduction as a final common pathway in the genesis of mania. Am J Psychiatry 1987;144:201.

33. Harvey AG. Sleep and circadian rhythms in bipolar disorder: seeking synchrony, harmony, and regulation. Am J Psychiatry 2008;165:820.

34. Pilcher JJ, Huffcutt AI. Effects of sleep deprivation on performance: a meta-analysis. Sleep 1996;19:318.

35. Yoo S, Gujar N, Hu P, et al. The human emotional brain without sleep: a prefrontal-amygdala disconnect? Curr Biol 2007;17:R877.

36. Zohar D, Tzischinsky O, Epsten R, et al. The effects of sleep loss on medical residents' emotional reactions to work events: a cognitive-energy model. Sleep 2005;28:47.

37. Carskadon MA. Patterns of sleep and sleepiness in adolescents. Pediatrician 1990;17:5.

38. Dickstein DP, Treland JE, Snow J, et al. Neuropsychological performance in pediatric bipolar disorder. Biol Psychiatry 2004;55:32.

39. Doyle AE, Wilens TE, Kwon A, et al. Neuropsychological functioning in youth with bipolar disorder. Biol Psychiatry 2005;58:540.

40. Van Dongen HP, Maislin G, Mullington JM, et al. The cumulative cost of additional wakefulness: dose-response effects on neurobehavioral functions and sleep physiology from chronic sleep restriction and total sleep deprivation. Sleep 2003;26:117.

41. Walker MP, Stickgold R. Sleep, memory, and plasticity. Annual Reviews in Psychology 2006;57:139.

42. Krishnan KR. Psychiatric and medical comorbidity of bipolar disorder. Psychosom Med 2005;67:1–8.

43. Jolin EM, Weller EB, Weller RA. The public health aspects of bipolar disorder in children and adolescents. Curr Psychiatry Rep 2007;9:106.

44. Elmslie JL, Silverstone JT, Mann JI, et al. Prevalence of overweight and obesity in bipolar patients. J Clin Psychiatry 2000;61:179.

45. Zimmermann U, Kraus T, Himmerich H, et al. Epidemiology, implications and mechanisms underlying drug-induced weight gain in psychiatric patients. J Psychiatr Res 2003;37:193.

46. Spiegel K, Tasali E, Penev P, et al. Brief communication: sleep curtailment in healthy young men is associated with decreased leptin levels, elevated ghrelin levels, and increased hunger and appetite. Ann Intern Med 2004;141:846.
47. Cappuccio FP, Taggart FM, Kandala NB, et al. Meta-analysis of short sleep duration and obesity in children and adults. Sleep 2008;31:619.
48. Wilens TE, Biederman J, Kwon A, et al. Risk of substance use disorders in adolescents with bipolar disorder. J Am Acad Child Adolesc Psychiatry 2004;43:1380.
49. Wilens TE, Biederman J, Adamson JJ, et al. Further evidence of an association between adolescent bipolar disorder with smoking and substance use disorders: a controlled study. Drug Alcohol Depend 2008;95:188.
50. Tynjala J, Kannas L, Levalahti E. Perceived tiredness among adolescents and its association with sleep habits and use of psychoactive substances. J Sleep Res 1997;6:189.
51. Johnson EO, Breslau N, Roehrs T, et al. Insomnia in adolescence: epidemiology and associated problems. Sleep 1999;22:s22.
52. Dahl RE, Ryan ND, Matty MK, et al. Sleep onset abnormalities in depressed adolescents. Biol Psychiatry 1996;39:400.
53. Liu X. Sleep and adolescent suicidal behavior. Sleep 2004;27:1351.
54. Liu X, Buysee DJ. Sleep and youth suicidal behavior: a neglected field. Current Opinion in Psychiatry 2005;19:288.
55. Arnedt JT, Owens J, Crouch M, et al. Neurobehavioral performance of residents after heavy night call vs after alcohol ingestion. J Am Med Assoc 2005;294:1025.
56. Carskadon MA. Risks of driving while sleepy in adolescents and young adults. In: Carskadon MA, editor. Adolescent sleep patterns: biological, social, and psychological influences. Cambridge (UK): Cambridge University Press; 2002. p. 148.
57. Haynes PL, McQuaid JR, Ancoli-Israel S, et al. Disrupting life events and the sleep-wake cycle in depression. Psychol Med 2006;36:1363.
58. Morin CM, Bootzin RR, Buysse DJ, et al. Psychological and behavioral treatment of insomnia: an update of recent evidence (1998–2004). Sleep 2006;29:1396.
59. Dahl RE. The consequences of insufficient sleep for adolescents: links between sleep and emotional regulation. Phi Delta Kappan 1999;354.
60. Minde K, Faucon A, Falkner S. Sleep problems in toddlers: effects of treatment on their daytime behavior. Journal of the American Academy of Child & Adolescent Psychiatry 1994;33:1114.
61. O'Brien LM, Gozal D. Neurocognitive dysfunction and sleep in children: from human to rodent. Pediatr Clin North Am 2004;51:187.
62. Sadeh A, Gruber R, Raviv A. The effects of sleep restriction and extension on school-age children: what a difference an hour makes. Child Dev 2003;74:444.
63. Bootzin RR, Stevens SJ. Adolescents, substance abuse, and the treatment of insomnia and daytime sleepiness. Clin Psychol Rev 2005;25:629.
64. Haynes PL, Bootzin RR, Smith L, et al. Sleep and aggression in substance-abusing adolescents: results from an integrative behavioral sleep-treatment pilot program. Sleep 2006;29:512.
65. Owens JA, Rosen CL, Mindell JA. Medication use in the treatment of pediatric insomnia: results of a survey of community-based pediatricicans. Pediatrics 2003;111(5 Pt 1):628.
66. Frank E, Swartz HA, Kupfer DJ. Interpersonal and social rhythm therapy: managing the chaos of bipolar disorder. Biol Psychiatry 2000;48:593.
67. Lam DH, Watkins ER, Hayward P, et al. A randomized controlled study of cognitive therapy for relapse prevention for bipolar affective disorder: outcome of the first year. Arch Gen Psychiatry 2003;60:145.

68. Patelis-Siotis I, Young LT, Robb JC, et al. Group cognitive behavioral therapy for bipolar disorder: a feasibility and effectiveness study. J Affect Disord 2001;65:145.
69. Miklowitz DJ, Goldstein MJ. Bipolar disorder: a family-focused treatment approach. New York: Guilford Press; 1997.
70. Craighead WE, Miklowitz DJ, Frank E, et al. Psychosocial treatments for bipolar disorder. In: Nathan PE, Gorman JM, editors. A guide to treatments that work. 2nd edition. London: Oxford University Press; 2002. p. 263.
71. Frank E, Kupfer DJ, Thase ME, et al. Two year outcomes for interpersonal and social rhythm therapy in individuals with bipolar I disorder. Arch Gen Psychiatry 2005;62:996.
72. Lam DH, Hayward P, Watkins ER, et al. Relapse prevention in patients with bipolar disorder: cognitive therapy outcome after 2 years. Am J Psychiatry 2005;162:324.
73. Miklowitz DJ, Simoneau TL, George EL, et al. Family-focused treatment of bipolar disorder: 1-year effects of a psychoeducational program in conjunction with pharmacotherapy. Biol Psychiatry 2000;48:582.
74. Weilburg JB, Sachs G, Falk WE. Triazolam-induced brief episodes of secondary mania in a depressed patient. J Clin Psychiatry 1987;48:492.
75. Sattar SP, Ramaswamy S, Bhatia SC, et al. Somnambulism due to probable interaction of valproic acid and zolpidem. Ann Pharmacother 2003;37:1429.
76. Saiz-Ruiz J, Cebollada A, Ibañez A. Sleep disorders in bipolar depression: hypnotics vs. sedative antidepressants. J Psychosom Res 1994;38:55.
77. Bersani G, Garavini A. Melatonin add-on in manic patients with treatment resistant insomnia. Progress in Neuro-Psychopharmacology and Biological Psychiatry 2000;24:185.
78. Leibenluft E, Feldman-Naim S, Turner EH, et al. Effects of exogenous melatonin administration and withdrawal in five patients with rapid-cycling bipolar disorder. J Clin Psychiatry 1997;58:383.
79. Calabrese JR, Guelfi JD, Perdrizet-Chevallier C. Agomelatine adjunctive therapy for acute bipolar depression: preliminary open data. Bipolar Disord 2007;9:628.
80. Frye MA, Grunze H, Suppes T, et al. A placebo-controlled evaluation of adjunctive modafinil in the treatment of bipolar depression. Am J Psychiatry 2007;164:1242.
81. Morin CM, Colecchi C, Stone J, et al. Behavioral and pharmacological therapies for late-life insomnia. JAMA 1999;281:991.
82. Sivertsen B, Omvik S, Pallesen S, et al. Cognitive behavioral therapy vs. zopiclone for treatment of chronic primary insomnia in older adults: a randomized controlled trial. JAMA 2006;295:2851.
83. Carskadon MA, Acebo C, Jenni OG. Regulation of adolescent sleep: implications for behavior. Ann N Y Acad Sci 2004;1021:276.
84. Miller WR, Rollnick S. Motivational interviewing: preparing people for change. 2nd edition. New York: Guilford Press; 2002.
85. Dahl RE, Harvey AG. Sleep in children and adolescents with psychiatric or emotional disorders. Sleep Medicine Clinics 2007;2:501.
86. Stepanski EJ, Wyatt JK. Use of sleep hygiene in the treatment of insomnia. Sleep Medicine Reviews 2003;7:215.
87. Lam D, Wong G. Prodromes, coping strategies and psychological interventions in bipolar disorders. Clinical Psychology Review. Special Issue. The psychology of bipolar disorder 2005;25:1028.
88. Biederman J, Faraone SV, Wozniak J, et al. Further evidence of unique developmental phenotypic correlates of pediatric bipolar disorder: findings from a large

sample of clinically referred preadolescent children assessed over the last 7 years. J Affect Disord 2004;82:S45.

89. Hyman SE. Goals for research on bipolar disorder: the view from NIMH. Biol Psychiatry 2000;48:436.

90. Cartwright R, Luten A, Young M, et al. Role of REM sleep and dream affect in overnight mood regulation: a study of normal volunteers. Psychiatry Res 1998; 81:1.

91. Perlis ML, Nielsen TA. Mood regulation, dreaming and nightmares: evaluation of a desensitization function for REM sleep. Dreaming 1993;3:243.

92. Kaplan KA, Harvey AG. Hypersomnia across mood disorders: a review and synthesis. Sleep Medicine Reviews, in press.

93. Staton D. The impairment of pediatric bipolar sleep: hypotheses regarding a core defect and phenotype-specific sleep disturbances. J Affect Disord 2008;108:199.

94. Bootzin RR. Stimulus control treatment for insomnia. Proceedings of the American Psychological Association 1972;7:395.

95. Johnson SL. Mania and dysregulation in goal pursuit: a review. Clin Psychol Rev 2005;25:241.

96. Morin CM, Espie CA. Insomnia: a clinical guide to assessment and treatment. New York: Kluwer Academic/Plenum Publishers; 2003.

97. Harvey AG, Payne S. The management of unwanted pre-sleep thoughts in insomnia: distraction with imagery versus general distraction. Behav Res Ther 2002;40:267.

98. Kupfer DJ, Himmelhoch JM, Swartzburgh M, et al. Hypersomnia in manic-depressive disease: a preliminary report. Dis Nerv Syst 1972;720.

99. Bennett-Levy JBG, Fennell M, Hackmann A, et al. The Oxford handbook of behavioural experiments. Oxford (UK): Oxford University Press; 2004.

100. Harvey AG, Schmidt DA, Scarna A, et al. Sleep-related functioning in euthymic patients with bipolar disorder, patients with insomnia, and subjects without sleep problems. Am J Psychiatry 2005;162:50.

101. Harvey AG. A cognitive theory of and therapy for chronic insomnia. An International Quarterly. J Cognitive Psychotherapy 2005;19:41.

102. Ree M, Harvey AG. Insomnia. In: Bennett-Levy J, Butler G, Fennell M, editors. Oxford guide to behavioural experiments in cognitive therapy. Oxford (UK): Oxford University Press; 2004. p. 287.

103. Espie CA. Insomnia: conceptual issues in the development, persistence, and treatment of sleep disorder in adults. Annu Rev Psychol 2002;53:215.

104. Harvey AG. Unwanted intrusive thoughts in insomnia. In: Clark DA, editor. Intrusive thoughts in clinical disorders: theory, research, and treatment. New York: Guilford Press; 2005. p. 86.

105. Ballenger JC, Reus VI, Post RM. The "atypical" clinical picture of adolescent mania. Am J Psychiatry 1982;139:602.

106. Faedda GL, Teicher MH. Objective measures of activity and attention in the differential diagnosis of psychiatric disorders of childhood. Essential Psychopharmacology 2005;6:239.

107. Ferreira Maia AP, Boarati MA, Kleinman A, et al. Preschool bipolar disorder: Brazilian children case reports. J Affect Disord 2007;104:237–43.

108. Findling RL, Gracious BL, McNamara NK, et al. Rapid, continuous cycling and psychiatric co-morbidity in pediatric bipolar I disorder. Bipolar Disord 2001;3:202.

109. Jerrell JM, Shugart MA. Community-based care for youths with early and very-early onset bipolar I disorder. Bipolar Disord 2004;6:299.

110. Lofthouse N, Fristad M, Splaingard M, et al. Parent and child reports of sleep problems associated with early-onset bipolar spectrum disorders. J Fam Psychol 2007;21:114.

111. Lofthouse N, Fristad M, Splaingard M, et al. Web survey of sleep problems associated with early-onset bipolar spectrum disorders. J Pediatr Psychol 2008;33:349.

112. Mehl RC, O'Brien LM, Jones JH, et al. Correlates of sleep and pediatric bipolar disorder. Sleep 2006;29:193.

113. Papolos D, Hennen J, Cockerham MS, et al. A strategy for identifying phenotypic subtypes: concordance of symptom dimensions between sibling pairs who met screening criteria for a genetic linkage study of childhood-onset bipolar disorder using the Child Bipolar Questionnaire. J Affect Disord 2007;99:27.

Suicidality in Pediatric Bipolar Disorder

Tina R. Goldstein, PhD

KEYWORDS

- Suicide • Suicidal behavior • Suicidal ideation
- Self-injurious behavior • Pediatric bipolar disorder

Risk for completed suicide in bipolar disorder (BP) is among the highest of all psychiatric disorders;[1] between 25% and 50% of adults with BP make at least one suicide attempt in their lifetime, and between 8% and 19% of individuals with BP will die from suicide.[2] Research indicates that between 20% and 65% of adults with BP experience onset in childhood,[3,4] and those adults with early illness onset are at higher risk for suicidal behavior.[4,5] Given the relative infancy of the field of clinical research examining the phenomenology and course of pediatric BP, it is not surprising that little is known about suicidal behavior in this population despite the apparent link between early illness onset and suicidality.

DEFINITIONS

To correct a history of inconsistent and unclear terminology regarding suicide-related behavior, O'Carroll and colleagues[6] developed a defined set of terms. According to these guidelines, "suicide" is a fatal self-inflicted destructive act with explicit or implicit intent to die. "Suicide attempt" refers to a nonfatal, self-inflicted destructive act (not necessarily resulting in injury) with explicit or implicit intent to die. "Suicidal ideation" refers to thoughts of harming or killing oneself. "Suicidality" refers to all suicide-related behaviors and thoughts. These terms and definitions will be used throughout this article.

EPIDEMIOLOGY
Completed Suicide

Evidence from case-control studies of adolescent suicide victims indicates that BP in adolescence imparts a particularly elevated risk for completed suicide.[7,8] Furthermore, reports from two longitudinal studies support significant mortality from suicide among pediatric BP patients. Srinath and colleagues[9] reported a 3% suicide rate among pediatric bipolar disorder I (BPI) patients 5 years after index episode

This work was supported by NIMH Grant #MH074581.
Department of Child and Adolescent Psychiatry, Western Psychiatric Institute and Clinic, University of Pittsburgh Medical Center, 3811 O'Hara Street, BFT #531, Pittsburgh, PA 15213, USA
E-mail address: goldsteintr@upmc.edu

Child Adolesc Psychiatric Clin N Am 18 (2009) 339–352
doi:10.1016/j.chc.2008.11.005   childpsych.theclinics.com

hospitalization, whereas Welner, Welner, and Fishman[10] documented a 25% suicide completion rate among a BP adolescent inpatient sample (compared with 6% among unipolar [UP] patients) at 10-year follow-up.

Suicide Attempt

Strober and colleagues[11] reported medically significant suicide attempts in 20% of an adolescent BPI sample over a 5-year follow-up. Goldstein and colleagues[12] documented a 32% lifetime suicide attempt rate among a large sample of youth diagnosed with BP; of these attempts, nearly 20% were rated to be moderate to severe medical lethality. Lewinsohn, Seeley, and Klein[13] reported a 44% lifetime suicide attempt rate among adolescents with BP spectrum disorders—significantly elevated compared with 22% of UP depressed teens and 1% of healthy controls. In this sample, BP attempters (compared with UP attempters) were younger at first attempt, made more lethal attempts, and were more likely to make multiple attempts. Bhangoo and colleagues[14] reported a 47% suicide attempt rate among BPI children and adolescents with an episodic pattern of mood symptomatology (one or more DSM-IV manic or hypomanic episodes), compared with a 15% attempt rate for patients with a chronic illness pattern (no discernable episodes).

Suicidal Ideation

Suicidal ideation can be thought of along a continuum from passive, nonspecific ideation (eg, "I wish I had never been born") to active, specific ideation with intent and/or plan. High rates of suicidal ideation have been documented among youth with BP. Cross-sectional data from Faedda and colleagues[15] indicate a 30% rate of suicidal ideation among BP youth assessed at an outpatient mood disorders clinic. Craney and Geller[16] reported a 25% rate of suicidal ideation at intake among youth with BP assessed as outpatients. With respect to lifetime rates of suicidal ideation, Lewinsohn and colleagues found that 72% of a community sample of youth with BP endorsed a lifetime history of suicidal ideation—significantly elevated compared with 52% of that of youth with UP and 41% of youth with subsyndromal BP. Similarly, in a large multisite investigation of BP in youth, Axelson and colleagues[17] reported a lifetime rate of suicidal ideation of more than 75%.

RISK FACTORS

Given preliminary studies documenting the elevated incidence of suicidal behavior among BP youth, Lewinsohn and colleagues[13] have called for comparative studies within the BP group to identify risk factors differentiating pediatric BP patients with a history of attempt from those without. This approach has been widely used in the adult literature, yielding a fairly consistent set of risk factors for suicidal behavior among BP adults. Yet little is known about the extent to which these risk factors for suicidal behavior among BP adults apply to youth with the illness. Identification of such risk factors may serve to inform the development of both preventive and therapeutic interventions for this high-risk group.

Sociodemographic Factors

Among adults with BP, males have higher rates of completed suicide than females, whereas males and females have similar rates of suicide attempt.[18] Multiple studies of BP adults failed to find racial differences in rates of suicidal behavior among BP adults. Among youth with BP, one study found no significant differences in terms of sex, race, or socioeconomic status between BP youth with a history of suicide attempt and those without.[19]

Clinical Factors

Age at illness onset

The adult BP literature indicates that earlier age of BP illness onset is associated with higher suicide risk.[5] It is important to note, however, that the general literature on youth suicide indicates that children are less likely to have attempted suicide than are adolescents,[20] likely due to a complex interaction of developmental, psychological, and family factors. In a sample of BP youth aged 7–17 years, a higher percentage of subjects with a history of suicide attempt (compared with subjects with no history of suicide attempt) reported illness onset after age 12.[12] It is, therefore, possible that a critical period for vulnerability to the development of suicidal behavior exists for pediatric onset, compared with adult-onset, BP.

Bipolar subtype

The literature on suicide attempts and bipolar subtypes among adults with BP is inconsistent, with some studies reporting higher attempt rates among BPII patients,[21] others associating a BPI diagnosis with higher risk,[22] and still others finding no differences between subtypes.[23] Goldstein and colleagues[12] found no differences in lifetime rates of suicide attempt between bipolar subtypes in a large clinical sample of BP youth.

Clinical state

Retrospective, cross-sectional, and prospective studies of adults with BP support a strong association between mixed states and suicidality.[24] In fact, of all phases of BP illness, rates of both suicidal ideation and suicide attempt are highest during mixed episodes.[25] One study reported an incidence of suicide attempt 37 times higher during mixed episodes.[26] Consistent with these findings are data from Dilsaver and colleagues,[27] indicating that of 82 BP adolescents in a mixed state, 67% reported suicidal ideation. Mixed states also independently contributed to increased risk for suicidal behavior for girls in this sample.[28] A history of mixed episodes was also significantly associated with a lifetime history of suicide attempt in a large sample of BP youth.[12]

Comorbid conditions

Comorbidity is the rule rather than the exception among youth who attempt and complete suicide, with up to 70% of suicidal youth meeting criteria for multiple psychiatric conditions.[29] Furthermore, as the number of comorbid conditions increases so does the risk for suicide attempt.[30] Only one study to date has examined comorbid conditions associated with suicidal behavior in pediatric BP. In this study, Goldstein and colleagues[12] showed that BP youth with a substance use disorder were three times more likely to report a history of suicide attempt than those without a comorbid substance use disorder. Additionally, a comorbid panic disorder was also associated with higher rates of suicidal behavior in youth with BP in this sample. Although no studies to date have expressly studied youth suicide completers diagnosed with BP, among mood-disordered youth who completed suicide, two studies reported high rates of comorbid substance abuse, particularly among males. In fact, more than 50% of mood-disordered male suicide completers in both samples had a comorbid substance abuse disorder.[31,32] Comorbid substance abuse increases the risk for attempted and completed suicide, both through the negative impact of substance use on mood disorder as well as the increased risk of lethal suicidal behavior while under the influence. This is particularly true among older adolescent males when coupled with disruptive behavior disorders. Although conduct disorder and related disruptive disorders are more likely to result in suicide and suicidal behavior when comorbid with substance use, disruptive disorders also independently contribute to suicide risk.[33]

Trauma history

Multiple studies demonstrate a strong link between a history of childhood maltreatment and suicidality. In a study of BP youth, Goldstein and colleagues[12] found a significant association between a history of abuse (physical and/or sexual abuse) and a history of suicide attempt. The relation between early maltreatment and suicidality is substantiated to a far greater degree among adults with BP, among whom a history of physical and/or sexual abuse is strongly associated with increased risk for suicide attempt.[34] In fact, the occurrence of both types of abuse appears to have an additive effect on risk for suicidal behavior.[5]

Psychosis

In adults, the risk associated with psychosis is unclear, with some studies documenting increased suicidal behavior among BP patients with psychotic features[35] and others finding no difference.[36] Among youth with BP, one study demonstrated an association between psychosis and a lifetime history of suicide attempt.[12]

Psychological Factors

Rucklidge[37] reported on several psychological factors differentiating BP youth with suicidal ideation from those without; namely, hopelessness, low self-esteem, external locus of control, and problems regulating anger were significantly greater among suicidal BP youth. Among BP adults, trait aggression[38] and impulsivity[39] are linked to increased risk for suicide attempt; however, these constructs have yet to be explored in a sample of youth with BP.

Suicidal ideation

In general, youth with frequent and severe suicidal ideation (ie, high levels of intent and/or planning) have about a 60% chance of making a suicide attempt within 1 year of ideation onset.[40]

Previous suicidal behavior

Among adults with BP, multiple studies indicate that one of the most potent predictors of future suicidal behavior is past suicidal behavior.[26] A history of suicide attempt in adults with BP increases the risk for subsequent attempt four-fold.[41] Follow-up studies of adolescent suicide attempters with a range of psychopathology report a re-attempt rate ranging from 6% to 15% per year, with the greatest risk occurring within 3 months of the initial attempt.[42] The period immediately following discharge from an inpatient psychiatric unit is associated with particularly high risk.[43]

Youth with a history of attempting suicide using methods high in medical lethality, such as hanging, shooting, or jumping, are at especially high risk for eventual completed suicide.[44] However, it is not necessarily the case that an attempt of low lethality reflects low suicidal intent, particularly among younger children who may overestimate the lethality of means.

Availability of lethal means

Evidence from case-control studies in youth indicates that firearms are much more common in the homes of suicide completers than attempters and controls. If a loaded gun is in the home, it is highly likely to be selected as a means of suicide and is associated with a 30-fold increased risk for completed suicide even among youth with no apparent psychopathology.[45]

Biological Factors

The neurobiology of suicide is a well-researched area, but little has been done in younger samples.[46] The most consistent biological finding is a relationship between altered central serotonin, as assessed by neuroendocrine challenge tests and cerebrospinal fluid (CSF) studies in attempters and by receptor binding in postmortem studies. Studies link low CSF 5-hydroxyindoleacetic acid (5-HIAA), a metabolite of serotonin, with impulsive aggression and suicidal behavior across psychiatric conditions in adults.[47] Greenhill and colleagues[48] found an association between serotonin measures and medically serious attempts within a small sample of depressed adolescent suicide attempter inpatients.

In a series of postmortem studies, Pandey and colleagues[49–51] showed that adolescent suicide completers, compared with deceased controls without disorder, have increased 5-HT2A binding, decreased protein kinase A (PKA) and C (PKC) activity, down-regulation of cAMP response element binding, and increased activity of brain-derived neurotropic factor in the prefrontal cortex and hippocampus (except PKA, which was not different in hippocampus). These findings are similar to those reported for adults, which suggest involvement of the serotonin system as well as systems involved in cell signaling and signal modulation.

Zalsman and colleagues[52] examined the allelic association of the serotonin transporter (5-HTTLPR) with suicidal behavior and related traits in a sample of Israeli suicidal inpatients and found no significant relationship. However, patients with the *ll* genotype were significantly different from patients with the *ls* genotype on a measure of trait violence. In a prospective longitudinal study of a New Zealand birth cohort, Caspi and colleagues[53] found that the *s* allele of 5-HTTLPR in the presence of stressful life events resulted in increased rates of depression and suicidality.

Family Factors

Research suggests both genetic and environmental mechanisms for the familial transmission of suicidal behavior in BP, and evidence suggests that suicidal behavior is transmitted in families distinct from its association with psychiatric illness.

Family history

Retrospective studies indicate that BP adults with a history of suicide attempt are more likely to report a positive family history of suicide.[54,55] Several studies also support an association between a family history of suicidal behavior and suicidal behavior in offspring.[56] Data from Brent and colleagues[57] indicate that offspring of mood-disordered suicide attempters have a significantly higher rate of suicidal behavior themselves compared with that of offspring whose parents had no history of suicidal behavior. Goldstein and colleagues[12] similarly found elevated rates of suicidal behavior in the families of BP youth who endorsed a lifetime history of suicide attempt.

Family environment

Youth who complete suicide are more likely than community controls to come from nonintact families of origin;[58,59] however, this question has not been expressly examined among youth with BP. Recent findings indicate no differences in the family constellation of BP youth who endorse suicidal ideation in the context of the current depressive episode, compared with nonsuicidal BP youth.[60]

Several studies have found that loss of a parent to death or divorce, or living apart from one or both biological parents, is a significant risk factor for completed suicide in youth.[61,62] Lewinsohn and colleagues[29] found an association between loss of a parent before age 12 years and multiple suicide attempts.

Similarly, in a sample of BP youth, Goldstein and colleagues[60] reported that suicidal BP youth endorsed a greater number of stressful family events over the prior year, including death of a family member as well as parental absence in the home.

There is a consistent literature linking family discord with youth suicide and suicide attempts.[59,63] The family environments of suicide attempters are characterized by high levels of discord and violence and are perceived as less supportive and more conflictual than those of nonattempters.[58,59] In one study of youth diagnosed with BP, those who endorsed suicidal ideation in the context of the current depressive episode reported greater conflict with their mother, increased arguments with parents over the past year, and rated their family environment as significantly less adaptable.[60]

ASSESSMENT

The best way to assess for suicidality is by asking the child/adolescent direct questions. Given that suicidality is so common among youth with BP, clinicians treating children and adolescents with the illness should evaluate for the presence of suicidality.[64] Assessment of the individuals' risk for suicidal behavior includes examining for the presence of specific known risk factors (see Risk Factors, above).

Self-administered scales are useful for screening with this population, since research indicates that adolescents disclose suicidality more readily on self-report than they do in a face-to-face interview. Similarly, adolescents are more likely to endorse suicidality if interviewed without a parent/guardian present. In the event that the teen endorses any item on a suicidality scale, it is strongly recommended that the clinician follow up with the patient regarding his/her safety. It is important to note that there is no evidence indicating that asking about suicidal thoughts or behaviors precipitates suicidality.

Thorough assessment of suicidal ideation includes questions regarding both severity (intent) and pervasiveness (frequency and intensity). Suicidal ideation characterized by a high degree of severity and pervasiveness is associated with a greater likelihood of suicide attempt in adolescents.[29] The clinician should also conduct a thorough and detailed review of prior suicidal behavior.

Suicidal Intent

Suicidal intent is the extent to which the individual wishes to die. Given findings that adolescents may disclose suicidal ideation on self-report ratings but deny this information during interview, assessment of suicidal risk should incorporate both means of assessment.

With regard to suicidal intent, the clinician should explore four components:[65] (1) belief about intent (ie, the extent to which the individual wished to die), (2) preparatory behavior (eg, giving away prized possessions; writing a suicide note), (3) prevention of discovery (ie, planning the attempt so that rescue is unlikely), and (4) communication of suicidal intent. High intent, as evidenced by expressing a wish to die, planning the attempt ahead of time, timing the attempt to avoid detection, and confiding suicide plans before the attempt, is associated with recurrent suicide attempts and with suicide completion.

Suicide Plan and Access to Means

Assessment should include inquiry regarding specific plans for inflicting self-harm as well as access to means considered (see Means Restriction, below).

Medical Lethality

Suicide attempts of high medical lethality (eg, hanging, shooting) are frequently characterized by high suicidal intent, and individuals who use more medically lethal means are at higher risk of completing suicide. However, evidence also indicates that an impulsive attempter with relatively low intent but ready access to lethal means may also engage in a medically serious, and even fatal, attempt.[30]

Precipitant

The most common precipitants for adolescent suicidal behavior are interpersonal conflict or loss, most often involving a parent or a romantic relationship. Legal and disciplinary problems also frequently precipitate suicidal behavior, particularly among youth with comorbid conduct disorder and substance abuse. Precipitants that are chronic and ongoing, especially recurrent physical or sexual abuse, are associated with poorer outcomes, including recurrence of suicidal behavior and even subsequent completion.[30]

Motivation

Motivation is the reason the individual cites for his/her suicidality. Individuals with high suicidal intent indicate that their primary motivation is either to die or to permanently escape an emotionally painful situation, and these youth are at elevated risk for reattempt.[66] Many youth who attempt suicide report that they are motivated by the desire to influence others or to communicate a feeling. Understanding the motivation for suicidal behavior has important implications for treatment, as intervention may focus on helping youth identify their needs more explicitly and find less dangerous ways to get their needs met.

Consequences

The consequences of suicidality refer to any environmental contingencies that occur in response to suicidality. Particularly salient are whether there are naturally occurring contingencies in the environment that reinforce suicidal behavior (eg, increased attention and support, decreased demands and responsibilities). However, positive reinforcement from the environment does not necessarily indicate that the individual acted purposefully to gain the reinforcement.

TREATMENT
Clinical Management

The clinical management of suicidality in BP includes the treatment of the underlying mood disorder and comorbid disorders (eg, substance abuse), minimizing risk factors, maximizing protective factors, and means restriction. Few clinical trials have examined the treatment of adolescent suicidality in general, and even less is known about suicidality in pediatric BP. In fact, many treatment studies exclude suicidal youth and do not report outcomes related to suicidality. Data from psychosocial and pharmacological studies among depressed youth suggest that the treatment of depression may not be sufficient to reduce suicidal risk; rather, specific treatments targeting suicidality may be required.[67]

Safety Planning

A safety plan is a hierarchically arranged list of strategies that the patient agrees to employ in the event of a suicidal crisis. The development of a safety plan is one of the most critical parts of the assessment and treatment of suicidal youth and involves collaboration between the clinician, patient, and family. On an outpatient basis, the clinician implements the safety plan once it is determined that the patient is safe to maintain as an outpatient; in fact, the clinician may use the safety plan to help determine the appropriate level of care (ie, the inability to collaborate on a safety plan may be indicative of the need for a higher level of care). However, the clinician should avoid the use of coercion when negotiating the safety plan, so as not to mask the adolescent's suicidal risk.

The first strategy is to eliminate the availability of lethal means in the patient's environment, including firearms, ammunition, and pills. Next, a no-harm agreement is negotiated between the adolescent, parents, and clinician that in the event the adolescent has suicidal urges, he/she will implement coping skills, inform a responsible adult, and/or call the clinician or emergency room. The clinician then works with the patient to develop a plan for coping with suicidal urges. The clinician asks the patient to identify the warning signs of a suicidal crisis; these may include specific thoughts (eg, "I hate my life"), emotions (eg, despair), and/or behaviors (eg, social isolation). Risk factors for that individual may also be identified (eg, not getting enough sleep). The safety plan involves a stepwise increase in the level of intervention from internal coping strategies to external strategies. Primarily, the clinician encourages the patient to consider internal strategies or coping skills he/she can employ without the assistance of other people (eg, distracting by playing a computer game). In the event that internal strategies are insufficient, patients should identify key figures who can be enlisted to help, including responsible adults. Their contact information should be made readily available to the patient.

Few studies have examined the effectiveness of safety plans. One quasi-experimental study showed a reduction in suicide attempts among youth at high risk for suicide after following a one-session intervention that included a written safety plan with a no-harm contract.[68] A recent review found that no-harm contracts alone are not a sufficient method for suicide prevention.[69]

Means Restriction

Few studies have evaluated the effectiveness of restriction of access to lethal means. Studies in psychiatric and pediatric outpatient settings have not found a significant effect of parental psychoeducation on securing access to lethal means.[70] However, treatment guidelines strongly recommend the removal of guns from the homes of at-risk youth. Specific elements of psychoeducation regarding access to lethal means may be critical in decreasing risk—insisting on removal of the gun (rather than merely securing it), speaking directly to the gun owner, and ascertaining the perceived risks of removing the gun. Some parents will be unwilling to remove guns but would be willing to secure them.[70] Therefore, clinicians may reduce risk by exploring alternatives to removal, including storing guns locked, unloaded, and/or disassembled.

Inpatient Hospitalization

Although psychiatric hospital admission is believed to provide a safe environment for suicidal patients to resolve acute suicidal crises, research has not demonstrated that inpatient hospitalization decreases suicide risk. In fact, one study conducted in Australia demonstrated no significant reduction in suicidal ideation or attempts over

3 years following hospitalization at a specialist inpatient child and adolescent mental health service.[71] Nonetheless, this can be a viable option to provide a safe environment during the short term as well as to stabilize and manage mood and medications. It is important to note that among individuals hospitalized for a suicide attempt, the highest risk period for suicide and reattempt occurs after discharge from the hospital,[43] making the transition particularly important.

Psychotherapy Approaches

Guidelines for the management of suicidality in adult BP indicate that adjunctive psychosocial intervention is a critical component of suicide risk reduction.[38,72,73] Such recommendations are largely based on studies demonstrating the efficacy of specific empirically supported psychosocial treatment models in delaying relapse, hastening recovery, and improving functioning in bipolar patients.[74,75] However, the extent to which these approaches influence suicidality in BP has not yet been expressly examined.

It is possible that "prevention of suicide in bipolar patients is…inextricably bound to the prevention of further affective episodes,"[76] such that affective symptoms and suicidality concurrently respond to treatment. However, data from psychosocial and pharmacological studies of suicidal individuals with an array of axis I and II pathology suggest that therapy targeting illness symptoms may not be sufficient to reduce suicidal risk.[77,78] If the same is true in BP, specific treatments targeting suicidality in this population may be required above and beyond standard treatments for mood disorder.[72,79]

Psychotherapy approaches for youth with BP are in various stages of treatment development. These include a multi-family psychoeducational group approach for families of school-aged BP children,[80] a modified version of family-focused treatment for adolescents with BP and their families (FFT-A),[81] a model combining FFT with cognitive-behavioral therapy for school-aged BP children,[82] and an adaptation of interpersonal and social rhythm therapy for adolescents.[83] Each model has shown promise in reducing mood symptoms. However, none of these models expressly targets suicidality, and outcomes related to suicidality in these trials are not reported. Specific psychosocial treatments that target the management of suicidality, such as dialectical behavior therapy (DBT),[84] have been recommended in the American Academy of Child and Adolescent Psychiatry (AACAP) treatment guidelines for pediatric BP. In an open pilot study, Goldstein and colleagues[19] demonstrated significant improvement in suicidal ideation and nonsuicidal self-injurious behavior from pre- to post-treatment with an adapted version of DBT for adolescents with BP and their families.

Pharmacological Approaches

Research supports the protective effects of lithium treatment against suicide among adults with BP,[85] with long-term lithium use associated with an eight-fold reduction in completed suicide and suicide attempts.[86] However, the literature on treatment of suicidality with other classes of medications, including antidepressants, anticonvulsants, and atypical antipsychotics, remains inconclusive.[87] No studies have been conducted to date examining the impact of any medication on suicidality in youth with BP.

FUTURE DIRECTIONS

The public health implications of suicidality among youth with BP are serious. Although some progress has been made in improving our understanding of risk factors for suicidality in BP youth, a great deal remains unknown about the effective prevention and treatment of suicidality in this population. Recommended directions for future research include increased inclusion of suicidal youth in research studies, treatment studies aimed at prevention, and studies examining the neurobiology associated with suicidality in BP youth.

SUMMARY

- Youth with BP exhibit high rates of suicidal ideation and behavior.
- Risk factors for suicidality in BP youth have begun to be identified, and they include psychosis, mixed episodes, history of abuse, family history of suicidal behavior, and comorbid substance use.
- Assessment of suicidal ideation should include attention to both severity (intent) and pervasiveness (frequency and intensity).
- Assessment of suicidal individuals should include explicit questions regarding plans for self-harm as well as determination of access to lethal means.
- Clinical management of suicidal youth includes safety planning with the adolescent and family members, means restriction, and inpatient hospitalization when warranted.
- Data from psychosocial and pharmacological studies suggest that treatment of the underlying mood disorder and comorbid conditions may not be sufficient to reduce suicidal risk in BP youth; rather, specific treatments targeting suicidality may be required and may include pharmacological and psychosocial interventions.

REFERENCES

1. Baldessarini RJ, Tondo L. Suicide risk and treatments for patients with bipolar disorder. J Am Med Assoc 2003;290(11):1517–8.
2. Goodwin FK, Jamison K. Manic-depressive illness. 21st edition. New York: Oxford University Press; 1990. p. 938.
3. Lish JD, Dime-Meehan S, Whybrow PC, et al. The National Depressive and Manic-Depressive Association (DMDA) survey of bipolar members. J Affect Disord 1994;31(4):281–94.
4. Perlis RH, Miyahara S, Marangell LB, et al. Long-term implications of early onset in bipolar disorder: data from the first 1000 participants in the systematic treatment enhancement program for bipolar disorder (STEP-BD). Biol Psychiatry 2004;55:875–81.
5. Leverich GS, Altshuler LL, Frye MA, et al. Factors associated with suicide attempts in 648 patients with bipolar disorder in the Stanley Foundation Bipolar Network. J Clin Psychiatry 2003;64(5):506–15.
6. O'Carroll PW, Berman AL, Maris RW, et al. Beyond the Tower of Babel: a nomenclature for suicidology. Suicide Life Threat Behav 1996;26:237–52.
7. Brent DA, Perper JA, Goldstein CE, et al. Risk factors for adolescent suicide: a comparison of adolescent suicide victims with suicidal inpatients. Arch Gen Psychiatry 1988;45:581–8.
8. Brent DA, Perper JA, Moritz G, et al. Psychiatric risk factors of adolescent suicide: a case control study. J Am Acad Child Adolesc Psychiatry 1993;32:521–9.
9. Srinath S, Reddy Y, Girimaji SR, et al. A prospective study of bipolar disorder in children and adolescents from India. Acta Psychiatr Scand 1998;98(6):437–42.

10. Welner A, Welner Z, Fishman R. Psychiatric adolescent inpatients: eight to ten-year follow-up. Arch Gen Psychiatry 1979;36(6):698–700.
11. Strober M, Schmidt-Lackner S, Freeman R, et al. Recovery and relapse in adolescents with bipolar affective illness: a five-year naturalistic, prospective follow-up. J Am Acad Child Adolesc Psychiatry 1995;34:724–31.
12. Goldstein TR, Birmaher B, Axelson D, et al. History of suicide attempts in pediatric bipolar disorder: factors associated with increased risk. Bipolar Disord 2005;7:525–35.
13. Lewinsohn PM, Seeley JR, Klein DN. Bipolar disorder in adolescents: epidemiology and suicidal behavior. In: Geller B, DelBello MP, editors. Bipolar disorder in childhood and early adolescence. New York: Guilford Press; 2003. p. 7–24.
14. Bhangoo RK, Dell ML, Towbin KE, et al. Clinical correlates of episodicity in juvenile mania. J Child Adolesc Psychopharmacol 2003;13(4):507–14.
15. Faedda GL, Baldessarini RJ, Glovinsky IP, et al. Pediatric bipolar disorder: phenomenology and course of illness. Bipolar Disord 2004;6:305–13.
16. Craney JL, Geller B. A prepubertal and early adolescent bipolar disorder-I phenotype: review of phenomenology and longitudinal course. Bipolar Disorder 2003;5:243–56.
17. Axelson DA, Birmaher B, Strober M, et al. Phenomenology of children and adolescents with bipolar spectrum disorders. Arch Gen Psychiatry 2006;63:1139–48.
18. Hawton K, Sutton L, Haw C, et al. Suicide and attempted suicide in bipolar disorder: a systematic review of risk factors. J Clin Psychiatry 2005;66(6): 693–704.
19. Goldstein TR, Axelson DA, Birmaher B, et al. Dialectical behavior therapy for adolescents with bipolar disorder: a one year open trial. J Am Acad Child Adolesc Psychiatry 2007;46(7):820–30.
20. Spirito A. Understanding attempted suicide in adolescence. In: Spirito A, Overholser JC, editors. Evaluating and treating adolescent suicide attempters. San Diego (CA): Academic Press; 2003. p. 1–18.
21. Rihmer Z, Pestality P. Bipolar II disorder and suicidal behavior. Psychiatr Clin North Am 1999;22(3):667–73.
22. Perugi G, Musetti L, Pezzica P, et al. Suicide attempts in primary major depression subtypes. Psychiatria Fennica 1988;19:95–102.
23. Slama F, Bellivier F, Henry C, et al. Bipolar patients with suicidal behavior: Toward the identification of a clinical subgroup. J Clin Psychiatry 2004;65(8):1035–9.
24. Oquendo MA, Waternaux C, Brodsky B, et al. Suicide behavior in bipolar mood disorder: clinical characteristics of attempters and nonattempters. J Affect Disord 2000;59:107–17.
25. Valtonen HM, Suominen K, Mantere O, et al. Suicidal behavior during different phases of bipolar disorder. J Affect Disord 2007;97:101–7.
26. Valtonen HM, Suominen K, Haukka J, et al. Differences in incidence of suicide attempts during phases of bipolar I and II disorders. Bipolar Disord 2008;10: 588–96.
27. Dilsaver SC, Benazzi F, Akiskal H. Mixed states: the most common outpatient presentation of bipolar depressed adolescents? Psychopathology 2005;38: 268–72.
28. Dilsaver SC, Benazzi F, Rihmer Z, et al. Gender, suicidality, and bipolar mixed states in adolescents. J Affect Disord 2005;87:11–6.
29. Lewinsohn PM, Rohde P, Seeley JR. Adolescent suicidal ideation and attempts: prevalence, risk factors, and clinical implications. Clin Psychol Sci Pract 1996; 3:25–46.

30. Brent DA, Baugher M, Bridge J, et al. Age and sex-related risk factors for adolescent suicide. J Am Acad Child Adolesc Psychiatry 1999;38(12): 1497–505.
31. Marttunen MJ, Aro HM, Henriksson MM, et al. Mental disorders in adolescent suicide: DSM-III-R axes I and II diagnoses in suicides among 13- to 19-year-olds in Finland. Arch Gen Psychiatry 1991;48:834–9.
32. Shaffer D, Gould MS, Fisher P, et al. Psychiatric diagnosis in child and adolescent suicide. Arch Gen Psychiatry 1996;53:339–48.
33. Fergusson DM, Horwood LJ, Lynskey MT. The stability of disruptive childhood behaviors. J Abnorm Child Psychol 1995;23(3):379–96.
34. Leverich GS, McElroy SL, Suppes T, et al. Early physical and sexual abuse associated with an adverse course of bipolar illness. Biol Psychiatry 2002;52(8): 288–97.
35. Axelsson R, Lagerkvist-Briggs M. Factors predicting suicide in psychotic patients. Eur Arch Psychiatry Clin Neurosci 1992;241(5):259–66.
36. Black D, Winokur G, Nasrallah A. Effect of psychosis on suicide risk in 1,593 patients with unipolar and bipolar affective disorders. Am J Psychiatry 1988; 145(7):849–52.
37. Rucklidge JJ. Psychosocial functioning of adolescents with and without paediatric bipolar disorder. J Affect Disord 2006;91:181–8.
38. Oquendo MA, Mann JJ. Identifying and managing suicide risk in bipolar patients. J Clin Psychiatry 2001;62(25):31–4.
39. Michaelis BH, Goldberg JF, Davis GP, et al. Dimensions of impulsivity and aggression associated with suicide attempts among bipolar patients: a preliminary study. Suicide Life Threat Behav 2004;34(2):172–6.
40. Kessler RC, Borges G, Walters EE. Prevalence of and risk factors for lifetime suicide attempts in the national comorbidity survey. Arch Gen Psychiatry 1999; 56(7):617–26.
41. Marangell LB, Bauer MS, Dennehy EB. Prospective predictors of suicide and suicide attempts in 1556 patients with bipolar disorder followed for up to 2 years. Bipolar Disord 2006;8:566–75.
42. Goldston DB, Daniel SS, Reboussin DM, et al. Suicide attempts among formerly hospitalized adolescents: a prospective naturalistic study of risk during the first 5 years after discharge. J Am Acad Child Adolesc Psychiatry 1999;38(6):660–71.
43. Kjelsberg E, Neegaard E, Dahl AA. Suicide in adolescent psychiatric inpatients: incidence and predictive factors. Acta Psychiatr Scand 1994;89:235–41.
44. Beautrais AL. Further suicidal behavior among medically serious suicide attempters. Suicide Life Threat Behav 2004;34(1):1–11.
45. Brent DA, Bridge J. Firearms availability and suicide: evidence, interventions, and future directions. Am Behav Sci 2003;46:1192–210.
46. Mann JJ. Neurobiology of suicidal behavior. Nat Rev Neurosci 2003;4:819–28.
47. Mann JJ. The neurobiology of suicide. Nat Med 1998;4(1):25–30.
48. Greenhill L, Waslick B, Parides M, et al. Biological studies in suicidal adolescent inpatients. Scientific Proceedings of the 42nd Annual Meeting of the American Academy of Child and Adolescent Psychiatry, New Orleans (LA); October 1995.
49. Pandey GN. Decreased catalytic activity and expression of protein kinase C isozymes in teenage suicide victims: a postmortem brain study. Arch Gen Psychiatry 2004;61(7):685–93.

50. Pandey GN, Conley RR, Pandey SC, et al. Benzodiazepine receptors in the post-mortem brain of suicide victims and schizophrenic subjects. Psychiatry Res 1997;71(3):137–49.

51. Pandey GN, Dwivedi Y, Rizavi HS, et al. Higher expression of serotonin 5-HT2A receptors in the postmortem brains of teenage suicide victims. Am J Psychiatry 2002;159:419–29.

52. Zalsman G, Frisch A, King RA, et al. Case control and family-based studies of tryptophan hydroxylase gene A218C polymorphism and suicidality in adolescents. Am J Med Genet 2001;105:451–7.

53. Caspi A, Sugden K, Moffitt TE, et al. Influence of life stress on depression: moderation by a polymorphism in the 5-HT gene. Science 2003;301:386–9.

54. Roy A. Genetic and biologic risk factors for suicide in depressive disorders. Psychiatr Q 1993;64:345–58.

55. Stallone F, Dunner DL, Ahearn J, et al. Statistical predictions of suicide in depressives. Compr Psychiatry 1980;21(5):381–7.

56. Gould MS, Greenberg T, Velting DM, et al. Youth suicide risk and preventative interventions: a review of the past 10 years. J Am Acad Child Adolesc Psychiatry 2003;42(4):386–405.

57. Brent DA, Oquendo M, Birmaher B, et al. Familial pathways to early-onset suicide attempt: risk for suicidal behavior in offspring of mood-disordered suicide attempters. Arch Gen Psychiatry 2002;59:801–7.

58. Brent DA, Perper JA, Moritz G, et al. Familial risk factors for adolescent suicide: a case-control study. Acta Psychiatr Scand 1994;89:52–8.

59. Gould MS, Fisher P, Parides M, et al. Psychosocial risk factors of child and adolescent completed suicide. Arch Gen Psychiatry 1996;53:1155–62.

60. Goldstein TR, Sinwell N, Birmaher B, et al. Family environment and suicidality among bipolar youth. Poster presented at the annual Pediatric Bipolar Disorder Conference. Cambridge (MA); March 28–29, 2008.

61. Agerbo E, Nordentoft M, Mortensen PB. Familial, psychiatric, and socioeconomic risk factors for suicide in young people: Nested case-control study. BMJ: British Medical Journal 2002;325(7355):74–7.

62. Shaffi M, Steltz-Lenarsky J, Derrick AM, et al. Comorbidity of mental disorders in the post-mortem diagnosis of completed suicide in children and adolescents. J Affect Disord 1998;15:227–33.

63. Fergusson DM, Lynskey MT. Childhood circumstances, adolescent adjustment, and suicide attempts in a New Zealand birth cohort. J Am Acad Child Adolesc Psychiatry 1995;34:612–22.

64. Kowatch R, Fristad MA, Birmaher B, et al. Treatment guidelines for children and adolescents with bipolar disorder. J Am Acad Child Adolesc Psychiatry 2005; 44(3):213–35.

65. Kingsbury SJ. Clinical components of suicidal intent in adolescent overdose. J Am Acad Child Adolesc Psychiatry 1993;32:518–20.

66. Cohen-Sandler R, Berman AL, King RA. Life stress and symptomatology: determinants of suicidal behavior in children. J Am Acad Child Adolesc Psychiatry 1982;21(2):178–86.

67. Emslie G, Kratochvil C, Vitiello B, et al. Treatment for Adolescents with Depression Study (TADS): safety results. J Am Acad Child Adolesc Psychiatry 2006;45(12): 1440–55.

68. Rotheram-Borus MJ, Bradley J. Triage model for suicidal runaways. Am J Orthop 1991;61(1):122–7.

69. Lewis LM. No-harm contracts: a review of what we know. Suicide Life Threat Behav 2007;37(1):50–7.
70. Brent DA, Baugher M, Birmaher B, et al. Compliance with recommendations to remove firearms by families participating in a clinical trial for adolescent depression. J Am Acad Child Adolesc Psychiatry 2000;39:1220–6.
71. McShane G, Mihalich M, Walter G, et al. Outcome of patients with unipolar, bipolar and psychotic disorders admitted to a specialist child and adolescent mental health service. Australas Psychiatry 2006;14(2):198–201.
72. Gray SM, Otto MW. Psychosocial approaches to suicide prevention: applications to patients with bipolar disorder. J Clin Psychiatry 2001;62:56–64.
73. Sachs GS, Yan LJ, Swann AC, et al. Integration of suicide prevention into outpatient management of bipolar disorder. J Clin Psychiatry 2001;62:3–11.
74. Miklowitz DJ. A review of evidenced-based psychosocial interventions for bipolar disorder. J Clin Psychiatry 2006;67(11Suppl):28–33.
75. Miklowitz DJ, Otto MW, Frank E, et al. Psychosocial treatments for bipolar depression: a 1-year randomized trial from the systematic treatment enhancement program. Arch Gen Psychiatry 2007;64:419–26.
76. Jamison KR. Psychotherapeutic issues and suicide prevention in the treatment of bipolar disorders. In: Hales RE, Frances AJ, editors, American Psychiatric Association annual review, Volume 6. Washington, DC: American Psychiatric Association; 1987. p. 108–24.
77. Brown GK, Have TT, Henriques GR, et al. Cognitive therapy for the prevention of suicide attempts. J Am Med Assoc 2005;294(5):563–70.
78. Linehan MM, Comtois KA, Murray A, et al. Two-year randomized controlled trial and follow-up of dialectical behavior therapy vs therapy by experts for suicidal behaviors and borderline personality disorder. Arch Gen Psychiatry 2005;63(7): 757–66.
79. Khan A, Warner HA, Brown WA. Symptom reduction and suicide risk in patients treated with placebo in antidepressant clinical trials: an analysis of the Food and Drug Administration database. Arch Gen Psychiatry 2000;57:311–7.
80. Fristad MA, Goldberg-Arnold JS, Gavazzi SM. Multi-family psychoeducation groups in the treatment of children with mood disorders. J Marital Fam Ther 2003;29(4):491–504.
81. Miklowitz DJ, George EL, Axelson DA, et al. Family-focused treatment for adolescents with bipolar disorder. J Affect Disord 2004;82:113–28.
82. Pavuluri MN, Graczyk P, Henry D, et al. Child- and family-focused cognitive behavioral therapy for pediatric bipolar disorder: development and preliminary results. J Am Acad Child Adolesc Psychiatry 2004;43(5):528–37.
83. Hlastala SA, Frank E. Adapting interpersonal and social rhythm therapy to the developmental needs of adolescents with bipolar disorder. Dev Psychopathol 2006;18:1267–88.
84. Linehan MM. Cognitive-behavioral treatment of borderline personality disorder. New York: Guilford Press; 1993.
85. Baldessarini RJ, Tondo L, Hennen J. Treating the suicidal patient with bipolar disorder. Reducing suicide risk with lithium. Ann N Y Acad Sci 2001;932:24–38.
86. Baldessarini RJ, Hennen J. Lithium treatment and suicide risk in major affective disorders; update and new findings. J Clin Psychiatry 2003;64(Suppl 5):44–52.
87. Ernst C, Goldberg JF. Antisuicide properties of psychotropic drugs: a critical review. Harv Rev Psychiatry 2004;12(1):14–41.

The Assessment of Children and Adolescents with Bipolar Disorder

Eric A. Youngstrom, PhD*, Andrew J. Freeman, BS,
Melissa McKeown Jenkins, MA

KEYWORDS

- Pediatric bipolar disorder • Children • Adolescents
- Diagnosis • Assessment • Outcome evaluation

There have been radical changes in our scientific understanding and clinical practices around the diagnosis of bipolar disorder in children and adolescents. Whereas the condition seldom used to be diagnosed before puberty, there has been a recent surge in rates of diagnosis such that a large proportion of psychiatrically hospitalized youths now carry clinical diagnoses of bipolar disorder,[1] and there has been a more than 40-fold increase in rates of diagnoses over a 10-year period.[2] There has been debate about whether the increase in diagnosis is primarily due to a correction of previous underdiagnosis versus concerns that it is now overdiagnosed or even a case of "disease mongering."[3] Discussion has also focused on whether bipolar disorder in youth is the same illness as in adults or represents a different condition or perhaps a pediatric subtype.[4–6] Although the topic is still portrayed as controversial in the popular media, at this point more than 350 peer-reviewed publications have investigated different aspects of pediatric bipolar illness.[7] Growing evidence from clinical and epidemiological studies around the world indicates that bipolar disorder often first manifests in adolescence or earlier,[8,9] and many apparent differences between adult and child presentations appear to be an artifact of definitional issues and not real variations in clinical presentation.[7] Prospective longitudinal studies are also documenting moderate to high levels of developmental continuity with adult bipolar disorder.[10–12] All lines of evidence strongly indicate that bipolar symptoms in youths are associated with considerable impairment and warrant clinical attention.

The goal of the present review is to provide a step-by-step, evidence-based approach to the assessment of bipolar disorder in children and adolescents. The

This work was supported in part by NIH R01 MH066647 (PI: E. Youngstrom). The authors have no other conflicts of interest to disclose.
Department of Psychology, University of North Carolina, CB #3270, Davie Hall, Chapel Hill, NC 27599-3270, USA
* Corresponding author.
E-mail address: eay@unc.edu (E.A. Youngstrom).

Child Adolesc Psychiatric Clin N Am 18 (2009) 353–390
doi:10.1016/j.chc.2008.12.002
1056-4993/08/$ – see front matter © 2009 Elsevier Inc. All rights reserved.

childpsych.theclinics.com

review is organized around clinical decision making and then monitoring progress over the course of treatment. The review does not discuss the potential merits of all the most commonly used instruments for psychological, educational, or psychiatric assessment; instead, it concentrates on those tools that have research supporting their validity with regard to pediatric bipolar disorder (PBD). The majority of the assessment tools routinely used for psychological[13] and psychiatric evaluation have not been validated for work with PBD.[14] Rather than using standardized assessment batteries out of convention or habit, we believe that the assessment endeavor will perform best when each component is chosen based on its demonstrated validity and relevance to clinical intervention. Evaluation strategies should address one of the "3 Ps" of clinical assessment: (1) *Predict* important criteria or developmental trajectories, (2) *Prescribe* a change in treatment choice, or (3) inform the *Process* of treating the patient or family.[15] Narrowing assessment batteries down in this manner has many benefits, which include creating a strong link between assessment and treatment, reducing time and expense by eliminating unnecessary testing, and improving decisions and treatment outcomes by reducing "information clutter" and providing more focused information that directly pertains to the individual patient. The three Ps provide a rubric to help navigate the assessment process from establishing risk of PBD confirming the diagnosis, informing treatment selection, measuring progress and outcome, and monitoring for relapse prevention.

DEFINITIONS: MOOD EPISODES AND BIPOLAR SPECTRUM

The diagnostic criteria for mood disorders are unusual in that they require a two-stage evaluation.[16,17] First, the clinician must evaluate the lifetime history of mood episodes, not just characterize the current presenting problem. Only after gathering data about the possible occurrence of each type of potential mood episode over the lifetime can the clinician proceed to establishing the formal diagnosis. Diagnosing bipolar disorder requires this complexity, because the presentation of the illness can change dramatically as it transitions into different episodes.

Mood Episodes

The diagnostic mood episodes include major depressive episodes, dysthymic episodes, hypomanic symptoms, hypomanic episodes, manic episodes, and mixed episodes. These categories are not exhaustive in terms of phenomenology. Additional mood presentations are possible and frequently encountered in clinical practice, including mild depressions, mixed hypomanias, and periods of mood dysregulation that are too brief or mild to meet current criteria for an index episode.[18] However, the formal diagnosis of mood disorder is anchored to the index episodes, not the other clinical presentations. It is only after ascertaining both the present and past lifetime mood episodes that the clinician can diagnose mood disorders accurately. **Table 1** shows how the combination of present and past episodes is often necessary to make a diagnosis on the bipolar spectrum. Unless the clinician inquires about past mood history, many cases of bipolar disorder will be misdiagnosed as unipolar depressive or dysthymic disorders—particularly given that people affected by bipolar disorders tend to spend more days depressed than manic and are much more likely to seek services for depression than mania.[19] The situation may be somewhat different with PBD, both because referrals are more often initiated by the parent rather than the youth in outpatient settings, and because mania and mixed episodes appear to be more common in younger cohorts and then decrease steadily with age.[8,20]

Table 1
Diagnoses as a function of past as well as current mood episode, according to DSM-IV criteria

Past Episode	Present Episode				
	No Mood	Major Depression	Dysthymic	Hypomanic	Manic/Mixed
No mood	No mood disorder[a]	Major depression, single episode[a]	Dysthymic disorder[a]	No diagnosis; rule out bipolar NOS[a]	Bipolar I[a]
Major depression	Major depression, in remission	Major depression, recurrent[b]	Depressive episode— mild or in partial remission	Bipolar II	Bipolar I
Dysthymic	Past dysthymic disorder	Major depression, past dysthymic disorder ("double depression")	Recurrent dysthymic disorder[b]	Cyclothymic disorder	Bipolar I
Hypomanic	No mood diagnosis	Bipolar II, current depressed	Cyclothymic disorder or bipolar NOS	Bipolar NOS (recurrent hypomanias)	Bipolar I
Manic/mixed	Bipolar I	Bipolar I, current depressed	Bipolar I	Bipolar I	Bipolar I

Abbreviations: DSM-IV, Diagnostic and Statistical Manual of Mental Disorders, 4th edition; NOS, not otherwise specified.

[a] Default diagnosis based on accurate identification of the presenting problem without consideration of past mood episodes.

[b] Note that Kraepelin considered recurrent depressive disorders as potentially on the manic-depressive spectrum, instead of lumping them with unipolar depressions. We suggest that recurrent depressions, along with early onset depressions, trigger careful evaluation of possible bipolar disorder.

Diagnoses

Bipolar I, often considered the most serious form of bipolar illness, has received the greatest attention from the research community. As **Table 1** makes evident, a bipolar I diagnosis only requires the presence of one manic or mixed lifetime episode.[16] Bipolar II disorder, in contrast, requires two distinct mood episodes to assign the diagnosis: at least one major depressive episode and a hypomanic episode. Without systematic assessment for lifetime hypomanic episodes, bipolar II is very likely to be misdiagnosed as a unipolar depression.[21]

The Diagnostic and Statistical Manual of Mental Disorders, 4th edition (DSM-IV) includes cyclothymic disorder as another condition to be considered in the bipolar family of disorders. The diagnostic criteria for cyclothymic disorder require long periods of moderate mood disturbance. The depressive symptoms cannot become too severe, or else the diagnosis would change to a major depressive episode or bipolar II disorder. Similarly, the hypomanic symptoms cannot become too extreme; otherwise, if they meet criteria for a full manic episode, then the diagnosis would change to bipolar I. Cyclothymic disorder is difficult to distinguish from temperament; indeed, much research in the area has used rating scales assessing cyclothymic temperament.[22] The diagnosis of cyclothymic disorder is rarely used in clinical practice[23] nor is it tracked in most large epidemiologic studies or clinical research samples.[8,10,24,25] However, studies that have investigated cyclothymic disorder have found that it is a highly impairing condition that warrants clinical attention.[26–33]

Bipolar disorder not otherwise specified (NOS) is a fourth diagnostic option in the bipolar section of DSM-IV. Bipolar NOS is a residual category, intended to be used when bipolar features are present, but the clinical presentation does not fit into any of the three above categories. DSM-IV provides some examples of presentations that would be appropriate to code as bipolar NOS. These include having recurrent hypomanias without any lifetime history of manic, mixed, or major depressive episodes;[34] having a disturbance in mood but with an insufficient number of the possible seven B-criteria symptoms (eg, elated mood plus one or two other symptoms; or irritable mood plus fewer than four other symptoms); or cases where the duration of the index mood episode is not long enough to satisfy the thresholds specified for hypomania (4 days) or mania or mixed episodes (1 week or else severe enough to necessitate psychiatric hospitalization). Both the "insufficient number of symptoms"[12,35,36] and the "insufficient duration" forms of bipolar NOS[29,37] have been documented in multiple studies in both children and adults. Although the definitions do not identify identical sets of cases, the cumulative evidence shows that either definition is associated with considerable chronicity and clinical impairment. If the core feature of episodic mood disturbance is present, then most evidence suggests that bipolar NOS falls on the bipolar spectrum. In short, bipolar NOS (a) appears to be at least as prevalent as bipolar I in epidemiologic and clinical samples, (b) has become well established as an impairing mood disorder, and (c) deserves clinical attention.

There is an important consideration about the potential overlap between bipolar NOS and cyclothymic disorder. In practice, most practitioners and researchers tend to lump cyclothymic disorder with the bipolar NOS category. Technically this is a departure from the official nosologies,[16,17] and it adds to the heterogeneity that is found under the rubric of bipolar NOS. The combination of short durations for mood states combined with long lengths of episode should trigger careful evaluation of the possibility of a cyclothymic disorder.

When making any of the bipolar diagnoses, the clinician must rule out the possibility that the mood symptoms are due to schizophrenia, a general medical condition, or induced by a substance.[16,17] Substance-induced exclusion criteria create the most challenges. Street drugs that have a strong dopaminergic effect can mimic the symptoms of mania, and hallucinogens can create symptoms that appear psychotic. A more subtle point is that manic symptoms secondary to the use of prescription medications, including antidepressant or stimulant medications, technically lead to diagnoses of "substance-induced mania." The literature on psychotropic medications inducing mania is complex,[38] but experts agree that manic symptoms emerging during the course of treatment always justify thorough evaluation of the possibility of bipolar diagnosis.

Additional Subtypes of Bipolar Disorder

In the pediatric literature, there has been much discussion about changes to criteria for youths or alternate definitions of bipolar subtypes.[5] Leibenluft and colleagues suggested the term "narrow phenotype" to indicate situations where the manic episode included symptoms of elated mood or grandiosity, consistent with the research operational definition of bipolar disorder used by Geller and colleagues.[5,39] People often think that the term "narrow" connotes strict adherence to DSM criteria, but actually the "narrow" definition is more restrictive than DSM criteria (which would include hypomania or mania with predominantly irritable mood, so long as there were sufficient numbers of B-criteria symptoms co-occurring). In many samples, there is substantial overlap between the cases that would meet DSM criteria that would also satisfy the narrow definition.[37,40] There is also considerably less research available based on the narrow criteria instead of the DSM criteria.[41] At the other extreme, the term "broad phenotype" has been used so widely and to refer to so many different things that it has become imprecise to the point of losing clinical utility. Because the evidence base is much stronger for DSM definitions than that of any alternate research definitions and DSM criteria guide clinical practice, the rest of this review concentrates on DSM definitions (bipolar I, bipolar II, cyclothymic disorder, and bipolar NOS—clarifying whenever possible if the NOS specification is due to insufficient symptoms or insufficient duration).

Course Specifiers: Definitions and Clinical Relevance

Course specifiers have considerable clinical value in the context of bipolar disorder. Notations such as "bipolar II disorder, current episode depressed" provide important information about the nature of the illness and change some of the treatment options (ie, prescription of different interventions for unipolar vs bipolar depression). There has been inconsistency about the use of the terms "cycling" and "rapid cycling." These are often used to connote polarity switches. However, the DSM definition of rapid cycling denotes the occurrence of at least four or more distinct mood episodes (not changes in mood state within an episode) within the same year. Thus, rapid cycling might be thought of as "rapid recurrence" or "rapid relapse." Indeed, when defined as four or more annual episodes, rapid cycling portends a much more chronic course, higher rates of comorbidity and substance use, greater treatment refractoriness, and potentially greater risk of suicide.[8] Thus, the phenomenon of rapid cycling/relapsing satisfies both the predictive and prescriptive litmus tests for inclusion in an assessment of bipolar disorder. If the rapid switching between mood polarities, which has been well described in children, is better construed as a mixed episode rather than multiple episodes, then the terms are being used consistently across the lifespan, and clinicians can better identify when there is a higher risk of relapse.

HOW COMMON IS PBD? BASELINE RISK AND PREVALENCE

The first question that must be answered is "How common is PBD, anyway?" At the time most practicing clinicians were trained, conventional wisdom was that bipolar disorder affected only adults and perhaps some adolescents; and the vast majority of training programs still do not provide formal didactics about the assessment or treatment of PBD.[42] The prevalence of the disorder is an important starting point for clinical evaluation.

The traditional figure has been that bipolar disorder affects 1% of the adult population. This figure was often based on rates of bipolar I and excluded all other DSM bipolar diagnoses. More recent epidemiologic studies have found lifetime prevalences of bipolar I and II to be closer to 3% or 4%,[24,25] and bipolar spectrum diagnoses appear to affect from 2.6% to 8.3% or more[36] of the general population (see Goodwin and Jamison for a review of 12 international studies).[8] Unfortunately, epidemiologic studies tend not to use strict DSM criteria for diagnoses, making it difficult to map findings directly onto clinical labels. Despite the varying definitions, it is clearly evident that (a) the bipolar spectrum is more common than is generally thought, (b) the "soft spectrum" cases occur at least as frequently as does bipolar I in both community and clinical samples, and (c) the soft spectrum is associated with both immediate impairment and long-term risk of poor outcomes on multiple measures.[10,36,37,43,44]

A major caveat for the clinician is that epidemiologic studies describe the incidence or prevalence of bipolar disorder in the general population. This is not the same thing as the frequency with which a practitioner encounters bipolar disorder in clinical settings. Bipolar disorder is more common in outpatient settings than in nonreferred community samples, and it is more frequent in settings providing more intensive services due to the acuity of the illness. **Table 2** lists prevalence rates from multiple settings. The table also includes information about how the diagnoses were made, whether both parents and youths were interviewed, and other features that might influence the comparability of the estimates. Another limitation is that different groups and settings use somewhat different definitions of bipolar disorder, which also change the rates and their generalizability to other clinical settings. However, these rates still provide meaningful benchmarks against which clinicians can compare the rate of their bipolar disorder diagnoses. They also offer some indication of whether bipolar disorder is likely to be rare or common in a given setting.

RISK FACTORS

Research has identified multiple risk factors that might pertain to bipolar disorder. In 2003 Tsuchiya and colleagues reviewed more than 100 studies evaluating more than 30 different risk factors. They concluded that family history of bipolar illness is the only sufficiently well-established risk factor for bipolar disorder to warrant clinical attention.[45] In studies of the offspring of bipolar parents, the risk of developing bipolar disorder appears to be at least 5 times higher than that in the comparison groups,[46] and estimates of the recurrence risk in adult samples indicate that the lifetime risk may be increased 10-fold.[47] A 2005 review recommended that clinicians treat a history of bipolar illness in a first-degree relative (biological mother, father, or full sibling) as increasing the risk of developing bipolar disorder by a factor of 5.0.[48,49] Bipolar history in a grandparent, aunt, uncle, or half sibling would confer half as much risk (ie, 2.5 times higher) based on the data suggesting that bipolar disorder is a polygenic illness. These changes in likelihood are large enough to be informative in clinical assessment. At the same time, they are not so large as to make a diagnosis of bipolar disorder automatic; in fact, most people with an affected relative will not have bipolar disorder themselves. **Table 3** lists other risk factors for PBD. These risk factors are less well established than family history but are sufficient to prompt additional assessment of the possibility of a bipolar diagnosis.

There are several concerns that arise with regard to family history as a risk factor relevant to diagnosing PBD. These include (a) the fact that the literature cannot yet disentangle genetic versus shared environmental familial factors, (b) the low diagnostic accuracy about bipolar diagnoses in general will undermine the sensitivity of family histories of bipolar disorder, and (c) bipolar disorder has historically been underdiagnosed in minority groups in the United States, with it often misdiagnosed as schizophrenia or antisocial behavior.[50,51] For the purposes of formulating a diagnostic impression, it is not necessary to tease apart genetic versus environmental contributions. The poor sensitivity of family history means that failure to report a bipolar history cannot be assumed to be accurate, whereas positive reports of family history may be given greater credibility. The historical inaccuracy of bipolar diagnoses in minority groups means that clinicians need to inquire about mood symptoms whenever they hear about other mental health issues in relatives. Learning about prior treatment

Table 2
Base rates of PBD in different settings

Setting	Base Rate (%)	Demography	Diagnostic Method
General outpatient practice[2]	1	All of United States	National Ambulatory Medical Care Survey
High school epidemiologic[43]	0.6	Northwestern USA high school	KSADS-PL[a]
Community nonreferred[142]	1.4	Upstate New York	—
United States epidemiologic[25]	1.59, child and adolescent onset; 4.5, adults	United States general population	CIDI
United States child/ adolescent (Lahey et al, unpublished, 1995 MECA)[8]	1.8	Eastern United States	DISC[a,b]
Community mental health center[23]	6	Midwestern urban, 80% non-white, low-income	Clinical interview and treatment[a,b]
General outpatient clinic[143]	6.3	Urban academic research centers	WASH-U-KSADS[a,b]
County wards (DCFS)[144]	11	State of Illinois	Clinical interview and treatment[a]
Specialty outpatient service[145]	15–17	New England	KSADS-E[a,b(only b young)]
Incarcerated adolescents[146]	2	Midwestern urban	DISC[a]
Incarcerated adolescents[147]	22	Texas	DISC[a]
Acute psychiatric hospitalizations, 1996–2004, children[1]	26	All of United States	CDC survey of discharge diagnoses
Inpatient service[97]	30, manic symptoms; <2, strict BP 1	New York City metro region	DICA; KSADS[a,b]
Acute psychiatric hospitalizations, 1996–2004, adolescents[1]	34	All of United States	CDC survey of discharge diagnoses

Abbreviations: DCFS, Division of Child and Family Services; CDC, Centers for Disease Control and Prevention; CIDI, World Health Organization's Composite International Diagnostic Interview; DICA, Diagnostic Interview for Children and Adolescents; DISC, Diagnostic Interview Schedule for Children; KSADS, Kiddie Schedule for Affective Disorders and Schizophrenia; KSADS-E, Epidemiologic version of the KSADS; MECA, Methods for Epidemiology of Child and Adolescent Mental Disorders Study; PBD, pediatric bipolar disorder; PL, Present and Lifetime version; WASH-U, Washington University version.[14]

[a] Youth interviewed as part of diagnostic assessment.
[b] Parent interviewed as component of diagnostic assessment.

Data from Youngstrom EA. Pediatric bipolar disorder. In: Mash EJ, Barkley RA, editors. Assessment of Childhood Disorders. 4th edition. New York: Guilford Press; 2007. p. 253.

Table 3		
Clinical interview red flags that should trigger thorough evaluation of possible PBD		
Red Flag	**Description**	**Reason**
Family history of bipolar disorder[a]	PBD most likely genetically driven	5×–10× increase for first-degree relative; 2.5×–5× for second-degree relative; 2× for "fuzzy" bipolar disorder in relative[47,49]
Antidepressant coincident mania	Manic symptoms while being treated with antidepressants	Undiagnosed PBD[38]
Episodic mood lability	Rapid switching between depressive and manic symptoms; depressive and manic symptoms at the same time	Common presentation; episodicity more suggestive of mood diagnosis[7]
Early onset depression	Onset < 25 years	First clinical episode is often depression; substantial portion of pediatric depressions ultimately show bipolar course[32,148]
Psychotic features	True delusions/hallucinations in the context of mood	Delusions/Hallucinations common during mood episode[40,149]
Episodic aggressive behavior	Episodic, high-energy; Not instrumental or planned, reactive	Not specific, but common[7,40]

Abbreviation: PBD, pediatric bipolar disorder.

[a] This is the risk factor that is currently most amenable to incorporation in actuarial or Bayesian methods.

history of family members will also provide valuable information about attitudes toward treatment and adherence and potentially about treatment response as well.[52]

COMBINING INFORMATION: IMPRESSIONISTIC VERSUS ACTUARIAL METHODS

How best can a clinician utilize information such as a positive family history of bipolar disorder or test results? Clinical decision making is usually done based on expertise and impressionistic synthesis of different pieces of information about the individual patient. Case formulation and diagnosis are highly technical skills that integrate multiple variables and involve considerable amounts of training. Within a typical assessment framework, knowledge about the family history becomes one more piece of data to blend into the global diagnostic impressions, increasing concern about the likelihood of bipolar disorder, yet not guaranteeing the diagnosis. Family history is a "red flag," ideally triggering other assessment procedures and helping build the case for a bipolar diagnosis when other confirming evidence emerges.

Using a Nomogram to Estimate Probabilities

It also is possible to use information about family history in a more quantitative manner. Evidence-based medicine (EBM) advocates the use of Bayesian approaches for assessing the probability of a patient having a diagnosis.[53] Bayesian methods

focus on combining new information with the prior probability of a diagnosis to estimate a revised, posterior probability. Bayesian approaches have been available for
centuries, but did not gain much popularity in clinical settings before the EBM movement. There are now a range of options for practitioners who want to use Bayesian
methods. In addition to doing the computations by hand, there are also applets available on the Web or for personal digital assistants, and there are also nomograms,
which function like a probability slide rule, facilitating estimation of probabilities
without requiring any computation, as shown in **Fig. 1**.

Youngstrom and Duax[48] provide a detailed description of how to use a nomogram
to estimate the probability of a youth having bipolar disorder when there is a family
history of the illness. One first determines a starting probability before considering
the other information that will be synthesized with it. In the absence of any other information, the base rate of the diagnosis, as contained in **Table 2**, provides a helpful
starting point.[54] The base rate anchors the clinical decision with an objective consideration of whether bipolar disorder is going to be uncommon or fairly frequent in a clinical setting. The clinician locates the starting probability on the left-hand scale of the
nomogram.

The middle line of the nomogram quantifies the impact of the new piece of assessment data, quantified as a diagnostic likelihood ratio (DLR).[53] Conceptually, the DLR
indexes the change in risk of a condition by comparing the rate at which the assessment event (such as a positive family history or a high test score) occurs in cases with

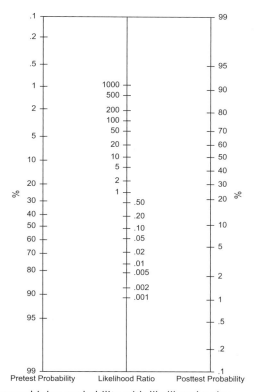

Fig. 1. Nomogram for combining probability with likelihood ratios.

bipolar disorder to the rate of occurrence for the same assessment event in cases without bipolar disorder. In other words, the DLR is the ratio of the sensitivity of the assessment to bipolar disorder (out of 100 cases with bipolar disorder, how many would obtain a positive assessment result), divided by the false alarm rate (out of 100 cases that do not have bipolar disorder, how many would also "falsely" obtain a positive assessment result—the opposite of the tool's specificity to the diagnosis). The DLR is the change in the odds of having a bipolar diagnosis. The nomogram obviates the clinician's need to perform calculations to combine the starting probability with the DLR. Instead, the clinician finds the DLR value on the middle column of the nomogram and then connects the dots between the first line (the starting probability) and the second line (the DLR) and extends the line across to the third, right-hand axis of the nomogram, which provides the revised probability estimate.

For example, a clinician evaluating a youth coming to an outpatient clinic whose mother has been diagnosed with bipolar II could use the nomogram in the following manner. First, the clinician would select the base rate of bipolar disorder, either using local historical information about the rate of diagnosis at his/her clinic or by finding a published estimate from a similar setting. The estimates listed in **Table 2** suggested the base rate of 6% for bipolar spectrum disorders in outpatient clinics. Thus, the clinician would put a dot at 6% on the left-hand line of the nomogram. Diagnosis of a bipolar disorder and a first-degree relative increases the risk of a bipolar diagnosis in the youth by a factor of five to 10. The clinician opts to use the more conservative estimate and marks the 5 on the middle line of the nomogram. Connecting the two dots and extending the line across the right-hand side of the nomogram yields a probability estimate in the vicinity of 24%, indicating that the youth has approximately a one in four chance of having bipolar disorder. Alternately, this value can be interpreted as meaning that roughly 24 out of 100 youths presenting to an outpatient clinic with a family history of bipolar disorder will themselves meet criteria for a bipolar spectrum diagnosis. If the clinician had picked the more liberal estimate of a tenfold increase due to family history, then the resulting risk estimate would have been roughly 39%. Comparing these two estimates illustrates several advantages of using the nomogram (or other Bayesian methods): (1) combining probabilities and risk factors is not an intuitive or linear process; (2) it is easy for clinicians to play "what if" scenarios by changing their starting assumptions or their choice of weight to assign to risk factors—referred to as "sensitivity analysis" in the EBM literature;[53] and (3) the results from the nomogram fall along a continuum and communicate more accurate information about the degree of diagnostic certainty. One of the major pitfalls of diagnostic testing is that results are prone to misinterpretation, especially when test findings are treated as black-and-white statements about the patient's status. The nomogram approach keeps the shades of gray. In this example, a black-and-white approach to testing would either focus on the test's positive result (family history) or on the posterior probability being less than 50%. Focusing only on the family history, or treating it as if it were synonymous with a bipolar diagnosis in the child, would be inaccurate in more than three out of four cases. The alternative would be to conclude that family history is not diagnostically useful in outpatient settings, because even when it is present, most youths will still not have bipolar disorder. Even when conducting a sensitivity analysis using two different estimates of risk, the results are consistent in showing that this particular combination of factors puts the youth at moderate risk (24%–39%) of having a bipolar spectrum illness. These numbers quantify the earlier statement that positive family history is a "red flag" that should initiate more comprehensive evaluation of a possible mood disorder.

How Does the Accuracy of Impressionistic Versus Statistical Methods Compare?

The actuarial/statistical approach to interpreting assessment information is unfamiliar to most clinicians and also contrasts sharply with more intuitive approaches to interpretation. However, the literature is unambiguous that simple statistical approaches, such as the nomogram method, consistently outperform typical clinical judgment.[54,55] The superiority of statistical approaches has been demonstrated more than 130 times, in disciplines spanning economics and education as well as clinical decision making.[56] Cognitive science is beginning to elucidate reasons why even simple statistical approaches perform better. The culprits often are "heuristics," cognitive shortcuts that facilitate the rapid identification and interpretation of information.[57,58] These heuristics help the brain process large volumes of complex information swiftly, but they also lead to systematic and predictable biases. The human brain has evolved to pay attention to cues of risk, for example, and to err on the side of high sensitivity at the expense of false alarms. Though highly adaptive in situations where a failure to detect risk could result in death, the high sensitivity to risk may lead to overestimates of rare but risky events in clinical settings.[59] A variety of other heuristics beset clinical judgment, including availability heuristics (such as noticing more bipolar symptoms in patients after repeatedly hearing about the rise in diagnosis in the popular press).

Many of these heuristics are likely to be relevant to the clinical diagnosis of bipolar disorder, suggesting that typical decision making would be vulnerable to at least as much bias and error as described in the larger decision-making literature. In fact, emerging evidence indicates that clinical diagnoses often have low accuracy with regard to bipolar disorder, including long delays between the emergence and recognition of symptoms,[60-62] cyclical trends where the diagnosis goes in and out of "fashion" compared to schizophrenia,[63] low agreement with systematic research diagnoses of bipolar disorders,[64] and large regional differences in the tendency to diagnose mania or in ratings of severity.[65-67] Coding videotaped interviews revealed a strong tendency for American clinicians to rate manic symptoms as more severe than British or Asian Indian clinicians,[67] and ratings of clinical vignettes showed that American psychiatrists were more likely to classify ambiguous clinical presentations as "bipolar" versus the rates identified by British clinicians.[65] More encouragingly, another vignette study has found that people can learn the nomogram approach quickly, and that applying the nomogram to the same clinical vignette results in significantly more accurate estimates of bipolar risk, greater consistency and agreement about the degree of risk (ie, much smaller range of opinion and smaller standard deviations), and a marked reduction in overdiagnosis of bipolar disorder.[66] Similar improvements in decision making have been documented in numerous other areas of medicine.[53]

QUESTIONNAIRES AND CHECKLISTS

Questionnaires and behavior checklists are an important tool in the kit of pediatric healthcare professionals. They offer an inexpensive, systematic way of gathering information, potentially from multiple sources (eg, teachers as well as parents or youths). The instruments can cover a broad range of areas of functioning and impairment, or they can drill deeper into more narrowly defined areas, helping to clarify diagnosis or establish the severity of problems. No single instrument will be equally suited to all of these diverse applications. What follows is a brief overview of the evidence pertaining to questionnaires and checklists with regard to PBDs.

Broadband Checklists

"Broadband" checklists cover a wide range of behavior problems. Both empirically derived versions (eg, the Achenbach System of Empirically Based Assessment, including the Child Behavior Checklist [CBCL])[68] and DSM-oriented versions (eg, child symptom inventory)[69] include subscales dealing with aggressive behavior, depression, anxiety, attention problems, social problems, and thought disorder or psychotic symptoms. The empirically derived versions also include superordinate scales that measure more global levels of externalizing and internalizing problems. Some versions provide scoring algorithms to map onto potential DSM diagnoses,[69] and others include age- and sex-based norms, comparing the level of behavior problems to typical levels of functioning for peers. Few of these instruments include a mania scale, reflecting the historical fact that most item pools were generated before there was concern about the possibility of PBD. The exceptions still tend to include the mania items only in the adolescent version[69] or only on the self-report (and not parent or teacher report) versions (Behavior Assessment System for Children).[70]

There are at least three major roles that a broadband instrument can play in the context of evaluating PBD: (1) high externalizing scores can trigger further assessment substituting other procedures for evaluating mania; (2) low scores can substantially reduce the probability that a case has PBD; and (3) broadband measures provide an inexpensive method of gauging the range of associated problems and comorbidities frequently seen with PBD. The CBCL is the most thoroughly investigated measure with regard to PBD, and evidence consistently shows that youths with PBD show elevated scores on multiple scales, including the externalizing problems broadband score.[71,72] However, in spite of PBD elevating average scores on several scales, from a diagnostic perspective it is the externalizing problems that convey the most information. After controlling for externalizing scores, no other scale or combination of scales provides incremental validity.[73] Most cases with PBD will show high externalizing scores (ie, they are sensitive to PBD), but high scores are also associated with many other conditions (ie, they are not specific to PBD). This sets up an asymmetry, where low externalizing scores are often decisive at ruling bipolar disorder out, but high scores are ambiguous.[74] Because of this, high scores should be treated as another warning sign, leading to deeper investigation of potential bipolar disorder. On the other hand, low scores will often decrease the risk enough to effectively rule bipolar disorder out, unless there are several countervailing risk factors and clinical signs. **Table 4** provides the DLRs associated with low, moderate, and high scores on the CBCL as well as the Achenbach Teacher's Report Form (TRF) and Youth Self-Report (YSR). More diagnostic information can be wrung from tests by estimating DLRs for multiple segments corresponding to low, medium, and high scores (as opposed to the common practice of setting a single threshold).[53] The low scores on the CBCL are more powerful at reducing probability of bipolar (DLR = .04) than extremely high scores are at increasing risk (DLR = four versus a 25 for a low score reducing risk).[53] Finally, regardless of whether the behavior problems represent true comorbid diagnoses, versus elements of a "core phenotype" of PBD or secondary consequences of the illness, the other clinical syndrome scales on broadband measures provide valuable information about functioning and other potential targets for treatment. For example, severe attention problems and chronic hyperactivity often require adjunctive treatment with stimulants even after mood stabilization has occurred,[75–77] and the social problems associated with PBD also respond well to targeted interventions.[78,79]

Mania-Specific Measures

Measures of mania for youths have proliferated over the last decade (see **Table 4**). They vary widely in terms of item content, reading level, and degree of validation. Although many are brief and most are in the public domain, the rarity of PBD and the false-positive rates produced by all of the tests preclude recommending the use of any mania checklist as a core component of outpatient assessment batteries. However, the best available measures are markedly more specific to PBD than the broadband instruments, suggesting a cost-effective, two-stage approach to assessment (**Fig. 2**).[49] First, clinicians would gather general developmental history and family history, which would include an assessment of several risk factors for PBD. Second, they would give a broadband measure as a way of getting a rapid scouting report about a wide array of clinical domains. If the family history and externalizing scores were both low risk, then bipolar disorder is effectively ruled out (see **Fig. 2**). If either the family history is significant for bipolar disorder or the externalizing score is high, then the clinician would supplement the assessment battery with a mania-specific measure. At present, the best validated and most discriminating instruments are the Parent General Behavior Inventory (Parent GBI)[33] and its 10-item mania form,[80] the Parent Mood Disorder Questionnaire (MDQ),[81,82] and the Child Mania Rating Scale (CMRS)[83] and its 10-item form.[84] Other instruments either have not performed as well or have not been validated under similarly generalizable clinical circumstances.[85] These three instruments produce functionally interchangeable results in terms of diagnostic assessment. As new articles are published, test users should compare the instruments not only on their area under the curve (AUC) in receiver operating characteristic analyses (which combines the diagnostic sensitivity and specificity into a single summary score) but also on the quality of the study, sample, and reporting.[86]

INTERPRETING TEST SCORES

The clinician can choose to interpret test scores from rating scales in a number of ways. The most common method is a categorical, impressionistic interpretation, where scores are grouped into "high" and "low" ranges. It is also possible to be more formal about the quantification of risk information conveyed by test results, using the same array of options as described earlier when interpreting family history. Current thinking in EBM is that the use of DLRs is a preferred strategy.[53] The DLR for a test result is the percentage of cases with bipolar disorder divided by the percentage of nonbipolar cases scoring in the same range. If a publication provides the sensitivity and specificity, then it is straightforward to convert these values into a pair of DLRs for scores above and below the threshold.[53] **Table 4** includes the DLRs for all available tests with regard to PBD at the time of writing.

Perusal of the DLR values leads to several observations. Many of the DLRs associated with low test scores are values lower than 1.0. A DLR of 1.0 indicates that the test result or risk factor did not change the probability of a bipolar diagnosis, because the score is equally likely to occur in both bipolar and nonbipolar reference groups. DLRs smaller than 1.0 reflect that the score is much more likely to occur in nonbipolar cases, thus reducing the likelihood that the current client has bipolar disorder. Whereas a value of 2.0 would signify a doubling of the odds of a bipolar diagnosis, a value of 0.5 would convey a similar change in odds in the opposite direction. DLRs greater than 10 or smaller than 0.1 are often decisive pieces of information:[53] They can change a prior probability of 50% (even odds) to more than 90% or less than 10% posterior probability. These benchmarks lead to the additional observation that available instruments are more powerful at decreasing the likelihood of bipolar disorder than at

Table 4
AUCs and likelihood ratios for potential screening measures for PBD

Screening Measure	AUC	DLR	Test Score	Clinical Generalizability
Adolescents (11–18 years)				
Parent general behavior inventory Hypomanic/biphasic[33]	.84 (N = 324)[73]	.1 .3 1.1 2.2 4.8 9.2	<9 9–15 16–24 25–39 40–48 49+	Moderate *Note:* Uses 0 to 3 scoring
CBCL externalizing T score[150]	.78 (N = 324)[73]	.04 .5 1.3 2.1 2.7 4.3	<54 54–56 65–69 70–75 76–80 81+	Moderate
Parent mood disorder questionnaire[81]	~ .84 (N<150)[81] .75 (N = 124)[82]	.3 3.9	<5[81] 5+	Moderate *Note:* required co-occurring and at least moderate impairment[81]
YSR externalizing T score[151]	.71 (N = 324)[73]	.3 .5 1.2 1.6 2.3 3.0	<49 49–55 56–62 63–69 70–76 77+	Moderate

---

Assessment of Pediatric Bipolar Disorder   367

Measure	Reliability	DLR	Score range	Clinical utility	Notes
TRF externalizing T score[152]	.70 (N = 324)[73]	.3 / .6 / 1.0 / 2.0 / 1.5 / 3.8	<46 / 46–53 / 54–60 / 61–68 / 69–76 / 77+	Moderate	
Parent young mania rating scale[153]	.80 (N = 324)[73]; .70 (N = 124)[82]	.2 / .3 / 1.0 / 2.0 / 4.1 / 7.4	<6[73] / 6–11 / 12–17 / 18–23 / 24–27 / 28+	High	Note: Uses 0 to 4 and 0 to 8 scoring[113]
Adolescent mood disorder questionnaire[154]	~.59 (N< 150)[81]; .63 (N = 124)[82]	.8 / 1.5	<5[81] / 5+	High	Note: Do not include co-occurring and at least moderate impairment items
Adolescent general behavior inventory Hypomanic/biphasic[34]	.62 (N = 324)[73]; .65 (N = 124)[82]	.3 / 1.0 / .8 / 1.2 / 2.0 / 3.9	<10[73] / 10–17 / 18–26 / 27–37 / 38–45 / 46+	High	Note: Uses 0 to 3 scoring
Adolescent young mania rating scale questionnaire[82]	.50 (N = 124)[82]	No better than chance	—	High	
Children (5–10 years)					
CBCL externalizing T score[150]	.82 (N = 318)[73]	.1 / .5 / 1.5 / 4.6 / 3.2 / 3.5	<58 / 58–67 / 68–72 / 73–77 / 78–81 / 82+	Moderate	

(continued on next page)

Table 4
(continued)

Screening Measure	AUC	DLR	Test Score	Clinical Generalizability
Parent general behavior inventory Hypomanic/biphasic[33]	.81 (N = 318)[73]	.1 .5 1.3 2.3 4.9 6.3	<11 11–20 21–30 31–42 43–50 51+	Moderate *Note:* Uses 0 to 3 scoring
Parent mood disorder questionnaire[81]	.72 (N = 141)[82]	—	—	High
Parent young mania rating scale[153]	.83 (N = 318)[73] .66 (N = 141)[82]	.1 .5 .9 2.8 6.9 8.9	<7[73] 7–13 14–21 22–29 30–34 35+	High *Note:* Uses 0 to 4, 0 to 8 scoring (Young et al., 1978)
TRF externalizing *T* score[152]	.57 (N = 318)[73]	.8 .9 1.2 1.7 1.3	<56 57–62 63–70 71–77 78+	Moderate *Note:* Not clinically useful
Combined samples (child and adolescent not reported separately)				
10-item parent child mania rating scale[83,84]	.91 (N = 150)[84]	.2 13.7	<20 20+	Low
2-Item screen[155]	.85 (N = 264)[155] .70 (N = 500)[85]	.31 5.2[a]	<9 for 7–8[155] <8 for 9–10 <6 for 11+ 9+ for 7–8 8+ for 9–10 6+ for 11+	Low[85]

General behavior inventory—teacher Depression scale[95]	.62	.7 1.3	<4 4+	High
General behavior inventory—teacher Hypomanic/biphasic scale[95]	Chance	No better than chance	—	High *Note:* Not clinically useful
Teacher report form[152]	Chance	No better than chance	—	High *Note:* Not clinically useful
Child mania rating scale—teacher[95]	Chance	No better than chance	—	High *Note:* Not clinically useful
Young mania rating scale—teacher[95]	Chance	No better than chance	—	High *Note:* Not clinically useful
Child bipolar questionnaire[156]	Not reported (N = 135)[157]	7.1	—	Low

Note: All studies used some version of KSADS interview by a trained rater combined with review by a clinician to establish consensus diagnosis. DLR refers to the change in probability associated with the test score. Likelihood ratios of 1 indicate that the test result did not change impressions. DLRs larger than 10 or smaller than 0.10 are frequently clinically decisive; 5 or 0.2 are helpful, and between 2.0 and 0.5 are small enough that they rarely result in clinically meaningful changes of formulation.[158] Generalizability was rated low, moderate, or high. Low generalizability meant that the sample was highly selected (eg, PBD, ADHD, healthy control). Moderate generalizability meant the sample was less highly selected (eg, few exclusion criteria). High generalizability meant that the sample did not exclude (eg, took everyone to the clinic).

Abbreviations: ADHD, attention-deficit/hyperactivity disorder; AUCs, areas under the curve; CBCL, Child Behavior Checklist; DLR, diagnostic likelihood ratio; KSADS, Kiddie Schedule for Affective Disorders and Schizophrenia; PBD, pediatric bipolar disorder.

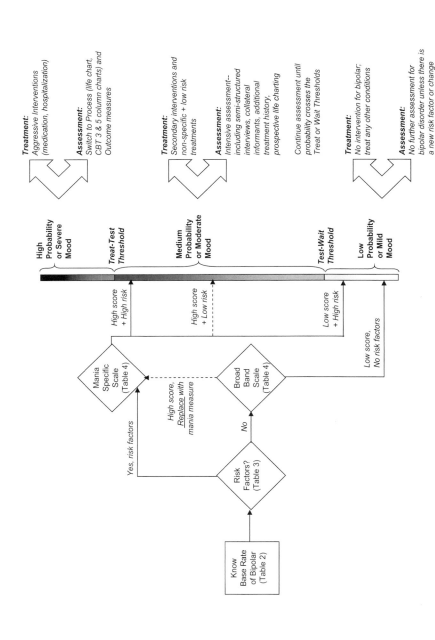

Fig. 2. Flow chart for assessment and treatment thresholds.

increasing it (ie, there are many test results yielding DLRs less than 0.1 but few with DLRs greater than 10 and none that have been validated in samples with a high degree of clinical generalizability). Small DLRs can actually play a valuable role by reducing the tendency to overdiagnose PBD.[1,2,66]

To use these DLRs with a nomogram, one follows the same procedure as that described with the interpretation of family history, only using the test score's DLR as the estimate on the middle line of the nomogram.[87] When multiple DLRs are available, such as when both family history information and a CBCL externalizing score are available, then all pieces of information can be combined within the nomogram framework. The sequence does not matter. Family history could be considered first, or the test score; or the DLRs could be multiplied together and the product used instead during a single pass through the nomogram. Algebraically, these are all equivalent scenarios. This degree of flexibility is extremely valuable clinically, though, because often it will not be possible to obtain some pieces of assessment information for a specific case, and the order with which clinical data become available often varies across cases. In contrast, other actuarial methods such as lookup tables, logistic regression, or decision trees require that all the component variables be measured for each case and that they be applied in a specified combination or sequence. Building on the earlier example, if a very high CBCL externalizing score ($T = 83$) was added to the case with a positive family history of bipolar disorder, then the current probability (24% based on a first-degree relative increasing the risk of a bipolar diagnosis by a factor of five) would be entered on the left-hand line of the nomogram. Table 4 provides the DLR associated with the T score (DLR = 4.3 for an adolescent scoring this high on the CBCL). Combining the prior probability and the DLR algebraically yields an estimate of 58%. Using the nomogram adds some imprecision, both because reference points need to be visually interpolated and because of error connecting the dots; but clinical estimates using the nomogram still wind up being centered around the best estimate and are dramatically more precise than when clinicians interpret the same information impressionistically.[66]

Either a high score on a broadband measure or a positive family history of bipolar disorder would justify the addition of one of the more specific mania scales to the assessment process. However, when the same person fills out two rating scales, only one of them should be incorporated into the formal assessment process, whether it be the nomogram or another method of combining risks.[14] The scores on the questionnaires will be highly correlated with each other by virtue of coming from the same source and thus will yield redundant information. Treating multiple questionnaire scores as if each were introducing new information will create bias in the probability estimates. The bias can be substantial when the scores are highly correlated ($r > .5$), which will often be the case when the same person fills out multiple instruments, even when the person measures different constructs.[88] As a result, the clinician should take the most valid piece of information available from the informant and substitute it into the nomogram cycle, ignoring other scores from the same source.[14] In our case example, the high CBCL score would cause the clinician to ask the caregiver to complete the Parent GBI. A very high score on this tool (eg, a raw score of 51; see Table 4) has a DLR of 9.2. This would replace the DLR of 4.3 from the CBCL completed by the same caregiver. Combining the DLR of 9.2 with a prior probability of 24% (based on the family history and the base rate of PBD in outpatient settings) generates an estimate of 58% risk.

Permuting the possible combinations of DLRs from the combination of family histories and test scores yields a range of eight to 24 probability estimates per test. When also accounting for the differences in base rate across clinical settings, the number of distinct probabilities will exceed 100 for each test × family history × setting combination. This reveals another advantage of the nomogram approach compared to generating tables of estimates for each configuration or versus trying to weight the information sources intuitively. The tandem of family history and rating scales is powerful enough to move the probability estimate of a PBD diagnosis to less than 1% (no family history plus a low score on a broadband) or as high as 85% (using a more aggressive estimate of a 10-fold increase in risk due to family history, plus a very high score on a Parent GBI or comparable tool). Thus, an evidence-based approach to assessment can rule PBD out in many cases and reduce the tendency to overdiagnose bipolar disorder; but even high-risk combinations do not create sufficiently high probabilities of diagnosis to replace a careful symptom-level assessment of bipolar disorder.

Cross-Informant Issues

There has been a substantial amount of research on the validity of YSR and teacher report as well as caregiver report (almost always mothers) about bipolar disorder. Findings consistently show the greatest validity for parent report, which shows significantly larger effect sizes than those in youth or teacher report in all published studies where the same instrument is available from multiple informants.[73,82,89,90] Examining **Table 4** reveals that the DLRs for parent report are consistently larger than the DLRs for youth or teacher report on the same instruments. The greater validity of parent report persists even when the parent has a diagnosed mood disorder.[91]

That parent report outperforms self-report contradicts conventional wisdom that self-report is a better source of information about mood disorders.[92] The lower validity of youth report appears to be due to a combination of mania compromising insight into one's own behaviors[93] and manic symptoms tending to disturb others before the affected individual perceives them as problematic.[94] The low validity of teacher report persists even when teachers complete mania-specific rating scales.[95] Notably, the agreement between parents and youths or parents and teachers is actually significantly higher than typical for cross-informant agreement,[91,96] and youths and teachers report significantly more behavior problems in PBD cases than would be predicted based on the parent's level of concern alone.[91] The challenge is the difficulty of intuitively appreciating what a cross-situational correlation of 0.2 or 0.3 might look like at a case level, so instances where dyadic agreement is actually good are often misinterpreted as one person having exaggerated concerns. Clinicians will often encounter families where the parent reports more mood issues than the teacher or youth. The evidence-based approach to these discrepancies is not to automatically discount the parent report but rather to systematically gather additional information to evaluate the possibility of PBD.[14] At a statistical level, youth and teacher report provide only modest, and often insignificant, incremental validity after controlling for parent report.[73,94] However, the correlation between parents and youths or teachers is sufficiently low for these to be treated as functionally separate sources of information and combined within the nomogram framework. Evidence also suggests that cases where mood symptoms are noticeable across informants and settings may have greater impairment,[97] also justifying the effort required to collect multiple perspectives. Teacher report can add useful information about the degree of problems in the school setting,[95] and youth report adds data about the degree of insight into problems and motivation for treatment, both providing helpful prescriptive information to guide intervention.

Deciding to Intervene: Crossing the Treatment Threshold

The clinical process has three different options with regard to diagnosis: "Ruled out," "sufficiently well established that treatment for the condition should begin," or else "possible, but not established." In EBM, the probability of diagnosis theoretically ranges from 0% to 100%, and there are two thresholds that separate the three different clinical options (see **Fig. 2**).[53] The Test-Wait threshold separates the low risk zone, where the diagnosis is effectively ruled out, from the indeterminate middle range. The Test-Treat threshold demarcates the zone where probability is high enough to initiate treatment. **Fig. 2** does not specify probability levels for these thresholds. In practice, the location of the threshold should take into consideration the risks and benefits associated with treatment as well as patient preferences. There is a formal framework for collecting and incorporating these utilities into adjusted thresholds,[98] with perhaps the easiest approach described in an EBM handbook.[53] As diagrammed in **Fig. 2**, the combination of family history and questionnaire data will be sufficient to rule bipolar disorder out when both indicate low risk. High-risk cases, with positive family history and high scores on mania measures, will still fall below the Test-Treat threshold, especially when considering the stigma, treatment burden, and potential side effects attendant on recommended treatments for PBD.[99] Within an EBM framework, probabilities falling between the Treat and Wait thresholds indicate the need for continued assessment. New assessment data then get combined with the current probability until the revised probability crosses the Wait threshold (ruling the diagnosis out) or the Treat threshold (ruling the diagnosis in).

Doses of Treatment Model

Psychology has long had a model of "levels of intervention," where primary preventions might be offered to everyone in order to avoid onset of an illness, secondary interventions might be offered only to targeted high-risk groups, and tertiary interventions would be deployed for cases already manifesting a disorder.[100] Preventive measures need to be low risk and low cost if they are going to be applied widely regardless of risk. Tertiary interventions can be higher risk and expense, because they have been reserved for cases with established diagnoses. This "levels-of-intervention" model can be mapped onto the EBM diagnostic threshold model,[15] as shown in **Fig. 2**, right-hand side. Synthesizing these two models creates a set of assessment and treatment recommendations for each of the three ranges of probability for a bipolar diagnosis. Instead of labeling cases having mid-range probabilities as "indeterminate," they can be called "moderate risk," and treatment using low-risk methods can start. Techniques such as psychotherapy, dietary supplementation, and improved sleep hygiene all might reasonably be tried for cases in this range. So long as the burden, risks, and costs are low, treatments that are nonspecific or potentially preventative can be used, even while assessment continues and clarifies diagnostic impressions.

LEAVING LIMBO: RULING BIPOLAR DISORDER IN OR OUT

Even when multiple risk factors are present, a clinician cannot assume that a PBD diagnosis has been established. How best should they proceed? The following suggestions provide an overview of strategies that help to confirm the diagnosis in high-risk cases or to rule a bipolar diagnosis in or out for cases that fall in the intermediate range of risk.

Diagnostic Interviews

Diagnostic interviews remain the standard of practice for determining clinical diagnosis. The typical unstructured diagnostic interview is prone to a variety of heuristics that render its reliability quite low.[101] For PBD, circumstances are likely to worsen the already typically poor degree of inter-rater reliability, due to issues such as the lack of formal training in recognition of PBD, the usage of different operational definitions, and the controversy around the diagnosis. Structured diagnostic interviews avoid some of the shortcomings of informal interviews, including systematic coverage of relevant symptoms and formal algorithms to make DSM diagnoses.[101] However, most structured interviews were designed before PBD was considered a serious possibility in youths, with the consequence that many pediatric structured interviews do not include a mania module, and those that do include few, if any, modifications to the probes or anchors to facilitate recognition in pediatric cases.[14]

For this reason, semistructured diagnostic interviews, such as the Kiddie Schedule for Affective Disorders and Schizophrenia (KSADS), have become the accepted standard for PBD research.[102] Different versions of the KSADS have demonstrated good reliability and validity with regard to PBD.[103,104] There are some obstacles hindering the widespread clinical adoption of semistructured interviews. These include the necessity for extensive training, or else the semistructured aspect opens the door for differences in clinical judgment to undermine the reliability[67] as well as the substantial amount of time required to administer and score the interview. A full KSADS can take anywhere from 2 to 8 hours to complete with a family, with administrations by experienced clinicians often averaging around 3 hours for typical cases. However, more streamlined versions of semistructured interviews deserve serious consideration as a potential component of clinical assessment.[105] The emerging literature around clinical diagnosis of PBD suggests that there may be great need for semistructured approaches despite the increased expense and burden involved. Medicaid and other providers will often reimburse for the diagnostic assessment time if medical necessity has been demonstrated. The framework described here—starting with a combination of rating scales and family history—provides strong documentation of medical necessity for such additional evaluation. Clinicians who want to adopt semistructured interviews as part of their assessment portfolio should pick an instrument that covers manic and depressive symptoms thoroughly, includes developmentally appropriate anchors, and supports the diagnosis of "spectrum" conditions (such as bipolar II, cyclothymic disorder, and bipolar NOS), as these will be more common than bipolar I, yet impairing enough to represent major clinical concerns.

"Handle" Symptoms

Not all symptoms carry equal weight toward making a diagnosis of mania. The DSM-IV and International Classification of Diseases criteria give greater emphasis to elated mood instead of irritable mood. Elated mood requires only three additional symptoms to support a diagnosis of mania, versus four additional symptoms for irritable mood.[16] This policy acknowledges that elated mood has greater diagnostic specificity to mania, whereas irritable mood is diagnostically nonspecific. Research suggests that decreased need for sleep, unstable self-esteem and grandiosity, hypersexuality, racing thoughts, and psychotic symptoms are all relatively specific to PBD.[7] The sensitivity of each of these symptoms is low enough that none should be required for making a diagnosis of bipolar disorder, or else somewhere between a quarter and two-thirds of bipolar cases might be excluded.[7] Each of these symptoms is also liable to occur in at least one other condition likely to be encountered in many clinical settings. For example, hypersexuality can be a sign of sexual abuse, and inflated self-esteem is frequently seen in conduct disorder.[7] However, a clinician can learn how these symptoms often manifest in the context of PBD,[106] and careful probing around these symptoms is an important component of refining diagnostic impressions. Evidence that any of the possible manic symptoms occur episodically, as opposed to chronically, or that they fluctuate with changes in mood and energy, heighten the suspicion that they are due to a mood disorder rather than a more chronic condition such as attention-deficit hyperactivity disorder (ADHD).[107] If the symptom occurs with an unusual *Frequency*, if the *Intensity* is excessive, if the *Number* of occurrences within an episode is extreme, or if the *Duration* is exceptional compared to age-appropriate behavior, that also helps build the case in favor of a mood diagnosis (the FIND mnemonic).[99,108]

Extending the Window of Assessment

Another crucial strategy to improve the detection of PBD is to extend the window of assessment beyond the conventional single session of intake assessment.[49] Relying on a single panel of information focused on the presenting problem will rarely be enough to allow a firm diagnosis of PBD.

Developmental history

Gathering a developmental history is a routine component of pediatric assessment. Its role is especially helpful when evaluating the possibility of PBD. In addition to gathering data about the family psychiatric history, pre- and perinatal risk factors and complications and temperamental characteristics all deserve consideration.[108] Developmental trajectories can help distinguish between chronic conditions such as ADHD (which is formally required to have onset before age seven) and episodic mood presentations.[107] Even though not all authorities concur that PBD will always have an episodic presentation, identifying episodic presentations still carries treatment utility by suggesting different intervention strategies.[52,109] The most intensive form of retrospective information gathering would be to complete a retrospective life chart.[110] The retrospective life chart is a tool that asks the family to reconstruct a week-by-week summary of the youth's past mood and energy levels, using a variety of anchors and techniques to facilitate accurate recall. The retrospective life chart can yield valuable information about the chronicity versus episodicity of mood presentation, and it can help to identify triggering events. However, the time and effort involved are substantial, and retrospective memory is subject to several sources of bias. Clinicians need to weigh the costs against the possible benefits on an individual-case basis before adding life charting.

Extending the Assessment Window Forward

The other way of moving beyond a single-session intake is by extending the window of assessment forward in time. There are many means of accomplishing this. They include starting with a diagnosis of "rule out bipolar disorder" based on the initial intake and following up with additional assessment to clarify the diagnosis. The EBM threshold model operationalizes this concept by indicating continued assessment for as long as the probability of PBD falls between the Wait and Treat thresholds.[53]

Another approach is to shift to a "dental model" of assessment, where ongoing "checkups" are scheduled to gauge mood and energy over the course of treatment.[49] At a minimum, these could consist of asking the patients at each visit about their mood and energy since the last visit. Alternately, the family could complete brief rating scales every few weeks over the course of treatment.[75,76] The clinician could also quantify impressions using ratings such as the Children's Global Assessment Scale (CGAS).[111] At the most intensive, the clinician could suggest doing prospective life charting.[110] In a prospective format, the patient records changes in mood and energy on a daily basis and also notes any coinciding events. There are free prospective life charts available on the web (Google "bipolar life chart" to find numerous examples) for use with youths, and sophisticated online versions are now available. If the family is willing and able to complete prospective life charts, then the information is highly useful for refining diagnosis and guiding treatment; but the demands of life charting exceed the resources and motivation of many families. The informal "mood and energy checkup" at each visit represents the minimum level of prospective information gathering that should be routine when working with mood disorders.

MEASURING SEVERITY

In addition to guiding diagnosis, a second crucial role of assessment tools is quantifying the severity of mood problems. More acute mood disturbance will require a different level of intervention services, with inpatient hospitalization providing the most intensive treatment for severest mood disturbance. Besides navigating the selection of treatment setting, the severity of the mood problems will help prescribe different treatment options. More severe mood problems will suggest the use of pharmacotherapy as a first-line treatment, and combination treatments with both psychotherapy and one or more pharmacologic agents may be needed to stabilize mood.[99] Moderate levels of mood symptoms may result in lower-dose interventions, including outpatient psychotherapy with longer intervals between sessions, or less aggressive dosing of medications. Assessments of severity are also crucial for establishing benchmarks against which to measure treatment response.

Clinician Ratings

Clinical ratings of the severity of mood problems steer the treatment of PBD. Typically, the assessment is informal, with all of the attendant limitations described in the discussion of informal diagnosis.[101] There are global rating scales, such as the Global Assessment of Functioning,[16] the CGAS,[111] and the Clinician Global Impressions Scale (CGI),[112] that assign a number to the clinician's overall impression of functioning. There is also a bipolar version of the CGI, where the clinician rates manic and depressive symptoms separately.[75]

The next level of sophistication would be to use a semistructured clinical rating scale. The two most widely used in research with PBD are the Young Mania Rating Scale (YMRS)[113] and the Children's Depression Rating Scale-Revised (CDRS-R).[114] Both have shown evidence of good reliability and acceptable validity in pediatric samples.[115–117] This is reassuring for the YMRS, which was not originally designed for use with children or as an interview.[113] The YMRS and CDRS-R both omit symptoms that are DSM-IV criteria for mania or depression, and they omit other associated features that can be important in assessing the severity of mood disturbance.[14] The YMRS does not include a grandiosity item, for example, nor does it measure threat of harm to self. There are newer rating scales designed specifically for use with children and adolescents, which provide more developmentally appropriate anchors, use consistent ratings across all items, and include all DSM symptoms of mood episodes. The KSADS-MRS and Depression Rating Scales (DRS) have all of these refinements and show good psychometrics.[118] Clinicians contemplating the use of mood rating scales should be aware that the interviews require a moderate amount of time (typically 15–45 minutes), and the semistructured format is both a blessing and a bane in terms of often leading to sizeable differences in scoring of the same interview by different clinicians.[67]

Checklists: A Reprise

Checklists can complement clinician ratings in measuring severity. Checklists are inexpensive, require virtually no training to use, and incorporate little or no clinical judgment in scoring; they are the mirror image of clinician ratings in each of these regards. Checklists also afford the assessment of a broader range of symptom domains than can generally be accomplished via clinician ratings. Parent checklists, in particular, have demonstrated a strong correlation with clinician-rated measures of severity, and they also show good sensitivity to treatment effects.[75,76]

Quality of Life

There is growing emphasis on quality of life as a vital aspect of the burden of illness and successful outcome of treatment. Several rating scales have been used to measure quality of life in the context of PBD.[119,120] The KINDL is especially attractive for clinical use because it has two parent and three youth report versions that are developmentally staged, and because it can be used free of charge (http://www.kindl.org/indexE.html).

Process Measures to Use During Treatment

Many of the assessment tools discussed above can contribute to process measurement during treatment. Prospective life charts, in-session mood and energy checkups, or repeated administrations of brief rating scales can chart response over the course of intervention. Of the various checklists available, the 10-item versions are generally preferable for repeated administration due to the reduced burden. An exception is the MDQ:[81] Although it is a good diagnostic aid, it does not capture information about the severity of current mood problems, so it is not useful as a process or outcome measure.

Prospective life charts can also provide information similar to that I three-column and five-column charts used in cognitive behavioral therapy.[121] All of these assessment devices ask the patients to chart fluctuations in mood as well as associated events. The three-column chart asks the patients to then also write down what they were thinking at the time, linking the cognition to the emotional response; and the five-column chart goes further by adding an alternative cognition and the emotional response it generates.[121,122] For those families that are able to do prospective life charting, it is possible to seamlessly weave the components of three- and five-column charting into the recording and in-session discussions of the data.

Other aspects of treatment process that are important to assess include adherence, risk of harm to self and others, and side effects. Measures of adherence can include regularity of kept appointments, completion rates of homework assignments, and compliance with prescribed dosing regimens. Because mood disorder is a major risk factor for suicide and self-harm, it is crucial to regularly assess potential suicidal ideation as well as the presence of a plan and means.[8] Similarly, the degree of aggression and irritability that often manifests with PBD requires regular, documented assessment of risk to others. Finally, the potential side effects for pharmacologic treatments are both numerous and potentially quite serious, so they need careful patient education and ongoing monitoring.[123] Although there are published rating scales for each of these domains, in general they are sufficiently cumbersome and it will usually be more practical to accomplish these goals via direct assessment by the clinician. At the same time, the clinician must follow through on assessing each of these domains and not fall into the trap of irregular assessment and poor documentation.

Measuring Outcomes

Many of the same questionnaires, checklists, and clinician rating scales used to evaluate severity can also provide good measures of outcome. The tools best suited for outcome assessment have good reliability, good content coverage of the relevant symptoms and key aspects of functioning, and are sensitive to treatment effects. Content that is useful for diagnosis may not be identical to the content most useful for outcome measures. For example, irritable mood is ambiguous when used for diagnostic purposes, but irritability is one of the most distressing and impairing features of PBD, and so it definitely merits a central role in outcome assessment. Conversely, two of the 11 items on the YMRS show weak validity when applied to pediatric cases (lack of insight and bizarre appearance),[117] and their inclusion probably dilutes the sensitivity of the YMRS to treatment effects. From a psychometric perspective, outcome measures can and should be longer than the process measures administered more frequently during treatment. The greater length improves reliability and thus the potential validity of the outcome measure,[124] and the length is more likely to be tolerable if administered infrequently. Counterintuitively, statistical power to detect change can be increased by shifting more items to the post-test instead of the pre-test.[125] Clinicians could take advantage of this by using more lengthy outcome measures as part of the termination assessment, where families would not also be spending substantial amounts of time on diagnostic evaluations or administrative paperwork (such as insurance forms). Of the available instruments, the CBCL, the Parent GBI, and Adolescent GBI have the most established track record as outcome measures. The CMRS also appears promising. Of the clinician rating scales, the YMRS and CDRS have by far the largest database in the literature, but the KSADS-MRS and DRS deserve consideration due to their advantages in terms of content coverage and developmental appropriateness.

Definitions of response, remission, and clinically significant change
In psychiatry outcome studies, treatment response has most commonly been defined using thresholds for percentage reductions in the severity of mood symptoms. For example, a 33% or 50% reduction in YMRS scores from baseline might define "response" to treatment.[126,127] Such definitions of response are convenient, but they also have some major shortcomings. These limitations include (a) the fact that different patients will need to show varying amounts of change to qualify as a responder, depending upon their initial level of severity; (b) the fact that mania and depression often show different responses to treatment, and sometimes one might worsen at the same time that the other mood symptoms are improving; (c) percentage reductions in symptoms do not necessarily translate into syndromal remission or improvements compared to normative benchmarks; and (d) percentage reductions ignore the degree of precision of an instrument, potentially penalizing more accurate instruments because they are more reliable. The vulnerability of definitions of "treatment response" to unreliability could be a factor contributing to the high rates of placebo response observed in clinical trials.

Multiple refinements have been developed to address these shortcomings of the percentage change approach. These include comparisons to "rules of thumb" about thresholds for mania, hypomania, or depression; the empirical definition of thresholds that distinguishes responders from nonresponders;[128] the use of compound definitions of remission that integrate improvement on mania and depression simultaneously;[75] and the articulation of formal clinical definitions of remission and recurrence.[129] None of these has achieved clear dominance in the research arena, and few have permeated into clinical practice yet.

Perhaps the most fully articulated framework for evaluating outcomes is the "clinically significant change" model proposed by Jacobson and Truax.[130] Their definition of clinically significant change requires achieving two goals: Demonstrating reliable improvement given the psychometric precision of the outcome measure and also passing one of three normative benchmarks defined by the range of scores observed in clinical and nonclinical reference samples. Reliable change is tied to the standard error of the difference score, which is a direct measure of the instrument's precision at measuring change. Jacobson and Truax advocated dividing the patient's raw change score by the standard error of the difference.[130] This would standardize the change score, converting it to a z score (with a mean of zero and standard deviation of one, the same metric as the familiar Cohen's d effect size). Jacobson and Truax called this standardized change score the "Reliable Change Index" (RCI). Two advantages of calculating the RCI are (a) that it facilitates comparison of the magnitude of treatment response across different measures (eg, a five-point reduction in the YMRS does not mean the same thing as a five-point reduction in a CDRS-R score, but converting both to RCIs would make clear whether the patient's mania or depression was responding more to treatment); and (b) that RCIs can be compared to established benchmarks drawn from the normal distribution. RCIs larger than 1.65 are big enough to be 90% certain that the patient is responding, and RCIs larger than 1.96 are enough to be 95% confident. Three drawbacks of the RCI are (a) that it is unfamiliar to most clinicians, (b) it involves computation, and (c) it requires knowledge of the standard error of the difference for the test, which is rarely available. However, all of these problems are tractable. A study in 2007 presents the standard error of the difference for several commonly used outcome measures relevant to PBD.[14] **Table 5** also includes "critical values" expressed in the raw or T score metric that clinicians normally use as a way of bypassing any computation. For example, if a patient shows at least 10 points of improvement on the YMRS, or six points on the CBCL externalizing score, then the clinician can be 90% sure that they are changing in this domain (or 95% sure that the patient is improving, one-tailed).

The second part of the definition of clinically significant change entails demarcating benchmarks based on reference clinical and nonclinical samples. Jacobsen defined three benchmarks, called simply A, B, and C. Youngstrom has suggested referring to them as *Away* from the clinical range, *Back* into the normal range, and *Closer* to the nonclinical than clinical mean.[14] The away threshold is set at two standard deviations below the mean for a clinical sample on the measure.[130] For PBD, estimating the away threshold would involve finding a sample of youths with PBD and then locating the score on the instrument that fell two standard deviations below the sample mean (roughly corresponding to the 2.5th percentile for cases with PBD). Similarly, the back into the nonclinical range is established by finding the score that falls two standard deviations above the mean for a nonclinical comparison group. The closer threshold is found by estimating the weighted mean of the clinical and comparison means, weighting by the sample standard deviations. The technical manuals for many tests include the needed information to calculate the three thresholds, and Cooperberg[131] calculated the thresholds for several other measures pertinent to PBD. **Table 5** includes the thresholds for several commonly used outcome measures.

Clinically significant change is frequently used to evaluate individual response in psychotherapy trials. It is a stringent definition of response, and it tends to produce lower estimates of response rates than the simple percentage symptom reduction approach.[132] The conservative definition should cause celebration when actually achieving any of the definitions of clinically significant change. Studying **Table 5** also reveals that some definitions are impossible given the distributional characteristics of a measure. The away threshold would frequently require obtaining negative scores, because the clinical mean falls within two standard deviations of the lowest possible score on the measure. Similarly, the back definition would accept high scores (eg, T scores of 70 on externalizing or internalizing problems) as potentially reflecting clinically significant change. This might make sense when coupled with reliable change—a seven-point reduction in internalizing problems from a 76 to a 69 could

				Table 5

Table 5
Clinically significant change benchmarks with common instruments and mood rating scales

	Cut Score			
Measure	Away	Back	Closer	90% Critical Change
BDI[159]				
BDI mixed depression	4	22	15	8
CBCL T scores (2001 Norms)[68]				
Total	49	70	58	4
Externalizing	49	70	58	6
Internalizing	a	70	56	7
Attention problems	a	66	58	7
TRF T scores (2001 Norms)[68]				
Total	a	70	57	4
Externalizing	a	70	56	5
Internalizing	a	70	55	7
Attention problems	a	66	57	7
YSR T scores (2001 Norms)[68]				
Total	a	70	54	6
Externalizing	a	70	54	8
Internalizing	a	70	54	8
Young mania rating scale (clinician rated)[113]	6	2	2	—
Child depression rating scale—revised[114]	a	40	29	7
Parent GBI—hypomanic/biphasic scale[33]	7	19	15	7
Parent GBI—depression scale[33]	a	18	13	6
Adolescent GBI—hypomanic/biphasic scale[27]	a	32	19	7
Adolescent GBI—depression scale[27]	a	47	27	9

Note: Away from the clinical range, Back into the nonclinical range, Closer to the nonclinical than clinical mean.

Abbreviations: BDI, Beck Depression Inventory; CBCL, Child Behavior Checklist; GBI, General Behavior Inventory; TRF, Teacher's Report Form; YSR, Youth Self-Report.

[a] These benchmarks would require impossible test scores, such as negative numbers.

constitute a substantial improvement, for example. Even so, the thresholds identified by the closer definition will often provide the most meaningful benchmarks for outcome evaluation.[14]

In summary, outcome evaluation is usually done informally, if at all.[101] However, a variety of assessment tools and definitions of outcome are now available for clinicians working with PBD. Using formal outcome assessment will help better gauge treatment response and enable comparisons between clinical practice and the outcomes described in the literature. The clinically significant change model addresses many of the technical shortcomings of other outcome definitions, and it can now be used with many, but not all, outcome measures relevant to PBD. The necessary benchmarks are not available for the CMRS or KSADS-MRS, for example. On the other hand, all of the different definitions could be applied to commonly used broadband and public domain measures of mania and depression using the information in **Table 5**.

Assessment Tools for Maintenance and Relapse Prevention

Longitudinal data indicate that PBD tends to show a recurrent course,[10,11] similar to the high rates of relapse observed in adult samples.[8,20] As treatment progresses, an important component will be planning strategies for monitoring against relapse. Reviewing the life charts and three- or five-column charts would expedite making a list of events likely to trigger exacerbation of mood. There are also normative developmental transitions that are likely to elicit major changes in mood, including the onset of puberty, leaving home, and major role changes such as graduating or failing out of school. Although not all events can be anticipated, many can; and a simple assessment strategy would be to list the likely events and then plan for ways of evaluating mood status when the events arise.

The later phases of treatment can also be a good time to identify warning signs of relapse, or "roughening" of mood.[133] It is helpful to have manic symptoms under control in order to increase insight into the illness. It is also desirable to have some experience working together with the patient, as many of the cues of relapse are not diagnostic symptoms per se, but rather idiosyncratic aspects of the person's functioning.[134,135] A major goal would be to develop warning signs that the patient would use and trust even when getting hypomanic, with the attendant feelings of wellness and loss of insight. An example would be how psychoeducation interventions often help the client learn to use the family or a trusted roommate as a "watchdog" who helps monitor mood.[136]

Given the geographic mobility of both patients and clinicians, a third assessment strategy worth considering is preparing a "care package" for the next clinician as part of the maintenance planning. This care package could be based on a review of the components of treatment, with the patient and practitioner candidly evaluating which were helpful and which were not. Preparing a list of medications tried and responses or adverse events and a list of therapeutic or lifestyle manipulations and their perceived effectiveness would avoid a lot of guesswork and missteps when resuming active treatment in the aftermath of relapse. Patients and practitioners could keep copies of the documentation to increase the chances that it would be available when needed.

Future Assessment Tools

A great deal of research investigates methods that could soon contribute to the diagnostic assessment of PBD. Some of the most exciting research includes neurocognitive testing, functional imaging techniques, and genetic testing. In spite of the promise, expert consensus is that none of these methods are currently ready for clinical use. Recent reviews of neurocognitive tests[137] and neuroimaging[138,139] have found that the replicated patterns of functioning in PBD tend not to be specific to bipolar disorder, but instead overlap with patterns of functioning seen in ADHD, schizophrenia, and other conditions.

Similarly, the present evidence indicates that bipolar disorder is a polygenic condition, with multiple genes, each contributing small increases in the risk of developing the disorder.[140] However, several companies are now marketing direct-to-consumer genetic testing, purportedly including tests for bipolar disorder (eg, https://psynomics.com/). This has provoked strong criticism from the academic community, arguing that it is premature to market tests for bipolar disorder and that the results are highly prone to misinterpretation.[141] The opportunity for misunderstanding is greatest when the results of any of these new methods are treated as yes/no, positive, or negative tests for bipolar disorder. This review has demonstrated that although family history, questionnaires, and rating scales are also imperfect measures, once their biases and limitations become known, it is still possible to assimilate them into an evidence-based framework for assessment.

SUMMARY

The diagnosis of PBD remains controversial. Evidence suggests that it is often diagnosed when not present, and yet many cases of bipolar disorder are also missed. Despite the aura of controversy, there is considerable consensus among experts about the validity of DSM-IV-based diagnoses in youth. Marked progress has also been made in validating and honing assessment strategies for PBD. As this review reveals, it is possible to use the literature to inform choices of assessment techniques that contribute to diagnosis, treatment selection, monitoring progress, evaluating outcomes, and long-term monitoring and relapse prevention. The review also synthesizes the available literature with the clinical decision-making framework advocated in EBM and in the clinically significant change literature in psychotherapy research. Both of these frameworks emphasize decision making about individuals, rather than groups of patients. In consequence, these models speak much more directly to individual clinical care than past research typically has done.

There is no aspect of the assessment of PBD that has been "perfected." Every assessment tool could be bettered, and each technique offers room for improvement. At the same time, the number of tools and ideas now available for clinicians to apply immediately in their clinical practice is impressively large and diverse. The potential gains from employing evidence-based strategies are only hinted at except for in the arena of diagnosis, where recent studies suggest that the contributions could be huge. The goal of clinical research is to answer gaps and uncertainties in clinical practice, and research in PBD is poised to support rapid advances in clinical assessment.

REFERENCES

1. Blader JC, Carlson GA. Increased rates of bipolar disorder diagnoses among U.S. child, adolescent, and adult inpatients, 1996–2004. Biol Psychiatry 2007; 62:107.
2. Moreno C, Laje G, Blanco C, et al. National trends in the outpatient diagnosis and treatment of bipolar disorder in youth. Arch Gen Psychiatry 2007;64:1032.
3. Healy D. The latest mania: selling bipolar disorder. PLoS Med 2006;3:e185.
4. Klein RG, Pine DS, Klein DF. Resolved: mania is mistaken for ADHD in prepubertal children. J Am Acad Child Adolesc Psychiatry 1998;37:1093.
5. Faraone SV, Glatt SJ, Tsuang MT. The genetics of pediatric-onset bipolar disorder. Biol Psychiatry 2003;53:970.
6. Geller B, Tillman R. Prepubertal and early adolescent bipolar I disorder: review of diagnostic validation by Robins and Guze criteria. J Clin Psychiatry 2005; 66(Suppl 7):21.
7. Youngstrom EA, Birmaher B, Findling RL. Pediatric bipolar disorder: validity, phenomenology, and recommendations for diagnosis. Bipolar Disord 2008;10:194.
8. Goodwin FK, Jamison KR. Manic-depressive illness. 2nd edition. New York: Oxford University Press; 2007.
9. Perlis R, Miyahara S, Marangell LB, et al. Long-term implications of early onset in bipolar disorder: data from the first 1000 participants in the systematic treatment enhancement program for bipolar disorder (STEP-BD). Biol Psychiatry 2004;55: 875.
10. Birmaher B, Axelson D, Strober M, et al. Clinical course of children and adolescents with bipolar spectrum disorders. Arch Gen Psychiatry 2006;63:175.

11. Geller B, Tillman R, Bolhofner K, et al. Child bipolar I disorder: prospective continuity with adult bipolar I disorder; characteristics of second and third episodes; predictors of 8-year outcome. Arch Gen Psychiatry 2008;65:1125.
12. Lewinsohn PM, Seeley JR, Buckley ME, et al. Bipolar disorder in adolescence and young adulthood. Child Adolesc Psychiatr Clin N Am 2002;11:461.
13. Camara W, Nathan J, Puente A. Psychological test usage in professional psychology: report of the APA practice and science directorates. Washington, DC: American Psychological Association; 1998. p. 51.
14. Youngstrom EA. Pediatric bipolar disorder. In: Mash EJ, Barkley RA, editors. Assessment of childhood disorders. 4th edition. New York: Guilford Press; 2007. p. 253.
15. Youngstrom EA. Evidence-based strategies for the assessment of developmental psychopathology: measuring prediction, prescription, and process. In: Miklowitz DJ, Craighead WE, Craighead L, editors. Developmental psychopathology. New York: Wiley; 2008. p. 34.
16. World Health Organization. The ICD-10 classification of mental and behavioural disorders: clinical descriptions and diagnostic guidelines. London: World Health Organization; 1992.
17. American Psychiatric Association. Diagnostic and statistical manual of mental disorders. 4th edition, Text Revision. Washington, DC: Author; 2001.
18. Ghaemi SN, Bauer M, Cassidy F, et al. Diagnostic guidelines for bipolar disorder: a summary of the International Society for Bipolar Disorders Diagnostic Guidelines Task Force Report. Bipolar Disord 2008;10:117.
19. Judd LL, Akiskal HS, Schettler PJ, et al. Psychosocial disability in the course of bipolar I and II disorders: a prospective, comparative, longitudinal study. Arch Gen Psychiatry 2005;62:1322.
20. Kraepelin E. Manic-depressive insanity and paranoia. Edinburgh: Livingstone; 1921.
21. Berk M, Dodd S. Bipolar II disorder: a review. Bipolar Disord 2005;7:11.
22. Akiskal HS, Pinto O. The soft bipolar spectrum: footnotes to Kraepelin on the interface of hypomania, temperament and depression. In: Marneros A, Angst J, editors. Bipolar disorders: 100 years after manic depressive insanity. Norwell (MA)/Netherlands: Kluwer Academic Publishers; 2000. p. 37.
23. Youngstrom EA, Youngstrom JK, Starr M. Bipolar diagnoses in community mental health: Achenbach CBCL Profiles and Patterns of Comorbidity. Biol Psychiatry 2005;58:569.
24. Merikangas KR, Akiskal HS, Angst J, et al. Lifetime and 12-month prevalence of bipolar spectrum disorder in the National Comorbidity Survey replication. Arch Gen Psychiatry 2007;64:543.
25. Grant BF, Stinson FS, Hasin DS, et al. Prevalence, correlates, and comorbidity of bipolar I disorder and axis I and II disorders: results from the National Epidemiologic Survey on Alcohol and related conditions. J Clin Psychiatry 2005;66: 1205.
26. Findling RL, Youngstrom EA, McNamara NK, et al. Early symptoms of mania and the role of parental risk. Bipolar Disord 2005;7:623.
27. Findling RL, Frazier TW, Youngstrom EA, et al. Double-blind, placebo-controlled trial of divalproex monotherapy in the treatment of symptomatic youth at high risk for developing bipolar disorder. J Clin Psychiatry 2007;68:781.
28. Kochman FJ, Hantouche E, Ferrari P, et al. Cyclothymic temperament as a prospective predictor of bipolarity and suicidality in children and adolescents with major depressive disorder. J Affect Disord 2005;85:181.

29. Hantouche EG, Akiskal HS. Toward a definition of a cyclothymic behavioral endophenotype: which traits tap the familial diathesis for bipolar II disorder? J Affect Disord 2006;96:233.
30. Klein DN, Depue RA, Slater JF. Inventory identification of cyclothymia. IX. Validation in offspring of bipolar I patients. Arch Gen Psychiatry 1986;43:441.
31. Alloy LB, Abramson LY, Walshaw PD, et al. Behavioral Approach System and Behavioral Inhibition System sensitivities and bipolar spectrum disorders: prospective prediction of bipolar mood episodes. Bipolar Disord 2008;10:310.
32. Danielson CK, Youngstrom EA, Findling RL, et al. Discriminative validity of the General Behavior Inventory using youth report. J Abnorm Child Psychol 2003;31:29.
33. Youngstrom EA, Findling RL, Danielson CK, et al. Discriminative validity of parent report of hypomanic and depressive symptoms on the general behavior inventory. Psychol Assess 2001;13:267.
34. Depue RA, Slater JF, Wolfstetter-Kausch H, et al. A behavioral paradigm for identifying persons at risk for bipolar depressive disorder: a conceptual framework and five validation studies. J Abnorm Psychol 1981;90:381.
35. Judd LL, Akiskal HS. The prevalence and disability of bipolar spectrum disorders in the US population: re-analysis of the ECA database taking into account subthreshold cases. J Affect Disord 2003;73:123.
36. Merikangas KR, Herrell R, Swendsen J, et al. Specificity of bipolar spectrum conditions in the comorbidity of mood and substance use disorders: results from the Zurich cohort study. Arch Gen Psychiatry 2008;65:47.
37. Axelson DA, Birmaher B, Strober M, et al. Phenomenology of children and adolescents with bipolar spectrum disorders. Arch Gen Psychiatry 2006;63: 1139.
38. Joseph M, Youngstrom EA, Soares JC. Antidepressant-Coincident Mania in Children and Adolescents Treated with Selective Serotonin Reuptake Inhibitors. Future Neurology Review, in press.
39. Leibenluft E, Charney DS, Towbin KE, et al. Defining clinical phenotypes of juvenile mania. Am J Psychiatry 2003;160:430.
40. Kowatch RA, Youngstrom EA, Danielyan A, et al. Review and meta-analysis of the phenomenology and clinical characteristics of mania in children and adolescents. Bipolar Disord 2005;7:483.
41. Youngstrom EA. Definitional issues in bipolar disorder across the life cycle. Clinical Psychology. Science & Practice, in press.
42. Stedman JM, Hatch JP, Schoenfeld LS. The current status of psychological assessment training in graduate and professional schools. J Pers Assess 2001;77:398.
43. Meyer SE, Carlson GA, Youngstrom E, et al. Long-term outcomes of youth who manifested the CBCL-pediatric bipolar disorder phenotype during childhood and/or adolescence. J Affect Disord 2008.
44. Lewinsohn PM, Klein DN, Seeley J. Bipolar disorder during adolescence and young adulthood in a community sample. Bipolar Disord 2000;2:281.
45. Tsuchiya KJ, Byrne M, Mortensen PB. Risk factors in relation to an emergence of bipolar disorder: a systematic review. Bipolar Disord 2003;5:231.
46. Hodgins S, Faucher B, Zarac A, et al. Children of parents with bipolar disorder. A population at high risk for major affective disorders. Child Adolesc Psychiatr Clin N Am 2002;11:533.
47. Smoller JW, Finn CT. Family, twin, and adoption studies of bipolar disorder. Am J Med Genet C Semin Med Genet 2003;123C:48.

48. Youngstrom EA, Duax J. Evidence based assessment of pediatric bipolar disorder, part 1: base rate and family history. J Am Acad Child Adolesc Psychiatry 2005;44:712.
49. Youngstrom EA, Findling RL, Youngstrom JK, et al. Toward an evidence-based assessment of pediatric bipolar disorder. J Clin Child Adolesc Psychol 2005; 34:433.
50. Strakowski SM, Flaum M, Amador X, et al. Racial differences in the diagnosis of psychosis. Schizophr Res 1996;21:117.
51. DelBello MP, Lopez-Larson MP, Soutullo CA, et al. Effects of race on psychiatric diagnosis of hospitalized adolescents: a retrospective chart review. J Child Adolesc Psychopharmacol 2001;11:95.
52. Duffy A, Alda M, Kutcher S, et al. Psychiatric symptoms and syndromes among adolescent children of parents with lithium-responsive or lithium-nonresponsive bipolar disorder. Am J Psychiatry 1998;155:431.
53. Straus SE, Richardson WS, Glasziou P, et al. Evidence-based medicine: how to practice and teach EBM. 3rd edition. New York: Churchill Livingstone; 2005.
54. Meehl PE. Clinical versus statistical prediction: a theoretical analysis and a review of the evidence. Minneapolis: University of Minnesota Press; 1954.
55. Dawes RM, Faust D, Meehl PE. Clinical versus actuarial judgment. Science 1989;243:1668.
56. Grove WM, Meehl PE. Comparative efficiency of informal (subjective, impressionistic) and formal (mechanical, algorithmic) prediction procedures: the clinical-statistical controversy. Psychology, Public Policy, and Law 1996;2:293.
57. Gigerenzer G, Hoffrage U. How to improve Bayesian reasoning without instruction: frequency formats. Psychol Rev 1995;102:684.
58. Davidow J, Levinson EM. Heuristic principles and cognitive bias in decision making: implications for assessment in school psychology. Psychology in the Schools 1993;30:351.
59. Gigerenzer G. The adaptive toolbox: toward a Darwinian rationality. Nebr Symp Motiv 2001;47:113.
60. Lish JD, Dime-Meenan S, Whybrow PC, et al. The National Depressive and Manic-Depressive Association (DMDA) survey of bipolar members. J Affect Disord 1994;31:281.
61. Hirschfeld RM, Lewis L, Vornik LA. Perceptions and impact of bipolar disorder: how far have we really come? Results of the national depressive and manic-depressive association 2000 survey of individuals with bipolar disorder. J Clin Psychiatry 2003;64:161.
62. Kessler RC, Rubinow DR, Holmes C, et al. The epidemiology of DSM-III-R bipolar I disorder in a general population survey. Psychol Med 1997;27:1079.
63. Zuckerman M. Vulnerability to psychopathology: a biosocial model. Washington, DC: American Psychological Association; 1999.
64. Youngstrom JK, Youngstrom EA. Bipolar disorder underdiagnosed in community mental health. Presented at the Biennial Meeting of the International Society of Bipolar Disorders. Delhi, India; February 2008.
65. Dubicka B, Carlson GA, Vail A, et al. Prepubertal mania: diagnostic differences between US and UK clinicians. Eur Child Adolesc Psychiatry 2008;17:153.
66. Mackin P, Targum SD, Kalali A, et al. Culture and assessment of manic symptoms. Br J Psychiatry 2006;189:379.
67. Jenkins M, Youngstrom JK, Perez Algorta G, et al. How the nomogram improves interpretation of assessment information by clinicians in the community. In

Annual Convention of the Association for Behavioral and Cognitive Therapy. Orlando (FL), November 2008.

68. Achenbach TM, Rescorla LA. Manual for the ASEBA school-age forms & profiles. Burlington (VT): University of Vermont; 2001.

69. Gadow KD, Sprafkin J. Child symptom inventories manual. Stony Brook (NY): Checkmate Plus; 1994.

70. Reynolds CR, Kamphaus R. BASC-2 behavior assessment system for children. Circle Pines (MN): AGS; 2004.

71. Mick E, Biederman J, Pandina G, et al. A preliminary meta-analysis of the child behavior checklist in pediatric bipolar disorder. Biol Psychiatry 2003;53:1021.

72. Kahana SY, Youngstrom EA, Findling RL, et al. Employing parent, teacher, and youth self-report checklists in identifying pediatric bipolar spectrum disorders: an examination of diagnostic accuracy and clinical utility. J Child Adolesc Psychopharmacol 2003;13:471.

73. Youngstrom EA, Findling RL, Calabrese JR, et al. Comparing the diagnostic accuracy of six potential screening instruments for bipolar disorder in youths aged 5 to 17 years. J Am Acad Child Adolesc Psychiatry 2004;43:847.

74. Sackett DL, Straus SE, Richardson WS, et al. Evidence-based medicine: how to practice and teach EBM. 2nd edition. New York: Churchill Livingstone; 2000.

75. Scheffer RE, Kowatch RA, Carmody T, et al. Randomized, placebo-controlled trial of mixed amphetamine salts for symptoms of comorbid ADHD in pediatric bipolar disorder after mood stabilization with divalproex sodium. Am J Psychiatry 2005;162:58.

76. Findling RL, McNamara NK, Gracious BL, et al. Combination lithium and divalproex in pediatric bipolarity. J Am Acad Child Adolesc Psychiatry 2003; 42:895.

77. Findling RL, McNamara NK, Stansbrey R, et al. Combination lithium and divalproex sodium in pediatric bipolar symptom restabilization. J Am Acad Child Adolesc Psychiatry 2006;45:142.

78. Miklowitz DJ, Chang KD. Prevention of bipolar disorder in at-risk children: theoretical assumptions and empirical foundations. Dev Psychopathol 2008;20:881.

79. Fristad MA. Psychoeducational treatment for school-aged children with bipolar disorder. Dev Psychopathol 2006;18:1289.

80. Youngstrom EA, Frazier TW, Findling RL, et al. Developing a ten item short form of the parent general behavior inventory to assess for juvenile mania and hypomania. Journal of Clinical Psychiatry 2008;69:831–9.

81. Wagner KD, Findling RL, Emslie GJ, et al. Validation of the mood disorder questionnaire for bipolar disorders in adolescents. J Clin Psychiatry 2006;67:827.

82. Youngstrom EA, Meyers OI, Demeter C, et al. Comparing diagnostic checklists for pediatric bipolar disorder in academic and community mental health settings. Bipolar Disord 2005;7:507.

83. Pavuluri MN, Henry DB, Devineni B, et al. Child mania rating scale: development, reliability, and validity. J Am Acad Child Adolesc Psychiatry 2006;45:550.

84. Henry DB, Pavuluri MN, Youngstrom E, et al. Accuracy of brief and full forms of the Child Mania Rating Scale. J Clin Psychol 2008;64:368.

85. Youngstrom EA, Meyers OI, Youngstrom JK, et al. Comparing the effects of sampling designs on the diagnostic accuracy of eight promising screening algorithms for pediatric bipolar disorder. Biol Psychiatry 2006;60:1013.

86. Bossuyt PM, Reitsma JB, Bruns DE, et al. Towards complete and accurate reporting of studies of diagnostic accuracy: the STARD initiative. Ann Intern Med 2003;138:40.

87. Youngstrom EA, Kogos Youngstrom J. Evidence based assessment of pediatric bipolar disorder, part 2: incorporating information from behavior checklists. J Am Acad Child Adolesc Psychiatry 2005;44:823.
88. Sechrest L, Davis MF, Stickle TR, et al. Understanding "method" variance. In: Bickman L, editor. Research design: Donald Campbell's legacy. Newbury Park (CA): Sage; 2000. p. 63–88.
89. Geller B, Warner K, Williams M, et al. Prepubertal and young adolescent bipolarity versus ADHD: assessment and validity using the WASH-U-KSADS, CBCL and TRF. J Affect Disord 1998;51:93.
90. Hazell PL, Lewin TJ, Carr VJ. Confirmation that Child Behavior Checklist clinical scales discriminate juvenile mania from attention deficit hyperactivity disorder. J Paediatr Child Health 1999;35:199.
91. Youngstrom EA, Meyers O, Youngstrom JK, et al. Diagnostic and measurement issues in the assessment of pediatric bipolar disorder: implications for understanding mood disorder across the life cycle. Dev Psychopathol 2006;18:989.
92. Loeber R, Green SM, Lahey BB. Mental health professionals' perception of the utility of children, mothers, and teachers as informants on childhood psychopathology. J Clin Child Psychol 1990;19:136.
93. Dell'Osso L, Pini S, Cassano GB, et al. Insight into illness in patients with mania, mixed mania, bipolar depression and major depression with psychotic features. Bipolar Disord 2002;4:315.
94. Youngstrom EA, Findling RL, Calabrese JR. Effects of adolescent manic symptoms on agreement between youth, parent, and teacher ratings of behavior problems. J Affect Disord 2004;82:S5.
95. Youngstrom EA, Joseph MF, Greene J. Comparing the psychometric properties of multiple teacher report instruments as predictors of bipolar disorder in children and adolescents. J Clin Psychol 2008;64:382.
96. Achenbach TM, McConaughy SH, Howell CT. Child/adolescent behavioral and emotional problems: implication of cross-informant correlations for situational specificity. Psychol Bull 1987;101:213.
97. Carlson GA, Youngstrom EA. Clinical implications of pervasive manic symptoms in children. Biol Psychiatry 2003;53:1050.
98. Kraemer HC, Lowe KK, Kupfer DJ. To your health: how to understand what research tells us about risk. New York: Oxford University Press; 2005.
99. Kowatch RA, Fristad MA, Birmaher B, et al. Treatment guidelines for children and adolescents with bipolar disorder. J Am Acad Child Adolesc Psychiatry 2005;44:213.
100. Mechanic D. Mental health and social policy. Englewood Cliffs (NJ): Prentice-Hall, Inc.; 1989.
101. Garb HN. Studying the clinician: judgment research and psychological assessment. Washington, DC: American Psychological Association; 1998.
102. Nottelmann E, Biederman J, Birmaher B, et al. National Institute of Mental Health research roundtable on prepubertal bipolar disorder. J Am Acad Child Adolesc Psychiatry 2001;40:871.
103. Kaufman J, Birmaher B, Brent D, et al. Schedule for Affective Disorders and Schizophrenia for School-Age Children-Present and Lifetime version (K-SADS-PL): initial reliability and validity data. J Am Acad Child Adolesc Psychiatry 1997;36:980.
104. Geller B, Zimerman B, Williams M, et al. Reliability of the Washington University in St. Louis Kiddie Schedule for Affective Disorders and Schizophrenia

(WASH-U-KSADS) mania and rapid cycling sections. J Am Acad Child Adolesc Psychiatry 2001;40:450.

105. Weller EB, Weller RA, Fristad MA, et al. Children's interview for psychiatric syndromes (ChIPS). J Am Acad Child Adolesc Psychiatry 2000;39:76.

106. Geller B, Zimerman B, Williams M, et al. Phenomenology of prepubertal and early adolescent bipolar disorder: examples of elated mood, grandiose behaviors, decreased need for sleep, racing thoughts and hypersexuality. J Child Adolesc Psychopharmacol 2002;12:3.

107. Galanter CA, Leibenluft E. Frontiers between attention deficit hyperactivity disorder and bipolar disorder. Child Adolesc Psychiatr Clin N Am 2008;17:325.

108. Quinn CA, Fristad MA. Defining and identifying early onset bipolar spectrum disorder. Curr Psychiatry Rep 2004;6:101.

109. Masi G, Perugi G, Millepiedi S, et al. Clinical implications of DSM-IV subtyping of bipolar disorders in referred children and adolescents. J Am Acad Child Adolesc Psychiatry 2007;46:1299.

110. Denicoff KD, Smith-Jackson EE, Disney ER, et al. Preliminary evidence of the reliability and validity of the prospective life-chart methodology (LCM-p). J Psychiatr Res 1997;31:593.

111. Shaffer D, Gould MS, Brasic J, et al. A children's global assessment scale (CGAS). Arch Gen Psychiatry 1983;40:1228.

112. National Institute of Mental Health. Rating scales and assessment instruments for use in pediatric psychopharmacology research. Psychopharmacol Bull 1985;21:839.

113. Young RC, Biggs JT, Ziegler VE, et al. A rating scale for mania: reliability, validity, and sensitivity. Br J Psychiatry 1978;133:429.

114. Poznanski EO, Miller E, Salguero C, et al. Preliminary studies of the reliability and validity of the children's depression rating scale. J Am Acad Child Psychiatry 1984;23:191.

115. Fristad MA, Weller EB, Weller RA. The mania rating scale: can it be used in children? A preliminary report. J Am Acad Child Adolesc Psychiatry 1992;31:252.

116. Fristad MA, Weller RA, Weller EB. The mania rating scale (MRS): further reliability and validity studies with children. Ann Clin Psychiatry 1995;7:127.

117. Youngstrom EA, Danielson CK, Findling RL, et al. Factor structure of the Young Mania Rating Scale for use with youths ages 5 to 17 years. J Clin Child Adolesc Psychol 2002;31:567.

118. Axelson DA, Birmaher BJ, Brent D, et al. A preliminary study of the Kiddie Schedule for Affective Disorders and Schizophrenia for School-Age Children mania rating scale for children and adolescents. J Child Adolesc Psychopharmacol 2003;13:463.

119. Rademacher J, DelBello MP, Adler C, et al. Health-related quality of life in adolescents with bipolar I disorder. J Child Adolesc Psychopharmacol 2007;17:97.

120. Freeman A, Youngstrom EA, Michalak EE, et al. Quality of life in pediatric bipolar disorder. Pediatrics, in press.

121. Danielson CK, Feeny NC, Findling RL, et al. Psychosocial Treatment of Bipolar Disorders in Adolescents: a Proposed Cognitive-Behavioral Intervention. Cogn Behav Pract 2004;11:283.

122. Newman CF, Leahy RL, Beck AT, et al. Bipolar disorder: a cognitive therapy approach. Washington, DC: American Psychological Association; 2002.

123. Wilens TE. Straight talk about psychiatric medications for kids. revised edition. New York: Guilford Press; 2004.

124. Streiner DL, Norman GR. Health measurement scales: a practical guide to their development and use. 2nd edition. New York: Oxford University Press; 1995.
125. Venter A, Maxwell SE. Maximizing power in randomized designs when N is small. In: Hoyle RH, editor. Statistical strategies for small sample research. Thousand Oaks (CA): Sage Publications; 1999. p. 31.
126. Kafantaris V. Treatment of bipolar disorder in children and adolescents. J Am Acad Child Adolesc Psychiatry 1995;34:732.
127. Kowatch RA, Sethuraman G, Hume JH, et al. Combination pharmacotherapy in children and adolescents with bipolar disorder. Biol Psychiatry 2003;53:978.
128. Patel NC, Patrick DM, Youngstrom EA, et al. Response and remission in adolescent mania: signal detection analyses of the Young Mania Rating Scale. J Am Acad Child Adolesc Psychiatry 2007;46:628.
129. Frank E, Prien RF, Jarrett RB, et al. Conceptualization and rationale for consensus definitions of terms in major depressive disorder. Remission, recovery, relapse, and recurrence. Arch Gen Psychiatry 1991;48:851.
130. Jacobson NS, Truax P. Clinical significance: a statistical approach to defining meaningful change in psychotherapy research. J Consult Clin Psychol 1991;59:12.
131. Cooperberg MD. Characterizing clinical change in youths with bipolar disorders. United States – Ohio: Case Western Reserve University; 2004.
132. Youngstrom EA, Cooperberg M, Findling RL, et al. Identifying the Most Sensitive Outcome Measure for Pediatric Bipolar Disorder. Presented at the Annual meeting of the American Academy of Child and Adolescent Psychiatry, Miami Beach, FL; October 2003.
133. Sachs GS. Strategies for improving treatment of bipolar disorder: integration of measurement and management. Acta Psychiatr Scand 2004;422.
134. Jamison KR. An unquiet mind: a memoir of moods and madness. New York: Vintage Books; 1995.
135. Hinshaw SP. Parental mental disorder and children's functioning: silence and communication, stigma and resilience. J Clin Child Adolesc Psychol 2004;33:400.
136. Miklowitz DJ, Biuckians A, Richards JA. Early-onset bipolar disorder: a family treatment perspective. Dev Psychopathol 2006;18:1247.
137. Joseph M, Frazier TW, Youngstrom EA, et al. A quantitative and qualitative review of neurocognitive performance in pediatric bipolar disorder. Journal of Child & Adolescent Psychopharmacology 2008:18:595–605.
138. Chang K, Adleman N, Wagner C, et al. Will neuroimaging ever be used to diagnose pediatric bipolar disorder? Dev Psychopathol 2006;18:1133.
139. DelBello MP, Kowatch RA. Neuroimaging in pediatric bipolar disorder. In: Geller B, DelBello MP, editors. Bipolar disorder in childhood and early adolescence. New York: Guilford; 2003. p. 158.
140. WTCCC. Genome-wide association study of 14,000 cases of seven common diseases and 3,000 shared controls. Nature 2007;447:661.
141. Braff DL, Freedman R. Clinically responsible genetic testing in neuropsychiatric patients: a bridge too far and too soon. Am J Psychiatry 2008;165:952.
142. Pine DS, Cohen P, Gurley D, et al. The risk for early-adulthood anxiety and depressive disorders in adolescents with anxiety and depressive disorders. Arch Gen Psychiatry 1998;55:56.
143. Geller B, Craney JL, Bolhofner K, et al. Two-year prospective follow-up of children with a prepubertal and early adolescent bipolar disorder phenotype. Am J Psychiatry 2002;159:927.
144. Naylor MW, Anderson TR, Kruesi MJ, et al. Pharmacoepidemiology of bipolar disorder in abused and neglected state wards. Presented at the National

Meeting of the American Academy of Child and Adolescent Psychiatry, San Francisco; October 2002.

145. Biederman J, Faraone S, Mick E, et al. Attention-deficit hyperactivity disorder and juvenile mania: an overlooked comorbidity? J Am Acad Child Adolesc Psychiatry 1996;35:997.

146. Teplin LA, Abram KM, McClelland GM, et al. Psychiatric disorders in youth in juvenile detention. Arch Gen Psychiatry 2002;59:1133.

147. Pliszka SR, Sherman JO, Barrow MV, et al. Affective disorder in juvenile offenders: a preliminary study. Am J Psychiatry 2000;157:130.

148. Birmaher B, Ryan ND, Williamson DE, et al. Childhood and adolescent depression: a review of the past 10 years. Part I. J Am Acad Child Adolesc Psychiatry 1996;35:1427.

149. Tillman R, Geller B, Klages T, et al. Psychotic phenomena in 257 young children and adolescents with bipolar I disorder: delusions and hallucinations (benign and pathological). Bipolar Disord 2008;10:45.

150. Achenbach TM. Manual for the child behavior checklist/4-18 and 1991 profile. Burlington: University of Vermont, Department of Psychiatry; 1991.

151. Achenbach TM. Manual for the Youth Self Report form and 1991 profile. Burlington: University of Vermont, Department of Psychiatry; 1991.

152. Achenbach TM. Manual for the Teacher's Report Form and 1991 profile. Burlington: University of Vermont, Department of Psychiatry; 1991.

153. Gracious BL, Youngstrom EA, Findling RL, et al. Discriminative validity of a parent version of the Young Mania Rating Scale. J Am Acad Child Adolesc Psychiatry 2002;41:1350.

154. Hirschfeld RM, Williams JBW, Spitzer RL, et al. Development and validation of a screening instrument for bipolar spectrum disorder: the mood disorder questionnaire. Am J Psychiatry 2000;157:1873.

155. Tillman R, Geller B. A brief screening tool for a prepubertal and early adolescent bipolar disorder phenotype. Am J Psychiatry 2005;162:1214.

156. Papolos DF, Papolos J. The bipolar child: the definitive and reassuring guide to childhood's most misunderstood disorder. 2nd edition. New York: Broadway Books; 2002.

157. Papolos DF, Hennen J, Cockerham MS, et al. The child bipolar questionnaire: a dimensional approach to screening for pediatric bipolar disorder. J Affect Disord 2006;95:149.

158. Sackett DL, Straus SE, Richardson WS, et al. Evidence-based medicine: how to practice and teach EBM. New York: Churchill Livingstone; 1998.

159. Beck AT, Steer RA. Beck depression inventory manual. San Antonio (TX): The Psychological Corporation; 1987.

Preschool Bipolar Disorder

Joan L. Luby, MD*, Mini Tandon, DO, Andy Belden, PhD

KEYWORDS

• Preschool • Bipolar • Mania

Despite significant progress over the last decade in the characterization and validation of numerous forms of preschool psychopathology, the area of bipolar disorder remains perhaps the most controversial. The difficulty of distinguishing normative extremes in mood intensity and lability known to characterize early childhood from those emotions and behaviors that cross the threshold into clinically significant psychopathology is a central issue. Further, another fundamental problem is the ongoing lack of clarity about the diagnostic criteria and validity of the diagnosis in older children, as phenotypes in older children are a key source for the downward extension of nosologies in the preschool period. Along this line, contrasting definitions of bipolar disorder in children and adolescents have been proposed and tested. This definitional debate remains a salient issue in the existing literature. Questions about the basic validity of the diagnosis in children, its temporal features, and continuity into adulthood, as well as treatment are only a few key areas debated in both the psychiatric literature and in public forums.[1]

While a growing body of empirical research is available to inform these issues in older children, studies in preschoolers remain scarce. Along this line, the studies that are available in preschoolers with suspected bipolar disorder are limited predominantly to case reports and chart reviews. There is a smaller body of systematic literature, but many of these studies are limited by retrospective designs with small sample size. In 2007, for example Danielyan and colleagues[2] reviewed 26 outpatient charts of preschoolers referred to a psychiatric clinic and diagnosed bipolar and found high recovery and relapse rates. Similarly, Ferreira Maia and colleagues[3] also retrospectively reviewed outpatient charts in a mood disorders clinic and found preschoolers to have classic symptoms of mania, but the reports were also limited by the small sample size of preschoolers who met Diagnostic and Statistical Manual of Mental Disorders, 4th edition (DSM-IV), bipolar disorder criteria (n = 8). Classic

---

Funding for the study of preschool depression and for preparation of this manuscript was provided by NIMH R01 MH64769-01 and 02 grant to Joan Luby, MD.

Washington University School of Medicine in St. Louis, Department of Psychiatry, 660 S. Euclid, Box 8134, St. Louis, MO 63110, USA

* Corresponding author.

E-mail address: lubyj@psychiatry.wustl.edu (J.L. Luby).

features of mania such as elation, grandiosity, psychomotor agitation, and decreased need for sleep were also observed by Dilsaver and Akiskal [4] over a 2-year period, and a family history notable for affective illness was described. Three presumptive cases of preschool bipolar disorder were also described, with subjects having classic symptoms or "cardinal features," by Luby and colleagues,[5] but these cases were from a specialty preschool mood disorders clinic and with potentially limited generalizability. One larger systematic study of preschoolers in a community-based sample investigated the presence of age-adjusted mania symptoms.[6] Ironically, there is a somewhat larger body of literature on treatment in preschoolers, although this is limited to case reports and retrospective chart reviews, with only a couple of open label investigations available to date.

REVIEW OF NOSOLOGY IN OLDER CHILDREN: IMPLICATIONS FOR STUDY OF PRESCHOOLERS

Amid the ongoing debate on the appropriate criteria for diagnosis in older children, the rate of clinical diagnosis of bipolar disorder in children has increased 40-fold between 1994 and 2003.[7] The precise source of this increase in diagnosis remain unclear. However, there is significant concern that the diagnosis may be liberally and nonspecifically applied in many cases. Multiple perspectives exist as to which primary symptoms best characterize the disorder and importantly how to distinguish it from other disruptive behavioral disorders, especially attention-deficit hyperactivity disorder (ADHD).[8–11] Geller and colleagues[12] have provided empirical data suggesting that all DSM-IV symptom criteria, but not standard discrete episode criteria, must be met to make the diagnosis in childhood. This group has provided data suggesting that the cardinal features of mania, elation, grandiosity, hypersexuality, flight of ideas (racing thoughts), and increased energy along with decreased need for sleep are the best discriminators from ADHD. While some argue that irritability is a highly nonspecific symptom in childhood psychopathology, others suggest that "extreme irritability" is a key marker of the disorder in childhood.[13,14] Others have suggested that the irritability is a nonspecific feature of many childhood psychiatric disorders and therefore cannot be used as a marker of childhood bipolar disorder.[12,15] Leibenluft and colleagues[16] have proposed another view, outlined below, in which a distinction between broad and narrow phenotypes is made.

SYMPTOM DURATION AND FREQUENCY CRITERIA IN OLDER CHILDREN

In addition to questions about the most sensitive and specific symptom criteria for diagnosis, the duration and related temporal features of these symptoms are also an area of debate. The question of whether the same duration criteria for adult bipolar disorder should be applied to children is currently unclear. Leibenluft and colleagues[16] have suggested that only those children who meet full symptom criteria and who demonstrate discrete episodes of mania would be designated as "bipolar," also referred to as the "narrow" phenotype. Alternatively, the "broad" phenotype encompasses those who have a chronic, nonepisodic illness characterized by irritability and hyperarousal but do not necessarily manifest cardinal features of mania (elation and grandiosity). In addition to the narrow and broad phenotypes, they suggested two intermediate groups: the first includes those with shorter duration criteria of 1–3 days including distinct manic episodes; the second incorporates distinct episodes of severe irritability but not "cardinal" mania symptoms of elation and grandiosity.[16]

Modification of duration criteria more appropriate for children has been suggested by several additional research groups who studied the disorder in school-age children.[15,17,18] More specifically, Tillman and Geller[18] have described and distinguished between *episodes* and *cycling*. *Episodes* are used to describe the entire duration of illness, whereas *cycling* refers to fluctuations of mood within an episode. Tilllman and Geller[18] adapted definitions from Kramlinger and Post[19] and redefined what was previously referred to as *rapid cycling* as four or more episodes in a year; *ultra-rapid* as mood fluctuations every few days to a few weeks, and fluctuation within 1 day as *ultradian cycling*. Their data suggest that children typically have a more none-pisodic, chronic course than that of older adolescents and adults who often have distinct episodes of fluctuation in mood.[15,18] This apparent developmental difference in the phenomenology of prepubertal bipolar disorder suggests that assuming that adult-based criteria can be simply extrapolated to children is unwise. Along this line, even greater caution in the generalization of adult-based phenomenology to the youngest of children is also advisable.

EMERGING LITERATURE IN PRESCHOOLERS

While there is a dearth of studies that have systematically studied mania symptoms in preschoolers as outlined above, the existing literature has begun to shed some light on this area of early psychopathology. Developmental manifestations of mania symp-toms among preschool-aged children have been described in case reports of preschoolers with suspected bipolar disorder. For example, common among these case reports are observations of excessive energy, decreased need for sleep, impair-ing elation, as well as hypersexuality although the latter appears perhaps less common than the others. Furthermore, these preschoolers were generally described as highly impaired and challenging to treat. Historically, case histories have depicted presumptively manic, impaired preschoolers as far back as the late 1880s.[20–24]

Between 2003 and 2007, increasing numbers of published case series describing mania manifestations during the preschool period have emerged.[2–5,25] Tumuluru and colleagues[25] described mania in six hospitalized preschoolers who had irritable but not elated mood and decreased need for sleep, with significant impairment leading to hospitalization. They further noted that all met DSM criteria for ADHD at some time point as well; further, all six children were described to have a strong family history of affective illness. Similarly, family history of affective illness was also noted in an additional open case series of community mental health clinic patients with mania, but in contrast to the former study, more classical features of mania were described, including elation.[4] Elation and other age-adjusted classical features of mania were described in a series of suspected bipolar disorder cases in several outpatient specialty mood disorders clinics;[3,5] these studies also reported family history of affec-tive illness in the affected preschoolers.

Conversely, aggression and irritability were the most common symptoms reported among presumptive bipolar preschoolers in a chart review of 26 outpatients.[2] This review contributed to the literature by noting high relapse rates defined as meeting hypomania or mania criteria along with moderate symptoms requiring intervention as rated by the Clinical Global Impression Severity-Scale (greater than or equal to five and minimally improved for at least 2 weeks) of these preschoolers with suspected bipolar disorder based on an outpatient record review.[2] The phenomenology of preschoolers with presumptive bipolar disorder has been detailed in a systematic investigation in 2006, outlined below.[6]

Luby and Belden[6] reported on a sub-group (n = 26) of preschoolers meeting symp-tom criteria for bipolar disorder I from a larger community-based sample (n = 306) that was over sampled for preschoolers with mood symptoms. An age-appropriate parent informant diagnostic measure was used to assess for mania symptoms. This specific mania module was developed in collaboration with the authors of the Preschool Age Psychiatric Assessment (PAPA)[26,27] to ascertain DSM-IV bipolar symptoms in a developmentally appropriate manner. Favorable test-retest reliability of the mania module of the PAPA have been established and reported elsewhere.[6] The characteristics of this group and the symptoms that distinguished them from both depressed and disruptive preschoolers were described. The study findings indicated that 5 out of 13 DSM-IV bipolar symptoms, including elation, grandiosity, hypertalkativeness, flight of ideas, and hypersexuality, could differentiate preschoolers with bipolar disorder from those with disruptive disorders (ADHD, oppositional defiant disorder [ODD], and/or conduct disorder [CD]) 92% of the time.[6] Most notably, the bipolar group was not only found to be more impaired than healthy but, notably, also more impaired than preschoolers with other Axis I psychiatric disorders (major depressive disorder (MDD) and DSM-IV disruptive groups). This finding emerged even after controlling for comorbid disorders (important due to high rates of comorbidity found and well known in childhood disorders). This sample has been followed longitudinally more than 2 years, and longitudinal stability of the bipolar diagnosis has been demonstrated. For example, results indicated that preschoolers diagnosed with bipolar disorder at wave one were at 12 times greater risk than non-bipolar preschoolers to be diagnosed with bipolar disorder when assessed 2 years later.[28] Longitudinal data pertaining to symptoms, psychosocial functioning, and family history of psychiatric disorders in this population assessed at preschool age are currently being obtained at school-age in the study population.

EVIDENCE FOR ALTERATIONS IN EMOTIONAL REACTIVITY

A key issue in investigating the question of whether bipolar disorder can manifest in preschool children is whether those who manifest symptoms of the disorder also demonstrate differences in patterns of emotional reactivity. Since the disorder is characterized by a fundamental impairment in mood and affect regulation, and related to this, by periods of extremely intense emotional responses, investigating the typical emotion reactivity characteristics (in response to incentive events) of this group relative to others is of interest. Building on the emerging body of data on atypical emotion development, the idea that early onset bipolar disorder may be characterized by alterations in patterns of emotional reactivity has been previously proposed.[29]

As a part of an ongoing National Institute of Mental Health (NIMH) funded longitudinal study focusing on preschool mood disorders (also described above), the assessment of emotional development and reactivity styles in the study population (and the mood-disordered groups in particular) was of interest. Standardized developmental measures of emotion recognition, regulation, and emotional display rules were obtained. However, to assess the child's typical pattern of emotionality, a novel parental report assessment of the intensity and duration of the child's characteristic emotional responses was developed. This measure was designed to elicit from the parent details of the timing and intensity of the childrens typical emotional reactions using a narrative depicting commonly experienced evocative events. This approach was thought to capture the child's typical emotional functioning by detailing quantifiable features of emotional response rather than global ratings, which are more vulnerable to reporter bias. This measure, titled "The Emotion Reactivity Questionnaire" (ERQ) was developed based on an emotional dynamic model of mood disorders described in detail in Luby and Belden.[29] This model posits that the temporal and dynamic features of emotional response may be key to identifying the emotional developmental precursors and characteristics of early onset mood disorders. Observational measures of emotional reactivity or temperament in the laboratory, which also quantify the child's emotional response to an evocative event, were obtained and will be reported elsewhere. Such objective measures, while potentially highly informative, are limited by lack of representativeness based on the cross-sectional nature of the observation.

The ERQ[30] is a 28-item measure that assesses the intensity of children's emotional reactions during a 24-hour period based on caregiver report. Four vignettes depicting situations that occur at the very beginning of the day and that are thought to elicit joy, sadness, guilt, or anger in young children are read to caregivers by an examiner. After hearing each vignette, caregivers are asked to rate the intensity of the emotional reactions they would expect their children to display. Caregivers are given an "emotion meter," which allows them to slide and place a red line on an exact intensity from 0 (no emotional reaction) to 100 (very intense emotional reaction). Caregivers are asked to rate their child's emotional reactions at seven time points as follows: immediately after the incentive event depicted in the narrative, 30 minutes after, 60 minutes after, at lunchtime, dinnertime, bedtime, and again the next morning when the child wakes up. Basic psychometric properties for this new measure have been tested and are described below.

Internal consistency for each of the four emotion subscales using Chronbach's alpha ranged from 0.87 to 0.89. The ability of the ERQ to assess emotionally specific reactions of children (versus global reactions) was evidenced by the results of a principal component analysis illustrating four predominant factors that represented each of the 4 emotions assessed in the ERQ. As described in the findings below, initial indicators are that the ERQ also has strong face validity. Additional analyses were conducted to examine convergent validity between the ERQ and the Child Behavioral Questionnaire (CBQ),[31] a well-established measure of children's dispositional temperament. It was hypothesized that caregivers' reports on the CBQ 1 year before completing the ERQ would predict mothers' reports of children's initial scores on each of the three ERQ emotions (the CBQ does not include a guilt subscale). As hypothesized, the CBQ sadness subscale was associated with ERQ initial sadness scores 1 year later ($r = .20$, $p<.01$), CBQ anger subscale scores were associated with ERQ initial anger scores 1 year later ($r = .25$, $p<.001$), and CBQ pleasure subscale scores were correlated with ERQ initial joy scores 1 year later ($r = .14$, $p<.05$).

Based on these preliminary findings suggesting the ERQ is a psychometrically acceptable measure, we tested whether bipolar preschoolers' ERQ scores differed significantly from those of same-age peers in healthy and psychiatric comparison groups. Analyses were also conducted to determine whether preschoolers with bipolar disorder versus comparison groups had longer emotional reaction durations, suggesting difficulty with emotion regulation. To address this question, nonparametric Mann-Whitney U tests (M-W test) were conducted because of the small sample sizes in two of three comparison groups.

Compared with healthy preschoolers, preschoolers with bipolar disorder were described by their parents as expressing significantly higher levels of joy after 30 (M-W test, $Z = -2.847$, $P<.01$) and 60 (M-W test, $Z = -2.831$, $P<.01$) minutes in response to a joy-inducing incentive event (**Fig. 1**). Preschoolers with bipolar disorder also retained higher levels of joy by lunch time (M-W test, $Z = -2.514$, $P<.05$) and by dinnertime (M-W test, $Z = -2.024$, $P<.05$) compared with those of healthy peers.*$P<.05$ **$P<.01$.

Bipolar preschoolers were also rated as having significantly higher levels of sadness after 30 minutes (M-W test, $Z = -2.439$, $P<.05$) compared with those of healthy preschoolers. Notably, in the domain of anger, bipolar preschoolers were also reported to have significantly higher initial levels of anger (M-W test, $Z = -3.400$,

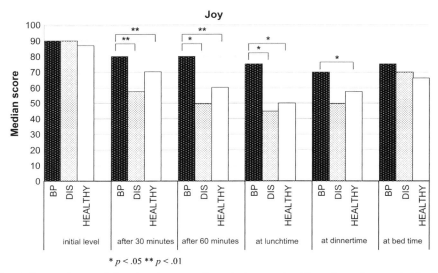

Fig. 1. Comparison of joy levels over time between healthy disruptive and bipolar preschoolers.

$P<.01$) and higher levels after 30 minutes (M-W test, $Z = -2.111$, $P<.05$) than those of healthy preschoolers. No other differences were found between bipolar and healthy preschoolers.* $P<.05$ ** $P< 01$.

Notably and in contrast to the findings above, preschoolers without bipolar disorder but who had a DSM-IV disruptive disorder were rated by parents as displaying significantly lower levels of sadness than those of healthy preschoolers after 60 minutes (M-W test, $Z = -1.997$, $P<.05$, **Fig. 2**). Preschoolers with disruptive disorder were also reported to display significantly lower levels of anger after 30 (M-W test, $Z = -2.129$, $P<.05$) and 60 (M-W test, $Z = -1.957$, $P=.05$) minutes compared with those of healthy peers (**Fig. 3**). Furthermore, in the area of guilt, they were reported to display significantly lower levels of guilt after 60 minutes (M-W test, $Z = -2.845$, $P<.01$), at lunch time (M-W test, $Z = -2.558$, $P<.05$), and at dinnertime (M-W test, $Z = -2.664$, $P<.01$) compared with those of healthy peers (**Fig. 4**).* $P<.05$ ** $P< 01$.

Comparing preschoolers with bipolar disorder to those with disruptive disorders, parents described bipolar preschoolers as expressing significantly higher levels of joy after 30 (M-W test, $Z = -2.865$, $P<.01$) and 60 (M-W test, $Z = -2.544$, $P<.05$) minutes, as well as at lunch time (M-W test, $Z = -2.510$, $P<.05$) compared with those of disruptive preschoolers. Bipolar preschoolers versus disruptive preschoolers were also reported to display significantly higher levels of sadness after 30 (M-W test, $Z= -3.090$, $P<.01$) and 60 (M-W test, $Z = -2.559$, $P<.05$) minutes as well as at bedtime (M-W test, $Z = -2.377$, $P<.05$). The bipolar group was also rated as having a significantly higher initial level of anger (M-W test, $Z = -2.177$, $P<.05$) and higher levels of anger after 30 (M-W test, $Z = -3.072$, $P<.01$) and 60 (M-W test, $Z = -2.168$, $P<.05$) minutes. Similar differences were also detected between the groups in the domain of guilt in which bipolar preschoolers had higher levels of guilt after 30 (M-W test, $Z = -2.010$, $P<.05$) and 60 (M-W test, $Z = -2.857$, $P<.01$) minutes, at lunch time (M-W test, $Z = -2.209$, $P<.05$), and at bedtime (M-W test, $Z = -2.146$, $P<.05$) compared to disruptive preschoolers.

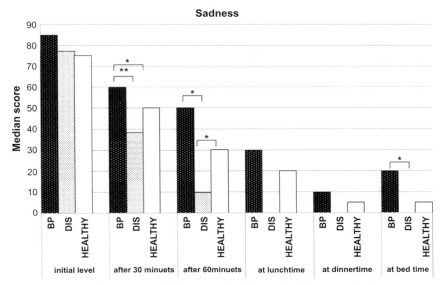

Fig. 2. Comparison of sadness levels between healthy and bipolar preschoolers.

These findings provide evidence that preschool children who meet DSM-IV symptom criteria for bipolar disorder display more intense emotional responses in the domains of joy, sadness, and anger than those of healthy peers, as would be expected. In addition, they also display higher intensities of these emotions (as well as guilt) than those of a key psychiatric comparison group of children with disruptive disorders. The latter group is of particular importance given that the differential diagnosis between early onset bipolar

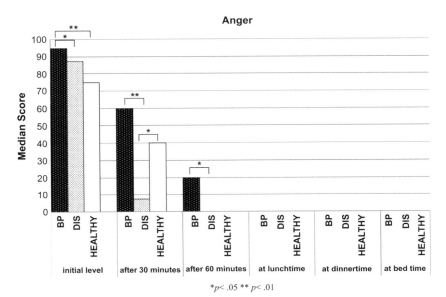

*p< .05 ** p< .01

Fig. 3. Comparison of anger levels between healthy and bipolar preschoolers.

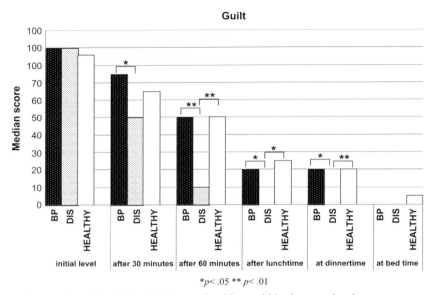

Fig. 4. Comparison of guilt levels between healthy and bipolar preschoolers.

disorder and disruptive disorders is particularly difficult clinically. Beyond elevations in intensity, these findings also provide support for the notion that bipolar preschoolers have more difficultly regulating their emotions over time. This is evidenced by sustained elevations in emotional intensity at periods several hours after the incentive event (eg, lunch and dinner) compared with healthy and disruptive peers. These findings suggest that an emotional reactivity model may be useful in the understanding and diagnosis of bipolar disorder in young children.

Findings are limited by the fact that they are based on parent report of typical emotional responses. Reporter biases, as well as the fact that diagnostic determinations were also based on parent report, are important issues to consider in the interpretation of these findings. However, this limitation may also be offset by the fact that the measure aimed to obtain an objective and quantitative estimate of the child's response through the use of an emotion meter and obtaining estimation at multiple fixed time points over a 24-hour period. Further investigation of emotional reactivity in groups of mood-disordered preschoolers using similar measures as well as observational measures is now indicated.

FAMILY HISTORY AND BIPOLAR DISORDER IN OLDER CHILDREN

Elevations in reported rates of bipolar disorder in the older offspring of bipolar parents compared with the offspring of healthy parents vary depending on study design. However, prior studies have suggested that the offspring of bipolar parents are at four to five times greater risk for any affective disorder (including bipolar disorder) compared with the offspring of parents without mental disorders.[32,33] One source of variation might be that some meta-analyses have included both adult and child offspring. In a review of studies involving only child and adolescent offspring of parents with bipolar disorder, Delbello and Geller[34] found rates of mood disorders ranging from 5% to 52%. Furthermore, these offspring were also at higher risk for disruptive and anxiety disorders than those from healthy parents.[34] Similarly, Chang and colleagues[35] reported that 51% of the offspring of bipolar parents had psychiatric disorders, including bipolar disorder. Parents with earlier onset symptomatology were more likely to have offspring with bipolar disorder.[35] This earlier age of symptom onset has been suggested to be a marker of heritability in a more recent study using genome-wide scanning.[36] In addition to the heritability of early age at onset, poor social functioning and comorbid conditions have also been suggested to be familial.[37]

IMPLICATIONS OF BIPOLAR FAMILY HISTORY IN PRESCHOOL CHILDREN

The notion that early onset of bipolar symptoms in a parent may increase the risk of heritability of the disorder suggests that such offspring would be an ideal group in which to search for prodromes or early markers of the disorder. Findings to date in preschool populations have suggested that preschoolers with MDD and family history of bipolar disorder have distinctive symptoms of MDD suggestive of mania precursors when compared with those of preschoolers with MDD but no family history of bipolar disorder. In particular, depression in this group was characterized by increased rates of agitation and restlessness.[38] Extrapolating from the work of Geller and colleagues[39,40] suggesting that prepubertal children with early onset MDD with a family history of bipolar disorder are at higher risk for later switching to mania, younger depressed children may be an important group to follow and assess for mania based on the hypothesis that they are at a particularly high risk for switching.

Unique behavioral features have been identified in studies of the young children of parents with bipolar disorder in at least one study.[41] More specifically, the rate of behavioral disinhibition among offspring of bipolar parents was significantly increased compared with that of offspring of parents with both panic disorder and unipolar depression, even after controlling for parental ADHD, substance use disorders, CD, and antisocial personality disorder. Although this pilot study was limited by the small sample size of the bipolar offspring, it proposes early intervention when markers of risk such as behavioral disinhibition are observed among high-risk offspring.[41] Similarly, difficulties in sharing and challenges in inhibiting aggressive impulses with peers were observed in 2-year-olds who had a bipolar parent, in a naturalistic observational study focusing on social and emotional functioning of offspring of bipolar parents. Conversely, these children were also noted to have a heightened sense of recognizing suffering in others, despite having difficulty in modulating their own emotions.[42,43]

DIFFERENTIAL DIAGNOSIS OF BIPOLAR DISORDER IN THE PRESCHOOL PERIOD

The prevailing controversy about the nosology of bipolar disorder in older children provides an uncertain framework for studies of nosology in preschoolers as outlined above. Amid these diagnostic uncertainties, clinicians are increasingly placed in the position of evaluating preschool children for suspected bipolar disorder. As evidenced by dramatic increases in the rates of clinical diagnosis of bipolar disorder in childhood more generally as mentioned above, clinicians appear to more readily consider the diagnosis of bipolar disorder in young children presenting with intense mood lability or bouts of extreme irritability associated with functional impairment. Because further scientific clarity of the clinical characteristics of the disorder in young children is still needed, proper consideration in the differential diagnosis for other more clearly understood disruptive disorders and/or ADHD is even more critical.

ADHD and ODD are disorders known and relatively well characterized in preschool children. ADHD has been reported to have a prevalence rate of 3.3% in preschoolers, and those with ADHD were reported to have an 8-fold greater rate of ODD.[44] Therefore, the occurrence of one of these more common disorders is more likely and must be considered first. Further, at least one report has suggested that preschoolers who meet symptom criteria for bipolar disorder have high rates of comorbid ODD and ADHD similar to those found in school-age bipolar samples.[6] In addition, extreme temper tantrums and irritability in young children may also be a marker of an autistic spectrum disorder (ASD), a group of disorders increasing in prevalence. Therefore, in preschool children presenting with extreme irritability, more commonly occurring diagnoses should be considered and ruled in or out before consideration of bipolar disorder.

Differentiating bipolar disorder from these more common disorders may be difficult in cases in which there is a complex comorbid and/or developmental delay clinical picture. Key features in differentiating bipolar disorder from ASD are that the latter is characterized by a core impairment in social relatedness, whereas bipolar preschoolers would be expected to have intact or often unusually high social interest. Further, stereotypes and perseverations that characterize ASDs are not a typical feature of bipolar disorder, although developmental delay and social rejection may be present.

One of the more challenging aspects of the differential diagnosis is distinguishing oppositional behaviors toward adults found in ODD from grandiosity found in bipolar disorder. It is important to determine whether the oppositional or extremely bossy behavior is generalized or relationship-specific; the latter would be associated with ODD rather than bipolar disorder. Perhaps even more important is whether this behavior is associated with a fixed and false elevated sense of powers and capabilities that is acted upon. Such behavior is an important manifestation of clinical level and delusional grandiosity, which appears to be a key feature of mania that may manifest as early as the preschool period.

TREATMENT CONSIDERATIONS

Although the diagnostic characteristics of bipolar disorder in the preschool period remain ambiguous as outlined, and much empirical work is needed, to date there has been relatively more scientific investigation of treatments for presumptive mania in this age group. Most of the available treatment literature has been descriptive and is composed of case reports and retrospective chart reviews. These reports provide some promising findings for the use of atypical antipsychotic agents and mood stabilizers, both singly and in combination.[13,45–49] Such observations in uncontrolled clinical settings suggest that systematic open-label studies of these agents should be pursued as a next step. An open-label study of olanzapine and risperidone was conducted in a sample of preschoolers with a form of bipolar disorder that might best be classified as bipolar disorder not otherwise specified.[13] Both medications rapidly decreased mania symptoms but residual symptoms remained. Similarly, case reports of open-label use of the mood stabilizers valproate, lithium, topiramate, and carbamazepine have described reduction in preschool mania symptoms, with atypical antipsychotics used for augmentation of residual symptoms when necessary.[45–49] At this time, reliance on these data for treatment decisions must be approached with caution due to the small sample sizes and lack of necessary controlled investigations. Although studies of psychotherapeutic interventions for preschool bipolar disorder have not been conducted to date, an age-appropriate parent–child dyadic treatment modality has been designed and described for treatment of preschool bipolar disorder for future testing in this population.[50]

SUMMARY

Although some empirical work has now been added to the larger body of case material, preschool bipolar disorder remains a highly ambiguous diagnostic area. This is notable in the context of the significant progress that has been made in many other areas of psychopathology in the preschool period. Although there is a need for well-controlled empirical investigations in this area, a small but growing body of empirical literature suggests that some form of the disorder may arise as early as age 3 years. The need for large-scale and focused studies of this issue is underscored by the high and increasing rates of prescriptions of atypical antipsychotics and other mood stabilizing agents for preschool children with presumptive clinical diagnosis of bipolar disorder or a related variant. Clarifying the nosology of preschool bipolar disorder may also be important to better understand the developmental psychopathology of the disorder during childhood. Data elucidating this developmental trajectory could then inform the design of earlier potentially preventive interventions that may have implications for the disorder across the lifespan.

REFERENCES

1. Ghaemi S, Martin A. Defining the boundaries of childhood bipolar disorder. Am J Psychiatry 2007;164(2):185–8.
2. Danielyan A, Pathak S, Kowatch RA, et al. Clinical characteristics of bipolar disorder in very young children. J Affect Disord 2007;97(1–3):51–9.
3. Ferreira Maia AP, Boarati MA, Kleinman A, et al. Preschool bipolar disorder: Brazilian children case reports. J Affect Disord 2007;104(1–3):237–43.
4. Dilsaver SC, Akiskal HS. Preschool-onset mania: incidence, phenomenology and family history. J Affect Disord 2004;82(Suppl 1):S35–43.
5. Luby J, Tandon M, Nicol G, et al. Cardinal symptoms of mania in clinically referred preschoolers: Description of three clinical cases with presumptive preschool bipolar disorder. J Child Adolesc Psychopharmacol 2007;17(2):237–44.
6. Luby J, Belden A. Defining and validating bipolar disorder in the preschool period. Dev Psychopathol 2006;18(4):971–88.
7. Moreno C, Laje G, Blanco C, et al. National trends in the outpatient diagnosis and treatment of bipolar disorder in youth. Arch Gen Psychiatry 2007;64(9):1032–9.
8. Geller B, Williams M, Zimmerman B, et al. Prepubertal and early adolescent bipolarity differentiate from ADHD by manic symptoms, grandiose delusions, ultra-rapid or ultradian cycling. J Affect Disord 1998;51(2):81–91.
9. Geller B, Zimerman B, Williams M, et al. DSM-IV mania symptoms in a prepubertal and early adolescent bipolar disorder phenotype compared to attention-deficit hyperactive and normal controls. J Child Adolesc Psychopharmacol 2002; 12(1):11–25.
10. Leibenluft E, Rich BA. Pediatric bipolar disorder. Annu Rev Clin Psychol 2008;4: 163–87.
11. Biederman J, Klein RG, Pine DS, et al. Resolved: mania is mistaken for ADHD in prepubertal children. J Am Acad Child Adolesc Psychiatry 1998;37(10):1091–6 [discussion 1096–9].
12. Geller B, Zimerman B, Williams M, et al. Phenomenology of prepubertal and early adolescent bipolar disorder: Examples of elated mood, grandiose behaviors, decreased need for sleep, racing thoughts and hypersexuality. J Child Adolesc Psychopharmacol 2002;12(1):3–9.

13. Biederman J, Faraone SV, Wozniak J, et al. Clinical correlates of bipolar disorder in a large, referred sample of children and adolescents. J Psychiatr Res 2005;39: 611–22.

14. Wozniak J, Biederman J, Kwon A, et al. How cardinal are cardinal symptoms in pediatric bipolar disorder? An examination of clinical correlates. Biol Psychiatry 2005;58(7):583–8.

15. Geller B, Tillman R, Craney JL, et al. Four-year prospective outcome and natural history of mania in children with a prepubertal and early adolescent bipolar disorder phenotype. Arch Gen Psychiatry 2004;61(5):459–67.

16. Leibenluft E, Charney DS, Towbin KE, et al. Defining clinical phenotypes of juvenile mania. Am J Psychiatry 2003;160(3):430–7.

17. Biederman J, Mick E, Faraone SV, et al. Pediatric mania: a developmental subtype of bipolar disorder? Biol Psychiatry 2000;48(6):458–66.

18. Tillman R, Geller B. Definitions of rapid, ultrarapid, and ultradian cycling and of episode duration in pediatric and adult bipolar disorders: a proposal to distinguish episodes from cycles. J Child Adolesc Psychopharmacol 2003;13(3):267–71.

19. Kramlinger KG, Post RM. Ultra-rapid and ultradian cycling in bipolar affective illness. Br J Psychiatry 1996;168(3):314–23.

20. Feinstein SC, Wolpert EA. Juvenile manic-depressive illness. Clinical and therapeutic considerations. J Am Acad Child Psychiatry 1973;12(1):123–36.

21. Thompson Jr RJ, Schindler FH. Embryonic mania. Child Psychiatry Hum Dev 1976;6(3):149–54.

22. Weinberg WA, Brumback RA. Mania in childhood: case studies and literature review. Am J Dis Child 1976;130(4):380–5.

23. Greves HE. Acute mania in a child of five years; recovery; remarks. Lancet 1884; ii:824–6.

24. Kraepelin E. Manic-depressive insanity and paranoia. Edinburgh, H.S. Livingson Ltd; 1921.

25. Tumuluru RV, Weller EB, Fristad MA, et al. Mania in six preschool children. J Child Adolesc Psychopharmacol 2003;13(4):489–94.

26. Egger HL, Ascher B, Angold A, et al. Preschool age psychiatric assessment (PAPA): version 1.1. In: Center for developmental epidemiology, department of psychiatry and behavioral sciences. Durham, NC: Duke University Medical Center; 1999.

27. Egger HL, Erkanli A, Keeler G, et al. Test-Retest Reliability of the Preschool Age Psychiatric Assessment (PAPA). Journal of the American Academy of Child & Adolescent Psychiatry 2006;45(5):538–49.

28. Luby J, Belden A, Tandon M, et al. Bipolar disorder in the preschool period: focus on development and differential diagnosis. In: Miklowitz DJ, Cicchetti D, editors. Bipolar disorder: a development psychopathology approach. Guilford Press, New York; in press.

29. Luby J, Belden A. Mood disorders: Phenomonology and a developmental reactivity model in. In: Luby J, editor. Handbook of Preschool Mental Health: Development Disorders and Treatment. New York: Guilford Press; 2006.

30. Belden A, Luby J. The emotion reactivity questionnaire unpublished measure. In: Early emotional development program; Washington University School of Medicine.

31. Rothbart MK, Ahadi SA, Hershey KL, et al. Investigations of temperament at three to seven years: the Children's Behavior Questionnaire. Child Dev 2001;72(5): 1394–408.

32. Lapalme M, Hodgins S, LaRoche C, et al. Children of parents with bipolar disorder: a metaanalysis of risk for mental disorders. Can J Psychiatry 1997; 42(6):623–31.

33. Todd RD, Reich W, Petti TA, et al. Psychiatric diagnoses in the child and adolescent members of extended families identified through adult bipolar affective disorder probands. J Am Acad Child Adolesc Psychiatry 1996;35(5):664–71.
34. DelBello MP, Geller B. Review of studies of child and adolescent offspring of bipolar parents. Bipolar Disord 2001;3(6):325–34.
35. Chang KD, Steiner H, Ketter TA. Psychiatric phenomenology of child and adolescent bipolar offspring. J Am Acad Child Adolesc Psychiatry 2000;39(4):453–60.
36. Faraone SV, Glatt SJ, Su J, et al. Three potential susceptibility loci shown by a genome-wide scan for regions influencing the age at onset of mania. Am J Psychiatry 2004;161(4):625–30.
37. Schulze TG, Hedeker D, Zandi P, et al. What is familial about familial bipolar disorder? Resemblance among relatives across a broad spectrum of phenotypic characteristics. Arch Gen Psychiatry 2006;63(12):1368–76.
38. Luby JL, Mrakotsky C. Depressed preschoolers with bipolar family history: a group at high risk for later switching to mania? J Child Adolesc Psychopharmacol 2003;13(2):187–97.
39. Geller B, Fox LW, Clark KA, et al. Rate and predictors of prepubertal bipolarity during follow-up of 6- to 12-year-old depressed children. J Am Acad Child Adolesc Psychiatry 1994;33(4):461–8.
40. Geller B, Zimerman B, Williams M, et al. Adult psychosocial outcome of prepubertal major depressive disorder. J Am Acad Child Adolesc Psychiatry 2001;40(6):673–7.
41. Hirschfeld-Becker D, Biederman J, Henin A, et al. Laboratory-observed behavioral disinhibition in the young offspring of parents with bipolar disorder. Am J Psychiatry 2006;136:265–71.
42. Zahn-Waxler C, Cummings EM, McKnew DH, et al. Altruism, aggression, and social interactions in young children with a manic-depressive parent. Child Dev 1984;55(1):112–22.
43. Zahn-Waxler C, McKnew DH, Cummings EM, et al. Problem behaviors and peer interactions of young children with a manic-depressive parent. Am J Psychiatry 1984;141(2):236–40.
44. Egger HL, Kondo D, Angold A, et al. The Epidemiology and diagnostic issues in preschool attention-deficit/hyperactivity disorder: a review. Infants & Young children. An Interdisciplinary Journal of Special Care Practices 2006;19(2):109–22.
45. Mota-Castillo M, Torruella A, Engels B, et al. Valproate in very young children: an open case series with a brief follow-up. J Affect Disord 2001;67:193–7.
46. Pavuluri MN, Janicak PG, Carbray J, et al. Topiramate plus risperidone for controlling weight gain and symptoms in preschool mania. J Child Adolesc Psychopharmacol 2002;12(3):271–3.
47. Pavuluri MN, Henry DB, Carbray JA, et al. A one-year open-label trial of risperidone augmentation in lithium nonresponder youth with preschool-onset bipolar disorder. J Child Adolesc Psychopharmacol 2006;16(3):336–50.
48. Scheffer RE, Niskala Apps JA. The diagnosis of preschool bipolar disorder presenting with mania: open pharmacological treatment. J Affect Disord 2004; 82(suppl 1):S25–34.
49. Tuzun U, Zoroglu SS, Savas HA, et al. A 5-year-old boy with recurrent mania successfully treated with carbamazepine. Psychiatry Clin Neurosci 2002;56(5):589–91.
50. Luby J, Stalets M, Blankenship S, et al. Treatment of preschool bipolar disorder: a novel parent-child interaction therapy and review of data on psychopharmacology. In: Geller B, DelBello M, editors. Treatment of childhood bipolar disorder. New York; Guilford Press; p. 270–86.

Affect Regulation in Pediatric Bipolar Disorder

Daniel P. Dickstein, MD[a],*, Alison C. Brazel, BS[a],
Lisa D. Goldberg, BA[a], Jeffrey I. Hunt, MD[b]

KEYWORDS

- Bipolar disorder • Child • Adolescent • Affect • Emotion
- Development

Bipolar disorder (BD) is among the most significant health problems for adults in America today, causing great morbidity and mortality and more than $40 billion in annual health care expenditures. We know far less about BD in children and adolescents.[1] Recent data indicate that pediatric BD (PBD) is a growing health problem whose incidence has risen 40-fold in the past decade, now accounting for 20% of all minors discharged from psychiatric hospitals.[2,3] It remains unknown if this increase represents greater awareness of a serious psychiatric disorder once thought not to exist in children or adolescents or if it represents the diagnosis being too broadly applied. Determining which of these possibilities is correct is further complicated by the fact that there is no laboratory test for BD or any other psychiatric disorder, whether in children or adults. Instead, establishing the diagnosis of BD (or any other psychiatric disorder) is based entirely on detailed clinical history, which is often more difficult to elicit from minors than from adults. Thus, there is a pressing need to identify biobehavioral markers of BD that could augment clinical history in the diagnostic and treatment process, especially for children and adolescents.

Toward that end, clinicians and researchers alike have been using the language of neuroscience to describe PBD patients as having "affect regulation problems." Although our understanding of PBD has advanced thanks to such neurobiological research, some researchers have suggested that thinking of BD youth as suffering from affect regulation problems may be an oversimplification, akin to stating that a febrile child is suffering from "temperature regulation problems"—that is, factually

Disclosures: Dr. Dickstein is supported by Bradley Hospital and NIMH K22 MH 74945 and a NARSAD Young Investigator Award. Dr. Hunt is supported by Bradley Hospital and NIMH R01 MH59691.
a Pediatric Mood, Imaging, & Neurodevelopment Program, EP Bradley Hospital, Bradley/Hasbro Children's Research Center, Warren Alpert Medical School of Brown University, 1 Hoppin Street, Coro West 2nd Floor, Providence, RI 02903, USA
b EP Bradley Hospital, 1001 Veterans Memorial Parkway, East Providence, RI 02915, USA
* Corresponding author.
E-mail address: daniel_dickstein@brown.edu (D.P. Dickstein).

true but not illuminating the situation sufficiently to render a diagnosis and a treatment.[4] Clinicians and parents may wonder, "does affect regulation improve what we know about the diagnosis and treatment of PBD, or does it further complicate matters?"

In a word, our answer is "yes:" although adding complexity and depth, we believe affect regulation does improve what we know about PBD. Affect regulation provides a framework for conducting biological research to identify the underlying mechanisms of BD, ultimately improving our care for these youth. Although numerous books, articles, and presentations have begun to address this topic, this article is intended to provide a concise and current guide to affect regulation in PBD, incorporating the latest in research as well as highlighting goals for the future. First, we review the basics of affect regulation.[5] Then, we discuss what is known about the 3 important affects in BD: irritability, euphoria, and depression. Finally, we review what is known about affect regulation in PBD.

AFFECT REGULATION BASICS

What is affect regulation? Clinicians and researchers alike often report BD youth as suffering from "affect regulation problems," including having abnormally high highs and low lows and frequently shifting between the two, without maintaining much stability. Moreover, the pharmaceutical industry has seized upon this notion by using the term "mood stabilizer" to refer to medications used to treat BD, despite the fact that such medications are incredibly heterogeneous in terms of their pharmacologic mechanisms.[6,7]

Further complicating matters is the fact that the terms "emotion," "feeling," "mood," and "affect" are used interchangeably. Clinically, mental health professionals routinely distinguish between "mood" and "affect" when evaluating and treating patients, whether child or adult, in their formal mental status examination. In this context, the term "mood" usually refers to the patient's self-assessment of the emotional state (eg, happy, sad, worried), whereas "affect" usually refers to the mental health professional's objective, observable assessment of the patient's emotional state and responsiveness (eg, emotional state: depressed, euphoric, euthymic; emotional responsiveness: blunted, flat, expansive). The term "feeling" is often used similarly to "mood" as describing an individual's conscious awareness of their emotional state (eg, I feel happy, sad, worried). Yet there is no universal agreement among clinicians or researchers on the distinction between the terms "emotion" and "affect." Some clinicians or researchers use these terms interchangeably. In contrast, others suggest that "affect" is a biological, innate, instinctive response, and "emotion" is the individual's memory of prior affects, which was summarized by Nathanson as "affect is biology, feeling is psychology, and emotion is biography."[8] Given the lack of consensus on distinctions between "affect" and "emotion," and to align with the field of studying the neurobiology of emotion, known as "affective neuroscience," we preferentially use the term "affect" but recognize that the two terms may be used similarly.

From an affective neuroscience perspective, "affect" may be defined as "an evoked response to an environmental stimulus with motivational salience."[9] Motivational salience may be parsed into two orthogonal dimensions: (1) "valence" and (2) "arousal." Valence refers to whether a stimulus is appetitively rewarding [positive valence] or aversive [negative valence]. Arousal refers to the amount of an organism's resources, such as energy, that are mobilized in response to a stimulus. In turn, affect regulation has been defined by Thompson as the "extrinsic and intrinsic processes responsible for monitoring, evaluating, and modifying emotional reactions, especially their intensive and temporal features, to accomplish one's goals."[10] To amplify several aspects of this definition, affect regulation is not just dampening or suppression of negative emotion (such as anger) but rather the dynamic balance between positively and negatively valenced emotions, which can involve increasing or decreasing the elicited arousal.[11] Moreover, affect regulation involves processes within the individual, both conscious and unconscious, as well as external influences, such as input from caretakers and experience from prior interactions with others. Lastly, affect regulation is not a solitary process that follows a one-way sequence from emotion to its regulation.[12] Instead, affect regulation requires the interplay between many separable subprocesses, such as attention and processing of emotional stimuli, memory for prior events, response to rewards and punishments, and decision making.

To exemplify these constructs, consider the scenario of a child tasting some chocolate ice cream (stimulus). The child finds the ice cream very positively rewarding (affect; moderate arousal, positive valence). The child is aware that the ice cream tastes good (feeling), and she or he giggles remembering the last time she or he had ice cream (emotion). The child then goes to obtain more ice cream (affect regulation).

It is beyond the scope of this article to fully describe all of the brain/behavior interactions underlying the subprocesses of affect regulation, as innumerable articles, presentations, and entire books have attempted this. However, we would like to discuss several that seem germane to BD.

By definition, affect regulation begins with the detection of an environmental stimulus and categorizing it. For example, is that a lion that I should avoid, or a housecat that I should pet? Is mom or dad happy … or angry? Making these determinations of object identity involves the fusiform gyrus, occipital cortex, and superior temporal gyrus among others.[13] These regions categorize stimuli as animate or inanimate and moving or not moving. Importantly, these regions seem especially geared to process faces, which are among the most important emotional stimuli in humans.[14–18]

The recognition of facial emotions is another subprocess of affect regulation. It can be probed using computerized behavioral tasks on their own or in conjunction with magnetic resonance imaging (MRI), whereby participants must identify the emotion (eg, happy, sad, angry) displayed by an actor. In addition to the above regions involved in stimulus detection and categorization, the amygdala has also been implicated in processing facial emotions. Many studies have linked the amygdala to negatively valenced emotional stimuli. For example, surgical resection of the amygdala results in impaired recognition of facial expressions of negatively valenced emotions, such as fear and sadness, but not of positively valenced emotions, such as happiness.[19,20] Compared with adults, adolescents have greater amygdala activation to negatively valenced emotional expressions, including fear, versus neutral stimuli.[21–23] Moreover, there is a significant association between increased activation to fearful or threatening faces and the short variant of the serotonin transporter gene that is thought to convey susceptibility to depression and anxiety.[24] Nevertheless, studies have also linked the amygdala to the processing of positively valenced emotional stimuli. For example, functional MRI studies have demonstrated increased amygdala activation to happy versus neutral faces in adult controls.[25]

Also by definition, affect regulation involves response to rewards (appetitive, pleasurable, positively valenced stimuli) and punishments (aversive, painful, negatively valenced stimuli). For example, do I finish my homework after I arrive home from school because it will make me happy? My parents happy? To get the 50 cents I was promised? To avoid getting my parents mad? If I do not do my homework, and my parents get mad, will I learn and tomorrow complete my homework when I arrive home from school? From an affective neuroscience perspective, response to rewards and punishment is integral to our understanding of BD, given clinical symptoms that potentially suggest mania to be a hyperhedonic period involving excessive goal-directed activity, involvement in pleasurable activities with high potential for painful consequences, and grandiosity, whereas depression may be a hypohedonic period involving anhedonia, worthlessness, and hopelessness. It appears that these behavioral/emotional manifestations of mood disorders are linked to three functionally connected brain regions involved in processing rewards and punishments: (1) the prefrontal cortex (PFC), (2) the amygdala, and (3) the striatum (**Fig. 1**).[26–29]

One example of the myriad subprocesses of affect regulation that involve response to rewards and punishment is cognitive flexibility, meaning the ability to adapt one's thinking and behavior in response to changing environmental conditions, including rewards.[30,31] In the laboratory, cognitive flexibility may be tested using reversal learning tasks, whereby participants try to win as many points as possible by first learning, through trial and error, which of two objects is rewarded (wins points) and which is punished (loses points), and then sticking with the rewarded stimulus. Then, without warning, the stimulus–reward association is reversed, that is, the previously rewarded stimulus is now punished, and the previously punished stimulus is now rewarded. For example, if a dog and cat are presented, through trial and error, the child figures out that the dog is rewarded initially. After a number of trials of successfully winning points by picking the dog, the child switches to now win points by picking the cat once the dog starts losing points.

Reversal learning is mediated by a distributed circuit encompassing (1) the PFC, including the orbitofrontal cortex (OFC), which mediates the reversal of stimulus–reward relationships;[30–32] (2) the striatum, including the accumbens area, caudate, and putamen, which transforms concrete stimulus–exemplar information into motor responses;[30,33] and (3) the amygdala, which encodes the salience of rewards and punishments.[27,34] Moreover, Blair and colleagues[35–38] suggest that reversal learning and the OFC tap into the regulation of aggression. In particular, the OFC has been linked to social response reversal, whereby people react to others' negatively valenced emotional states, such as anger, by displaying aggression, including frustration and irritability.

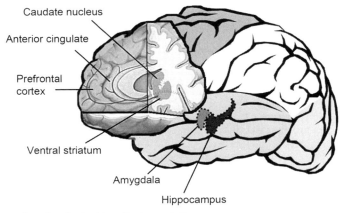

Fig. 1. Brain regions implicated in affect regulation.

Two additional and related subprocesses of affect regulation are attentional control and conflict monitoring. To illustrate these related processes, do I direct my attention to the teacher at the head of the class, or the student whispering next to me? Attentional control refers to the top-down process of devoting attentional resources and planning to stimuli and is most often linked to the dorsolateral PFC (DLPFC).[39–41] Conflict monitoring refers to the process of adjusting behavior to override 1 response in favor of another and is most often associated with the anterior cingulate cortex (ACC).[42] Attentional control can be tested by tasks involving planning, problem solving, and executive function. Conflict monitoring can be tested by tasks such as the Stroop paradigm, whereby participants have more difficulty with incongruous stimuli (eg, reading the word "RED" printed in blue ink) than with control items (eg, the word "RED" printed in red ink).[43] Go/No-go paradigms are also used to probe conflict monitoring and response inhibition, whereby participants are instructed to press a button as fast as they can if they see a word (eg, "ZEBRA") but not to press the button if they see a non-word (eg, "QWERT"). Most trials on a go/no-go task are go responses (words), so that pressing the button becomes the "prepotent" response, with not pressing (to non-words) requiring response inhibition.

AFFECT REGULATION IN TYPICAL DEVELOPMENT

What do we know about affect regulation in typically developing children and adolescents? The field of affective neuroscience aims to answer this question using a number of techniques, including behavioral experiments, neuroimaging, genetics, and temperament.

From infancy, affect regulation begins as the interplay between interactions with caregivers and an infant's temperament, the latter of which includes individual differences in (a) reactivity (the speed and intensity of emotional activation) and (b) self-regulation (the capacity to modify the intensity and duration of an emotion through behaviors, such as self-sucking or approaching/avoiding contact with caregivers).[44,45] Such early affect regulation can be observed and studied using constructs, such as behavioral inhibition [the tendency of a child to become fearful and withdraw from novel situations].[46] With time, cognitive development and emotional experience enable the infant to exert greater affect self-regulation.[47] Affect regulation is inherited to some degree, as demonstrated by identical twins performing more similarly than fraternal twins on parental reports of emotion regulation.[48,49]

Adolescence is also a time of great change, including not only physical changes and growth but also the development of the many subprocesses of affect regulation. Paradoxically, adolescence involves both greater ability to self-regulate as well as greater tendency to engage in risk-taking behavior, including driving, unprotected sex, and experimentation with illegal substances.[50] Recent longitudinal structural MRI studies have demonstrated that as children become young adults, there is a loss of cortical gray matter in prefrontal and temporal cortices and increase in white matter volume.[51,52] Functional MRI (fMRI) studies have shown age-related changes in recruitment of the PFC during tasks of working memory, response inhibition, and verbal fluency.[53–57] With all of this change and development, how does affect regulation account for the seeming inconsistency between adolescence as a time of cognitive development and a time of increased risk taking? Recently, Casey has proposed a neurobiological model of adolescence to account for these inconsistencies. According to this model, during adolescence affect regulation represents a dynamic balance between (a) bottom-up processing of rewards by subcortical limbic regions, including the amygdala and accumbens area, and (b) top-down processing of cognitive control by the PFC, with limbic structures maturing earlier than the PFC.[58]

AFFECTS IN BIPOLAR DISORDER: KEY QUESTIONS
Irritability

Although irritability is one of the most common symptoms spurring parents to bring their children and adolescents for psychiatric treatment, the diagnosis and treatment of irritability remain a major challenge for clinicians and researchers alike. In part, this is due to the fact that irritability is a nonspecific symptom in current psychiatric nosology. Irritability is an explicit diagnostic criterion according to the Diagnostic and Statistical Manual of Mental Disorders, 4th edition, text revision (DSM-IV-TR), for a manic episode, generalized anxiety disorder, post-traumatic stress disorder, and, for children or adolescents, for a major depressive episode. Irritability is an associated symptom for pervasive developmental delay-spectrum disorders (autism, Asperger's disease), attention-deficit hyperactivity disorder (ADHD), and oppositional defiant disorder.[59]

Despite its inclusion in the above diagnoses, there is no widely accepted definition of irritability. Moreover, there is no uniform assessment measure of irritability, as standardized diagnostic interviews employed both clinically and in research use different prompts to probe for irritability.[60] For example, irritability is defined as (a) "anger; crankiness; bad temper; short-tempered; resentment or annoyance, whether overtly expressed or not; easily lose temper; touchy or easily annoyed" (Kiddie Schedule for Affective Disorders and Schizophrenia [K-SADS]),[61] (b) "cranky; angry toward people you had no reason to; talk back; temper tantrum" (Diagnostic Interview Schedule for Children),[62] and (c) "grumpy, crabby, talked back, sassy, wouldn't do something your parents asked you to do" (Children's Depression Rating Scale).[63] Thus, the challenge for all those involved is to determine whether the irritability is a manifestation of normal childhood or adolescence or if it is a symptom of an underlying psychiatric disorder, including BD.[64]

Moreover, there is no solitary biological cause of irritability, whether brain region, neurotransmitter, or gene. The brain region most frequently implicated is the OFC, dating back to notable case reports such as Phineas Gage, whose personality was transformed from good-natured and hardworking to angry and labile after an iron tamping rod was blown through his skull and OFC, as shown by modern reconstruction of the incident.[65] Imbalances in virtually every major neurotransmitter, including serotonin, glutamate, γ-aminobutyric acid, and catecholamines, also play a role.[66] Moreover, recent studies have begun to explore the link between irritability and the genotype related to these neurotransmitters.[67,68]

Euphoria

Although irritability is a nonspecific, yet impairing, symptom of BD, the elevated and expansive mood (euphoria) found during mania is a specific symptom of BD. From an affective neuroscience perspective, euphoric mania may represent a hyperhedonic period of increased responsivity, or seeking out, of rewards. In BD adults, this position is supported by several lines of research. From a temperament perspective, two studies have found that those with a history of mania, although in remission, are more likely to endorse items reflecting perfectionism and the need to achieve goals including "If I try hard enough, I should be able to excel at anything I attempt."[69,70] Moreover, a longitudinal study using the Behavioral Inhibition System Behavioral Activation System (BIS/BAS), a scale designed to measure individual differences in the avoidance of punishment (BIS) or approach toward reward (BAS),[71] has shown that BAS hypersensitivity (ie, hypersensitivity to rewards) predicted shorter time to onset of manic and hypomanic episodes.[72] Neuroimaging studies also support the potential alteration in reward processing in BD adults, with a recent study showing that whereas schizophrenic or control adults have activation of dopaminergic brain areas, including ventral tegmentum areas, to the expectation of monetary rewards and accumbens area to receipt versus omission of rewards, manic BD adults did not.[73] Moreover, genetic studies have demonstrated that carriers of the short (S) polymorphism of the serotonin transporter gene have been associated with an increased risk for antidepressant-associated mania in BD adults.[74]

Depression

Whether called "BD" or "manic-depressive illness," BD is not just about mania, as it involves depression, too. As is the case with irritable and euphoric mania, we know far more about depression in BD adults than in minors. In adults, only 25% to 33% of those with a lifetime history of mania deny episodes of depression.[75] Moreover, several large prospective studies have shown that BD adults often spend more time depressed than manic in approximately a 3:1 ratio.[76] For example, Post and colleagues[77] showed that 258 BD adults followed prospectively for 1 year spent 33.2% of their time depressed, whereas only 10.8% spent their time manic. Anger attacks were more common in depressed BD adults (62%) than in those with unipolar depression (26%).[78]

With respect to pediatric patients, there are several important questions. For example, do BD youth spend the majority of their time depressed as has been shown in BD adults? If not, does this potentially reflect differences in affect regulation? In addition, can treatments resolve the depression found in PBD, given the risk for medication-induced mania, especially with serotonergic medications? At present, there is a great need to understand the neurobiology of depression in PBD subjects.

AFFECT REGULATION IN PEDIATRIC BIPOLAR DISORDER

Against this backdrop of the basics of affect regulation in normal development and in BD, what do we know about affect regulation in PBD? The short answer is that the past 8 to 10 years have seen great progress in PBD research. However, there is still a great deal to learn about the pathophysiology, phenomenology, and treatment of PBD, and this work is being conducted at a number of sites around the country and worldwide (**Table 1**).

Returning to the abovementioned subprocesses of affect regulation, several studies have evaluated face processing in PBD. Several of these have used the Diagnostic Analysis of Non-Verbal Accuracy, which requires participants to view and categorize sets of child and adult faces displaying high- and low-intensity expressions of happiness, sadness, anger, or fear.[79] These studies have shown that PBD youth were significantly more likely to miscategorize child images of happiness, sadness, and fear as anger compared with minors with either anxiety disorders or controls.[80] A second study found that an expanded sample of PBD participants made more errors on child and adult faces than an expanded sample of controls, with secondary analyses suggesting that PBD participants were less sensitive to anger and happiness in children's faces and less sensitive to anger and sadness in adults' faces than controls.[81] Functional neuroimaging studies have followed up on these behavioral studies. PBD youth had greater activation of the amygdala and striatum than controls when they were attending to emotional aspects of faces.[82] These same PBD youth had greater neural activation in the striatum and ACC when successfully encoding happy faces into

Table 1
Affect regulation in pediatric bipolar disorder

Function/Task	Study (Author, Year)	Major Finding
Face/emotion processing	McClure et al, 2003	PBD youth more likely to miscategorize happy, sad, and fearful faces compared with anxious and control youth
	McClure et al, 2005	PBD youth less sensitive to angry/happy child faces and angry/sad adult faces versus controls
	Rich et al, 2006	Greater amygdala/striatum activation when processing emotional faces in PBD youth than that in controls
	Dickstein et al, 2007	Greater ACC/striatum activation when encoding happy faces and greater OFC activation when encoding angry faces in PBD youth compared with that in controls
	Rich et al, 2008	NPBD and SMD youth required higher intensity of emotion to correctly identify emotional faces
	Guyer et al, 2007	NPBD and SMD youth made more errors identifying emotions compared with those by anxious, depressed, ADHD, CD, and control youth
Cognitive flexibility–reversal learning	Dickstein et al, 2004	PBD youth made more errors and required more trials/time on reversals compared with those by controls
	Gorrindo et al, 2005	PBD youth made more errors on probabilistic trials compared with those by controls
	Dickstein et al, 2007	NPBD youth performed worse than SMD and controls on reversal trials, with SMD performing worse than controls
Attentional control and conflict monitoring	Blumberg et al, 2003	Greater activation in left putamen and thalamus during incongruent trials compared with congruent trials of the Stroop Task
	Leibenluft et al, 2007	Reduced striatal activation during failed motor inhibition in PBD vs controls on the stop-signal task
	Nelson et al, 2007	Greater activation in DLPFC and primary motor cortex when correctly inhibiting a prepotent motor response and executing an alternative response in PBD youth vs controls
Response to reward and punishment	Rau et al, 2008	No difference in performance on reward decision-making task between NPBD and SMD
Electrophysiology/ERP response to reward and frustration	Rich et al, 2007	NPBD and SMD showed more arousal compared with controls during frustration and nonfrustration events
	Rich et al, 2005	No differences in magnitude of arousal found between NPBD, SMD, and controls during reward, punishment, or neutral conditions

Abbreviations: ACC, anterior cingulate cortex; ADHD, attention-deficit/hyperactivity disorder; CD, conduct disorder; DLPFC, dorsolateral prefrontal cortex; ERP, event-related potential; NPBD, narrow phenotype bipolar disorder; OFC, orbitofrontal cortex; PBD, pediatric bipolar disorder; SMD, severe mood dysregulation.

memory and greater activation of the OFC when successfully encoding angry faces into memory.[83]

Specifically with regard to cognitive flexibility, studies have shown that PBD participants are impaired compared with typically developing controls on reversal learning tasks. PBD youth make more errors, require more trials to achieve minimal competence, and require more time to complete the simple reversal stage of the intradimensional/extradimensional shift task (IDED), a computerized version of the Wisconsin card sorting task (Cambridge Neuropsychological Test Automated Battery, Cambridge, UK).[84] Four prior studies found similar results in BD adults with this task in both mania and euthymia, suggesting that this may be a trait deficit in BD, rather than a mood–state-dependent phenomenon.[85–88] In a separate study, PBD participants made more errors than those of controls on a probabilistic response reversal task that further manipulates reward and punishment by adding probabilistic trials (eg, for stimulus pair dog/cat, during initial acquisition trials, dog is rewarded 80% and punished 20%, whereas cat is rewarded 20% and punished 80%; subsequent reversal trials have dog rewarded 20% and punished 80%, whereas cat is now rewarded 80% and punished 20%).[89,90]

Studies of attentional control and conflict monitoring have demonstrated the following. Using a Stroop color-naming task, PBD adolescents had increased activation in the left putamen and thalamus during incongruent (the word "BLUE" written in red ink) versus congruent (the word "BLUE" written in blue ink) trials.[91] Using a stop-signal task that required participants to inhibit a prepotent motor response, PBD participants had a reduced striatal "error signal" (thought to cause avoidance of similar mistakes on subsequent trials) during failed motor inhibition compared with controls.[92] In a related study that used a change-signal task requiring participants to inhibit a prepotent response and substitute an alternative response, PBD participants had significantly more # neural activation in the DLPFC and primary motor cortex than healthy controls during correctly performed change trials compared with correctly performed go trials.[93]

Several important studies have begun to address the controversy regarding irritability versus euphoria in PBD. Although there is no rating instrument that is sensitive to and specific for irritability found in BD, a consensus has emerged that the development of such an instrument is vital. In this regard, the K-SADS Mania Rating Scale is designed to measure mania in children, and unlike other measures, has specific anchors for the irritability item.[94] However, many investigators assert that it is unlikely that a single item can capture the complexity of irritability in PBD.[60,95] For example, more than 50% of consecutive adolescents admitted to an inpatient psychiatric unit were judged to have moderate to severe irritability using the K-SADS Mania Rating scale, but the consensus diagnoses given to each of these admitted adolescents were quite varied.[96] Ongoing PBD studies from around the country report high rates of irritability in their samples but differing rates of euphoria. The Course and Outcome of Bipolar Youth (three sites: University of Pittsburgh, Brown University, University of California, Los Angeles) found that 84.5% of their BD type I youth (N = 220) had irritability or anger, and 91.8% had elevated or expansive mood during their most severe lifetime manic episode.[97] The research group at Massachusetts General Hospital found that of N = 86 PBD subjects, 94% had irritable mood, whereas only 51% had euphoria.[98] Geller and colleagues[99] at Washington University in St. Louis found that of N = 93 PBD subjects, 97.9% had irritable mood, whereas 89.3% had elated mood.

Leibenluft and colleagues[100] have proposed a classification system of PBD to facilitate research about irritability versus elation in PBD. At the heart of this system is a definition of irritability grounded in affect regulation, which consists of "marked reactivity to negative emotional stimuli manifest verbally or behaviorally—ie, temper tantrums out of proportion to the inciting event and/or child's developmental stage occurring >3 times per week during the past 4 weeks." Building on this definition, "broad phenotype" youth (also known as "severe mood dysregulation" [SMD]) have functionally impairing (1) irritability (as defined above), (2) baseline sad or angry mood, and (3) hyperarousal (≥ 3 of insomnia, agitation, distractibility, racing thoughts/flight of ideas, pressured speech, or intrusiveness) that are chronic and non-episodic (symptoms present for ≥ 12 months without ≥ 2 months symptom free). These SMD youth do not have euphoria, and they do not have distinct mood episodes. At the other extreme, "narrow phenotype BD" (NPBD) youth have (1) clearly defined episodes of euphoric mania accompanied by ≥ 3 DSM-IV-TR "B" symptoms of mania and (2) symptoms of euphoric mania present for most of the day, every day for ≥ 4 days for hypomania or ≥ 7 days for mania. Thus, NPBD and SMD groups are orthogonal to one another, to separate out issues of irritability versus euphoria and chronic course versus distinct episodes that have been controversial in PBD.[101,102]

Studies probing differences in affect regulation using these constructs are in their early stages. Thus far, epidemiologic samples of children have shown that SMD may have a prevalence of 3.3% among those 9 to 19 years, although when these same youth are followed into adulthood, they were significantly more likely to be diagnosed with unipolar depression than those without SMD.[103] Several lines of ongoing research are probing the brain/behavior interactions mediating affect regulation in NPBD versus SMD youth, including the processing of emotional faces and also processing of rewards/punishments. With respect to face processing, both NPBD and SMD youth required greater emotion intensity to correctly identify facial images (including those of happiness, surprise, fear, sadness, anger, and disgust) compared with that in controls.[104] Moreover, NPBD and SMD youth made more errors in the identification of facial emotions than those with anxiety and/or depression, those with ADHD and/or conduct disorder, and controls.[105] With respect to rewards and punishments and cognitive flexibility, although both NPBD and SMD youth performed worse than controls on the compound reversal stage of IDED, NPBD youth were specifically impaired on the simple reversal stage compared with both SMD and controls.[106] The same study also demonstrated that NPBD youth performed worse than both SMD and controls on a task requiring subjects to inhibit a prepotent motor response and substitute a new response (ie, press "1" if you see an "X," press "2" if you see an "O," and press "3" if you see a blue square after either an "X" or "O" are presented). In contrast, there was no difference between NPBD and SMD youth in a decision-making task requiring subjects to select from differentially rewarded and punished stimuli.[107] In an attempt to study differential response to frustration elicited via rigged feedback, a recent electrophysiology study found that, although both NPBD and SMD youth reported more arousal than controls, NPBD subjects had lower P3 event-related potential (brain wave) amplitude than that of either, reflecting impaired executive attention, whereas SMD youth had lower N1 event-related potential amplitude than that of either NPBD or controls during both frustration and nonfrustration events, suggesting impaired initial orientation.[108] In a separate study, there was no difference between NPBD, SMD, and controls in magnitude of startle response during reward, punishment, or neutral conditions.[109]

THE FUTURE

In summary, the past 8 to 10 years have shown great progress in what we know about affect regulation, including the brain/behavior interactions that differentiate PBD youth from typically developing youth without psychopathology. Affective neuroscience techniques, such as behavioral tasks, neuroimaging, and electrophysiology and event-related potentials, have advanced what is known about affect regulation in PBD. In particular, these studies have shown that PBD involves alterations in several subprocesses involved with affect regulation, including emotional face processing, cognitive flexibility, and response to reward and punishment. These deficits are mediated by alterations in several brain regions, including a distributed neural circuit encompassing the PFC, striatum, and amygdala. Ongoing and future studies will examine the diagnostic specificity of such impairments versus other psychiatric disorders. They will also probe the relationship between such processes and underlying neural, genetic, and developmental mechanisms and mediators. Lastly, they will evaluate the potential for treatments, including medications and/or computerized tasks, to improve affect regulation in children and adolescents with BD. More and more, the future will likely involve the integration of affective neuroscience into clinical practice.

REFERENCES

1. Kessler RC, Akiskal HS, Ames M, et al. Considering the costs of bipolar depression. Behav Healthc 2007;27:45–7.
2. Blader JC, Carlson GA. Increased rates of bipolar disorder diagnoses among U.S. child, adolescent, and adult inpatients, 1996–2004. Biol Psychiatry 2007; 62:107–14.
3. Moreno C, Laje G, Blanco C, et al. National trends in the outpatient diagnosis and treatment of bipolar disorder in youth. Arch Gen Psychiatry 2007;64:1032–9.
4. Forbes EE, Dahl RE. Neural systems of positive affect: relevance to understanding child and adolescent depression? Dev Psychopathol 2005;17:827–50.
5. Dickstein DP, Leibenluft E. Emotion regulation in children and adolescents: boundaries between normalcy and bipolar disorder. Dev Psychopathol 2006; 18:1105–31.
6. Bauer MS, Mitchner L. What is a "mood stabilizer"? An evidence-based response. Am J Psychiatry 2004;161:3–18.
7. Keck PE Jr, McElroy SL, Richtand N, et al. What makes a drug a primary mood stabilizer? Mol Psychiatry 2002;7(Suppl 1):S8–14.
8. Nathanson DL. Shame and pride. New York: W.W. Norton & Company, Inc.; 1992.
9. Lang PJ, Bradley MM, Cuthbert BN. Emotion, motivation, and anxiety: brain mechanisms and psychophysiology. Biol Psychiatry 1998;44:1248–63.
10. Thompson RA. Emotion regulation: a theme in search of definition. Monogr Soc Res Child Dev 1994;59:25–52.
11. Fox NA. Definitions and concepts of emotion regulation. Introduction. Monogr Soc Res Child Dev 1994;59:3–6.
12. Campos JJ, Frankel CB, Camras L. On the nature of emotion regulation. Child Dev 2004;75:377–94.
13. Haxby JV, Hoffman EA, Gobbini MI. Human neural systems for face recognition and social communication. Biol Psychiatry 2002;51:59–67.
14. Gauthier I, Behrmann M, Tarr MJ. Can face recognition really be dissociated from object recognition? J Cogn Neurosci 1999;11:349–70.
15. Gauthier I, Tarr MJ, Anderson AW, et al. Activation of the middle fusiform 'face area' increases with expertise in recognizing novel objects. Nat Neurosci 1999;2:568–73.

16. Tarr MJ, Gauthier I. FFA: a flexible fusiform area for subordinate-level visual processing automatized by expertise. Nat Neurosci 2000;3:764–9.
17. Lehmann C, Mueller T, Federspiel A, et al. Dissociation between overt and unconscious face processing in fusiform face area. Neuroimage 2004;21:75–83.
18. Bukach CM, Gauthier I, Tarr MJ. Beyond faces and modularity: the power of an expertise framework. Trends Cogn Sci 2006;10:159–66.
19. Adolphs R, Damasio H, Tranel D, et al. Cortical systems for the recognition of emotion in facial expressions. J Neurosci 1996;16:7678–87.
20. Adolphs R, Tranel D. Impaired judgments of sadness but not happiness following bilateral amygdala damage. J Cogn Neurosci 2004;16:453–62.
21. Hariri AR, Bookheimer SY, Mazziotta JC. Modulating emotional responses: effects of a neocortical network on the limbic system. Neuroreport 2000;11:43–8.
22. Williams MA, Morris AP, McGlone F, et al. Amygdala responses to fearful and happy facial expressions under conditions of binocular suppression. J Neurosci 2004;24:2898–904.
23. Phillips ML, Williams LM, Heining M, et al. Differential neural responses to overt and covert presentations of facial expressions of fear and disgust. Neuroimage 2004;21:1484–96.
24. Hariri AR, Drabant EM, Munoz KE, et al. A susceptibility gene for affective disorders and the response of the human amygdala. Arch Gen Psychiatry 2005;62: 146–52.
25. Breiter HC, Etcoff NL, Whalen PJ, et al. Response and habituation of the human amygdala during visual processing of facial expression. Neuron 1996;17: 875–87.
26. Bechara A, Damasio H, Damasio AR, et al. Different contributions of the human amygdala and ventromedial prefrontal cortex to decision-making. J Neurosci 1999;19:5473–81.
27. Baxter MG, Parker A, Lindner CC, et al. Control of response selection by reinforcer value requires interaction of amygdala and orbital prefrontal cortex. J Neurosci 2000;20:4311–9.
28. Amiez C, Joseph JP, Procyk E. Anterior cingulate error-related activity is modulated by predicted reward. Eur J Neurosci 2005;21:3447–52.
29. Bellebaum C, Koch B, Schwarz M, et al. Focal basal ganglia lesions are associated with impairments in reward-based reversal learning. Brain 2008;131:829–41.
30. Cools R, Clark L, Robbins TW. Differential responses in human striatum and prefrontal cortex to changes in object and rule relevance. J Neurosci 2004;24: 1129–35.
31. Clark L, Cools R, Robbins TW. The neuropsychology of ventral prefrontal cortex: decision-making and reversal learning. Brain Cogn 2004;55:41–53.
32. O'Doherty J, Dayan P, Schultz J, et al. Dissociable roles of ventral and dorsal striatum in instrumental conditioning. Science 2004;304:452–4.
33. Matsumoto N, Hanakawa T, Maki S, et al. Role of [corrected] nigrostriatal dopamine system in learning to perform sequential motor tasks in a predictive manner. J Neurophysiol 1999;82:978–98.
34. Baxter MG, Murray EA. The amygdala and reward. Nat Rev Neurosci 2002;3: 563–73.
35. Blair RJ, Colledge E, Mitchell DG. Somatic markers and response reversal: is there orbitofrontal cortex dysfunction in boys with psychopathic tendencies? J Abnorm Child Psychol 2001;29:499–511.
36. Blair RJ. Neurocognitive models of aggression, the antisocial personality disorders, and psychopathy. J Neurol Neurosurg Psychiatr 2001;71:727–31.

37. Blair RJ. The roles of orbital frontal cortex in the modulation of antisocial behavior. Brain Cogn 2004;55:198–208.
38. Finger EC, Marsh AA, Mitchell DG, et al. Abnormal ventromedial prefrontal cortex function in children with psychopathic traits during reversal learning. Arch Gen Psychiatry 2008;65:586–94.
39. Goldman-Rakic PS. Development of cortical circuitry and cognitive function. Child Dev 1987;58:601–22.
40. Fuster JM. Prefrontal neurons in networks of executive memory. Brain Res Bull 2000;52:331–6.
41. Casey BJ, Tottenham N, Fossella J. Clinical, imaging, lesion, and genetic approaches toward a model of cognitive control. Dev Psychobiol 2002;40:237–54.
42. Botvinick MM, Cohen JD, Carter CS. Conflict monitoring and anterior cingulate cortex: an update. Trends Cogn Sci 2004;8:539–46.
43. MacLeod CM, MacDonald PA. Interdimensional interference in the Stroop effect: uncovering the cognitive and neural anatomy of attention. Trends Cogn Sci 2000;4:383–91.
44. Rothbart MK, Ahadi SA, Evans DE. Temperament and personality: origins and outcomes. J Pers Soc Psychol 2000;78:122–35.
45. Cole PM, Martin SE, Dennis TA. Emotion regulation as a scientific construct: methodological challenges and directions for child development research. Child Dev 2004;75:317–33.
46. Fox NA, Henderson HA, Marshall PJ, et al. Behavioral inhibition: linking biology and behavior within a developmental framework. Annu Rev Psychol 2005;56:235–62.
47. Calkins SD. Origins and outcomes of individual differences in emotion regulation. Monogr Soc Res Child Dev 1994;59:53–72.
48. Goldsmith HH, Buss KA, Lemery KS. Toddler and childhood temperament: expanded content, stronger genetic evidence, new evidence for the importance of environment. Dev Psychol 1997;33:891–905.
49. Van Hulle CA, Lemery-Chalfant K, Goldsmith HH. Genetic and environmental influences on socio-emotional behavior in toddlers: an initial twin study of the infant-toddler social and emotional assessment. J Child Psychol Psychiatry 2007;48:1014–24.
50. Eaton DK, Kann L, Kinchen S, et al. Youth risk behavior surveillance–United States, 2005. MMWR Surveill Summ 2006;55:1–108.
51. Giedd JN, Lenroot RK, Shaw P, et al. Trajectories of anatomic brain development as a phenotype. Novartis Found Symp 2008;289:101–12.
52. Gogtay N, Giedd JN, Lusk L, et al. Dynamic mapping of human cortical development during childhood through early adulthood. Proc Natl Acad Sci U S A 2004;101:8174–9.
53. Monk CS, McClure EB, Nelson EE, et al. Adolescent immaturity in attention-related brain engagement to emotional facial expressions. Neuroimage 2003; 20:420–8.
54. Nelson EE, McClure EB, Monk CS, et al. Developmental differences in neuronal engagement during implicit encoding of emotional faces: an event-related fMRI study. J Child Psychol Psychiatry 2003;44:1015–24.
55. McClure EB, Monk CS, Nelson EE, et al. A developmental examination of gender differences in brain engagement during evaluation of threat. Biol Psychiatry 2004;55:1047–55.
56. Ernst M, Nelson EE, Jazbec S, et al. Amygdala and nucleus accumbens in responses to receipt and omission of gains in adults and adolescents. Neuroimage 2005;25:1279–91.

57. Yurgelun-Todd D. Emotional and cognitive changes during adolescence. Curr Opin Neurobiol 2007;17:251–7.
58. Casey BJ, Jones RM, Hare TA. The adolescent brain. Ann N Y Acad Sci 2008; 1124:111–26.
59. American Psychiatric Association. Diagnostic and statistical manual of mental disorders. Text Revision (DSM-IV-TR). 4th edition. Washington, DC: American Psychiatric Association; 2000.
60. Leibenluft E, Blair RJ, Charney DS, et al. Irritability in pediatric mania and other childhood psychopathology. Ann N Y Acad Sci 2003;1008:201–18.
61. Kaufman J, Birmaher B, Brent D, et al. Schedule for Affective Disorders and Schizophrenia for School-Age Children-Present and Lifetime Version (K-SADS-PL): initial reliability and validity data. J Am Acad Child Adolesc Psychiatry 1997;36:980–8.
62. Shaffer D, Fisher P, Lucas CP, et al. NIMH Diagnostic Interview Schedule for Children Version IV (NIMH DISC-IV): description, differences from previous versions, and reliability of some common diagnoses. J Am Acad Child Adolesc Psychiatry 2000;39:28–38.
63. Poznanski O, Freeman LN, Mokros HB. Children's depression rating scale-revised. Psychopharmacol Bull 1985;21(4):979–84.
64. Pavuluri MN, Birmaher B, Naylor MW. Pediatric bipolar disorder: a review of the past 10 years. J Am Acad Child Adolesc Psychiatry 2005;44:846–71.
65. Damasio H, Grabowski T, Frank R, et al. The return of Phineas Gage: clues about the brain from the skull of a famous patient. Science 1994;264:1102–5.
66. Siever LJ. Neurobiology of aggression and violence. Am J Psychiatry 2008;165: 429–42.
67. Gonda X, Rihmer Z, Zsombok T, et al. The 5HTTLPR polymorphism of the serotonin transporter gene is associated with affective temperaments as measured by TEMPS-A. J Affect Disord 2006;91:125–31.
68. Kang JI, Namkoong K, Kim SJ. The association of 5-HTTLPR and DRD4 VNTR polymorphisms with affective temperamental traits in healthy volunteers. J Affect Disord 2008;109:157–63.
69. Scott J, Stanton B, Garland A, et al. Cognitive vulnerability in patients with bipolar disorder. Psychol Med 2000;30:467–72.
70. Lam D, Wright K, Smith N. Dysfunctional assumptions in bipolar disorder. J Affect Disord 2004;79:193–9.
71. Carver CS, White TL. Behavioral inhibition, behavioral activation, and affective responses to impending reward and punishment: the BIS/BAS scales. J Pers Soc Psychol 1994;67:319–33.
72. Alloy LB, Abramson LY, Walshaw PD, et al. Behavioral Approach System and Behavioral Inhibition System sensitivities and bipolar spectrum disorders: prospective prediction of bipolar mood episodes. Bipolar Disord 2008;10: 310–22.
73. Abler B, Greenhouse I, Ongur D, et al. Abnormal reward system activation in mania. Neuropsychopharmacology 2008;33:2217–27.
74. Ferreira AD, Neves FS, da Rocha FF, et al. The role of 5-HTTLPR polymorphism in antidepressant-associated mania in bipolar disorder. J Affect Disord 2009; 112:267–72.
75. Kessler RC, Rubinow DR, Holmes C, et al. The epidemiology of DSM-III-R bipolar I disorder in a general population survey. Psychol Med 1997;27:1079–89.
76. Thase ME. STEP-BD and bipolar depression: what have we learned? Curr Psychiatry Rep 2007;9:497–503.

77. Post RM, Denicoff KD, Leverich GS, et al. Morbidity in 258 bipolar outpatients followed for 1 year with daily prospective ratings on the NIMH life chart method. J Clin Psychiatry 2003;64:680–90.
78. Perlis RH, Smoller JW, Fava M, et al. The prevalence and clinical correlates of anger attacks during depressive episodes in bipolar disorder. J Affect Disord 2004;79:291–5.
79. Nowicki S, Duke M. Individual differences in the nonverbal communication of affect: the diagnostic analysis of nonverbal accuracy scale. J Nonverbal Behav 1994;18:9–35.
80. McClure EB, Pope K, Hoberman AJ, et al. Facial expression recognition in adolescents with mood and anxiety disorders. Am J Psychiatry 2003;160: 1172–4.
81. McClure EB, Treland JE, Snow J, et al. Deficits in social cognition and response flexibility in pediatric bipolar disorder. Am J Psychiatry 2005;162:1644–51.
82. Rich BA, Vinton DT, Roberson-Nay R, et al. Limbic hyperactivation during processing of neutral facial expressions in children with bipolar disorder. Proc Natl Acad Sci U S A, 2006;103:8900–5.
83. Dickstein DP, Rich BA, Roberson-Nay R, et al. Neural activation during encoding of emotional faces in pediatric bipolar disorder. Bipolar Disord 2007;9:679–92.
84. Dickstein DP, Treland JE, Snow J, et al. Neuropsychological performance in pediatric bipolar disorder. Biol Psychiatry 2004;55:32–9.
85. Rubinsztein JS, Michael A, Paykel ES, et al. Cognitive impairment in remission in bipolar affective disorder. Psychol Med 2000;30:1025–36.
86. Sweeney JA, Kmiec JA, Kupfer DJ. Neuropsychologic impairments in bipolar and unipolar mood disorders on the CANTAB neurocognitive battery. Biol Psychiatry 2000;48:674–84.
87. Clark L, Iversen SD, Goodwin GM. A neuropsychological investigation of prefrontal cortex involvement in acute mania. Am J Psychiatry 2001;158: 1605–11.
88. Clark L, Iversen SD, Goodwin GM. Sustained attention deficit in bipolar disorder. Br J Psychiatry 2002;180:313–9.
89. Gorrindo T, Blair RJ, Budhani S, et al. Deficits on a probabilistic response-reversal task in patients with pediatric bipolar disorder. Am J Psychiatry 2005; 162:1975–7.
90. Budhani S, Blair RJ. Response reversal and children with psychopathic tendencies: success is a function of salience of contingency change. J Child Psychol Psychiatry 2005;46:972–81.
91. Blumberg HP, Martin A, Kaufman J, et al. Frontostriatal abnormalities in adolescents with bipolar disorder: preliminary observations from functional MRI. Am J Psychiatry 2003;160:1345–7.
92. Leibenluft E, Rich BA, Vinton DT, et al. Neural circuitry engaged during unsuccessful motor inhibition in pediatric bipolar disorder. Am J Psychiatry 2007; 164:52–60.
93. Nelson EE, Vinton DT, Berghorst L, et al. Brain systems underlying response flexibility in healthy and bipolar adolescents: an event-related fMRI study. Bipolar Disord 2007;9:810–9.
94. Axelson D, Birmaher BJ, Brent D, et al. A preliminary study of the Kiddie Schedule for Affective Disorders and Schizophrenia for School-Age Children mania rating scale for children and adolescents. J Child Adolesc Psychopharmacol 2003;13:463–70.

95. Carlson GA, Meyer SE. Phenomenology and diagnosis of bipolar disorder in children, adolescents, and adults: complexities and developmental issues. Dev Psychopathol 2006;18:939–69.

96. Hunt JI, Dyl J, Armstrong L, et al. Frequency of manic symptoms and bipolar disorder in psychiatrically hospitalized adolescents using the K-SADS Mania Rating Scale. J Child Adolesc Psychopharmacol 2005;15:918–30.

97. Axelson D, Birmaher B, Strober M, et al. Phenomenology of children and adolescents with bipolar spectrum disorders. Arch Gen Psychiatry 2006;63:1139–48.

98. Wozniak J, Biederman J, Kwon A, et al. How cardinal are cardinal symptoms in pediatric bipolar disorder? An examination of clinical correlates. Biol Psychiatry 2005;58:583–8.

99. Geller B, Zimerman B, Williams M, et al. DSM-IV mania symptoms in a prepubertal and early adolescent bipolar disorder phenotype compared to attention-deficit hyperactive and normal controls. J Child Adolesc Psychopharmacol 2002;12:11–25.

100. Leibenluft E, Charney DS, Towbin KE, et al. Defining clinical phenotypes of juvenile mania. Am J Psychiatry 2003;160:430–7.

101. Biederman J, Klein RG, Pine DS, et al. Resolved: mania is mistaken for ADHD in prepubertal children. J Am Acad Child Adolesc Psychiatry 1998;37:1091–6.

102. Biederman J, Faraone SV, Wozniak J, et al. Further evidence of unique developmental phenotypic correlates of pediatric bipolar disorder: findings from a large sample of clinically referred preadolescent children assessed over the last 7 years. J Affect Disord 2004;82(Suppl 1):S45–58.

103. Brotman MA, Schmajuk M, Rich BA, et al. Prevalence, clinical correlates, and longitudinal course of severe mood dysregulation in children. Biol Psychiatry 2006;60:991–7.

104. Rich BA, Grimley ME, Schmajuk M, et al. Face emotion labeling deficits in children with bipolar disorder and severe mood dysregulation. Dev Psychopathol 2008;20:529–46.

105. Guyer AE, McClure EB, Adler AD, et al. Specificity of facial expression labeling deficits in childhood psychopathology. J Child Psychol Psychiatry 2007;48: 863–71.

106. Dickstein DP, Nelson EE, McClure EB, et al. Cognitive flexibility in phenotypes of pediatric bipolar disorder. J Am Acad Child Adolesc Psychiatry 2007;46: 341–55.

107. Rau G, Blair KS, Berghorst L, et al. Processing of differentially valued rewards and punishments in youths with bipolar disorder or severe mood dysregulation. J Child Adolesc Psychopharmacol 2008;18:185–96.

108. Rich BA, Schmajuk M, Perez-Edgar KE, et al. Different psychophysiological and behavioral responses elicited by frustration in pediatric bipolar disorder and severe mood dysregulation. Am J Psychiatry 2007;164:309–17.

109. Rich BA, Bhangoo RK, Vinton DT, et al. Using affect-modulated startle to study phenotypes of pediatric bipolar disorder. Bipolar Disord 2005;7:536–45.

Magnetic Resonance Imaging Studies in Early Onset Bipolar Disorder: An Updated Review

Janine Terry, BA[a], Melissa Lopez-Larson, MD[a,b,*],
Jean A. Frazier, MD[c,d]

KEYWORDS

- Bipolar disorder • Child psychiatry
- Magnetic resonance imaging • Mood disorders
- Functional neuroimaging • Spectroscopy

BD (occurring before 18 years) is a severe psychiatric disorder that is associated with an earlier age of onset, higher rates of psychosis, more frequent suicidality, and greater genetic loading than is the adult-onset form of the illness.[1–4] Although the pathophysiology of early onset BD is unknown, magnetic resonance imaging (MRI) studies of affected children and adolescents are advancing the understanding of the neurodevelopmental processes that may give rise to this disorder. Our prior review article published in 2005 in the *Harvard Review of Psychiatry* on neuroimaging studies in youths with BD found that early onset BD was associated with functional, anatomic, and biochemical abnormalities in structures that are hypothesized to be involved in the neuroanatomic circuits of emotion processing and regulation, including the limbic-thalamic-prefrontal circuit and the limbic-striatal-pallidal thalamic circuit.[5] Specifically, structural neuroimaging studies reported differences in total cerebral volumes (TCVs), cortical gray matter, superior temporal gyrus (STG), putamen, thalamus, amygdala, and hippocampal volumes compared with healthy children. An increase in white matter hyperintensities (WMH) was also noted in youths with BD. Magnetic resonance

[a] The Brain Institute, University of Utah, 383 Colorow Drive, Salt Lake City, UT 84108, USA
[b] University of Utah Medical School, Salt Lake City, UT, USA
[c] Child and Adolescent Neurodevelopment Initiative, University of Massachusetts Medical School, 55 Lake Avenue North, Worcester, MA 01655, USA
[d] Department of Psychiatry, UMASS Memorial Medical Center, 55 Lake Avenue North, Worcester, MA 01655, USA
* Corresponding author. The Brain Institute, University of Utah, 383 Colorow Drive, Salt Lake City, UT 84108, USA.
E-mail address: melissa.lopez-larson@hsc.utah.edu (M. Lopez-Larson).

Child Adolesc Psychiatric Clin N Am 18 (2009) 421–439
doi:10.1016/j.chc.2008.12.004
1056-4993/08/$ – see front matter © 2009 Elsevier Inc. All rights reserved.

childpsych.theclinics.com

spectroscopy (MRS) abnormalities were reported in the dorsolateral prefrontal cortex (DLPFC), anterior cingulate cortex (ACC), and basal ganglia (BG). Studies with fMRI found increased activation in the putamen and thalamus of youths with BD and another found abnormal prefrontal-subcortical activation in familial pediatric BD during a cognitive and emotion-based task, respectively.

Advantages of MRI investigations in youths include the possibility of identifying the earliest presence, nature, and extent of brain changes that occur during development. In addition, neuroimaging studies of youths are relatively free of some of the confounding variables that frequently confront research in adults, including the effects of illness duration and chronicity, repeated illness episodes, heterogeneous samples (including childhood- and adolescent-onset BD), chronic stress, institutionalization, long-term substance and medication use, and exposure to electroconvulsive therapy. Furthermore, studies of children and adolescents with BD may help uncover endophenotypic markers or biomarkers of illness in the brain, which could lead to improvements in early identification and treatment as well as in prevention efforts.

Over the past 5 to 10 years, there has been an explosion in neuroimaging technology that has begun to emerge in the literature of early onset BD. For instance, investigators are using higher-resolution imaging scanners and newer imaging protocols such as diffusion-tensor imaging (DTI) and implementing whole brain analysis, automated or semiautomated segmentation, and cortical and subcortical parcellation methodologies. Furthermore, neuroimaging study design has also improved by including increased sample sizes, longitudinal studies, pre- and postillness onset studies, and the study of youths at genetic risk of BD, including those with and without illness. This article provides an update to our previous review of the literature regarding neuroimaging in youths with BD,[5] highlighting important new study designs and techniques. Such information may provide a foundation from which to form hypotheses for future MRI studies of child and adolescent onset BD.

METHODS

A PubMed literature search was performed to identify all original research articles that used neuroimaging methods to study pediatric BD published between January 1990 and October 2008 in any language. The search terms used included MRI, MRS, fMRI, DTI, and childhood-, adolescent-, pediatric-, or early onset, followed by BD, affective disorder, or mania. No methodological inclusion criteria were applied, and all child and adolescent neuroimaging studies were included for discussion and critical review in this article.

RESULTS OF THE LITERATURE REVIEW
Anatomic Neuroimaging

Manually traced region of interest (ROI) measurements continue to be the gold standard for structural evaluation of MRI scans. The major disadvantages of manual ROI measurements include significant time burden (including training staff and slice-by-slice tracing), a prior knowledge regarding the structures of interest, and the need to evaluate structures of interest according to defined anatomic landmarks (such as sulci or gyral patterns), which can be highly variable between individuals. Newer methodologies such as voxel-based morphometry (VBM) and optimized VBM allow unbiased whole-brain assessments of density/volume changes in white and gray matter. Optimized VBM helps to improve segmentation and also allows for the investigation of true gray matter volume instead of gray matter density.[6] VBM is relatively simple, automated (requires little to no intervention), and is sensitive to both small and large differences. The major disadvantages of VBM include susceptibility to registration and segmentation errors and its sensitivity to image quality and artifacts.[6] These disadvantages are particularly important when assessing youths, as they are particularly prone to movement, resulting in poor image quality. Furthermore, the gray matter changes detected with this method may not necessarily be due to reduced thickness or atrophy, but rather, misaligned gyri or sulci or a variation in gyral patterns.[7]

Another new methodology that has recently begun to appear in the early onset BD literature is DTI. This novel imaging technique allows for the study of the anatomic architecture of brain networks in vivo. DTI measures the diffusion of water molecules across tissues and can provide information about the integrity or organization of the major WM tracts.[8] A measure of this uniform diffusion, fractional anisotropy, is calculated and used to make group comparisons. Decreased fractional anisotropy values indicate more random water diffusion and suggest a reduction in the integrity of WM tracts. Another measure that is used in DTI is the apparent diffusion coefficient (ADC), which is a scalar representation of the total net water diffusion; fractional anisotropy and the ADC typically correlate negatively. Given its sensitivity to WM changes, DTI offers considerable potential in early onset BD, as it can facilitate the evaluation of early brain development, including both regressive (pruning) and progressive (myelination) events. Furthermore, it provides the capability to track disruption in WM maturation that may occur with disease progression.[8]

Our prior review[5] of the anatomic MRI literature from January 1990 to January 2005 in children and adolescents with BD reported volumetric differences in a number of brain structures when youths with BD were compared with healthy controls (HC), including smaller TCV,[9–11] increased number of WMH,[12–14] smaller limbic structures (amygdala and hippocampus),[9,10,15,16] larger putamen,[9] and smaller superior temporal gyri.[16] These studies were ROI studies performed on a 1.5 Tesla (T) scanner. However, one study performed by Wilke and colleagues[17] was conducted on a 3T scanner and used an optimized VBM protocol. This study reported cortical gray matter volume increases in the basal ganglia and deficits in the medial temporal lobe, orbital frontal cortex (OFC), and left anterior cingulate gyrus (ACG) in youths with BD (n = 10) compared with those in HC (n = 52).

A review of recent structural neuroimaging studies (dating from January 2005 to October 2008) in early onset BD is outlined below and compared and contrasted to older studies, as indicated. A review of WM pathology is followed by cortical gray matter and major lobes and gyri, and then subcortical structures, including the thalamus, amygdala, and hippocampus.

White matter

An increase in WMH is a consistent, although nonspecific, finding in MRI studies of adults and youths with BD.[12–14,18–21] The cause of the hyperintensities is unknown. Of the four studies considering WMH in youths with BD, three reported an increase in WMH in youths with BD compared with that in HC, whereas the most recent one, which used a higher-resolution scanner (3T as opposed to 1.5T used in the other studies) and a standardized protocol for WMH evaluation, did not find a difference in WHM.[22] This was a study of 20 adolescents with BD (age, 14.5 ± 2.8 years) who were at genetic risk for BD (based on having a parent with BD) compared with 20 age- and gender-matched HC. The authors postulated that based on their findings, WMH may be a later sequelae of BD.[22]

The inability to observe and isolate the major WM fiber systems with current imaging techniques has resulted in few WM ROI studies in the psychiatric literature. However, the corpus callosum (CC) is one exception, as it can be easily visualized and has well-defined boundaries. In fact, the CC has been studied extensively in psychiatric disorders, including in adults with BD. For example, a meta-analysis of 5 studies of adults with BD, by McIntosh and colleagues,[23] found that adults with BD had smaller CC in the anterior and middle regions in comparison with that in HC. In addition, abnormal growth trajectories for the CC have also been reported.[24] Unfortunately, to date, there has been only one ROI MRI investigation of the CC in youths with BD. These authors reported a shape difference marked by reduced splenium circularity in youths with BD compared with that in HC, but did not find differences between groups in the length or area of the CC.[25]

DTI has recently been applied to youths with BD to further investigate underlying WM abnormalities. For instance, Adler and associates[26] found that 11 medication-naïve adolescents with BD experiencing their first manic or mixed episode had a reduction in fractional anisotropy in the superior frontal WM tracts compared with that in 17 HC. Frazier and colleagues[27] compared 10 children with BD, eight HC, and seven healthy youths at risk for BD (family history of first-degree relative) on a 1.5 T scanner using DTI. They found that compared with HC, youths with BD had decreased fractional anisotropy in the left orbital frontal WM, the right CC body, and the right and left superior frontal tracts, including the superior longitudinal fasciculus I and the cingulate-paracingulate WM.[27] Compared to the at-risk BD group, children with BD showed reduced fractional anisotropy in the right and left cingulate-paracingulate WM.[27] Both the BD and at-risk BD groups showed reduced fractional anisotropy relative to that in HC in the bilateral superior longitudinal fasciculus I.[27] The authors suggested that the bilateral superior longitudinal fasciculus I finding in both the BD and at-risk BD groups may represent a trait-based marker or endophenotype of the disorder, whereas the decreased FA in the right and left cingulate-paracingulate WM in children with BD only may represent a disease-state finding.[27]

Cerebral cortex, lobes, and gyri

Before 2005, there had been only a few studies that looked at the cerebral cortex, individual lobes, or gyri in youths with BD. This included a study by Wilke and colleagues,[17] using an optimized VBM protocol, that found gray matter deficits in the medial temporal lobe, OFC, and ACC and increased gray matter in regions of the basal ganglia in youths with BD compared with those in HC, and two ROI studies that found smaller left total STG volumes[16] and no volumetric differences in the subgenual PFC[28] in children and adolescents with BD compared with those in HC.

More recently, there have been several ROI studies evaluating the cerebral cortex, lobes, and gyri. In addition, there have been three VBM studies, including 2 longitudinal studies that have looked at cerebral gray matter in youths with BD. For instance, Chang and colleagues[22] evaluated 20 adolescents with familial (first-degree relative with BD) BD (age, 14.5 ± 2.8 years) compared with 20 age- and gender-matched HC adolescents on a 3T scanner and found no differences in TCV and total cerebral gray matter or WM in youths with BD. Furthermore, no differences in frontal, prefrontal, parietal, temporal, or occipital lobes were found between groups. In contrast, another study by Frazier and colleagues[29] compared HC (n = 15; age, 11.2 ± 2.8 years) to youths with BD (n = 35) and found reduced bilateral parietal lobe and left temporal lobe in the BD group. On further analysis of the parietal lobe and temporal lobe, smaller volumes were noted in the bilateral postcentral gyri, left STG, and left fusiform gyrus, whereas the parahippocampal gyri were bilaterally increased in the BD group. Exploratory analysis of the frontal lobe found that the right middle frontal gyrus was smaller in the BD group. Differences in the findings of these 2 studies may be related to methodological differences, such as differences in MRI strength (1.5 versus 3 T), parcellation methods, and age of youths (11.2 versus 14.5 years) (Parcellation is a way of looking at the brain in three dimensions).

Newly published ROI studies have also targeted specific areas of interest, including the cingulate gyrus, the OFC, and the cerebellum. For instance, the ACC volume has been found to be smaller in youths with BD (n = 16) compared with that in youths with autism spectrum disorder (n = 24) and HC (n = 15).[30] Furthermore, Kaur and colleagues[31] found that youths with BD (n = 16) had significantly smaller left ACC and bilateral posterior cingulate gyri compared with that in HC (n = 21). Najt and colleagues[32] looked at OFC subdivisions and found gender-specific differences in subregion volumes for males and females (mean age, 15.5 ± 3.2 years) in youths with BD (n = 14) compared with those in HC (n = 20), with female subjects with BD having larger OFC subregion volumes and males having smaller OFC subregion volumes compared with those in HC (n = 20). In another study considering the cerebellum, no significant differences in the cerebellum or vermis measures were found between BD (n = 16) and HC (n = 21); however, there was a trend toward smaller vermis V2 areas in BD consistent with findings from studies in adult bipolar patients.[33]

An optimized VBM study followed by secondary selection of a priori ROIs, including the amygdala, accumbens, hippocampus, DLPFC, and OFC, was performed by Dickstein and colleagues in 2005.[34] These authors found that 20 youths with BD had reduced gray matter volume in the left DLPFC compared with that in 20 HC. With more liberal statistical analysis, the left accumbens and left amygdala were also noted to have gray matter reductions in the BD group compared with those in HC. In a longitudinal VBM study of an older group of adolescents and young adults, Farrow and associates[35] looked at 25 youths with schizophrenia and eight subjects with BD first-episode (mean age 19 ± 3 years) who had MRI scans at first presentation and 2 years later and 22 HC who had one set of MRI scans. Youths with BD compared with HC had decreased gray matter volumes in the frontal lobe (right inferior frontal/precentral gyrus), temporal lobe (bilateral inferior temporal gyrus/uncus, left insula, left posterior inferior/middle temporal gyrus), and parietal lobe (left posterior cingulate gyrus). In addition, the BD group also had reduced WM in the left frontal lobe and bilateral posterior parietotemporal junction. Follow-up MRI scans compared with initial scans in youths with BD found a reduction in gray matter volume over time in the frontal lobe (bilateral ACG). Furthermore, reductions in WM were found in the time two scans relative to the time one scan in the BD group in regions of the right posterior frontal/parietal cortex, left temporoparietal junction, right parietooccipital junction, left parietal lobe, and right cerebellum. When initial MRI scans of youths with schizophrenia and BD were compared, youths with BD had smaller gray matter volumes in regions of the temporal lobe, whereas those with schizophrenia had reduced gray matter volumes in regions of the frontal lobe. A comparison of follow-up MRI scans between these two groups (BD and schizophrenia) found similar differences.

In one of the only pre-post BD conversion longitudinal imaging studies to date, Gogtay and colleagues[36] followed and obtained neuroimaging scans on a group of 32 multidimensionally impaired (MDI) youths defined as youths with transient hallucinations, comorbid attention-deficit/hyperactivity disorder (ADHD), and prominent mood lability over several years. Twelve of these youths converted to BD (had their first manic episode), and nine of these youths had MRI scans both before and after BD conversion. These nine youths were subsequently compared with eight youths with MDI who did not convert to BD and to 18 HC. All subjects in this study were male. Total gray matter and total cerebral volume TCV were not different between the BD, MDI, or HC groups either initially or with age. On comparison between pre– and post–first manic episode MRI scans, youths with BD were found to have cortical gray matter gains in the left temporal lobe (middle and inferior temporal gyri), OFC, and ventrolateral PFC (VLPFC) compared with those in HC, which was most prominent after illness onset. Furthermore, youths with BD were found to have gray matter losses on the right temporal lobe, right OFC, bilateral anterior and subgenual cingulate cortices, and left posterior cingulate gyrus compared with those in HC. Youths with MDI showed a similar but more widespread pattern of cortical gray matter changes compared with that in HC. There were no significant differences between the MDI and BD groups; therefore, the authors suggested that these overall developmental trajectory abnormalities in youths with BD and MDI might more generally reflect affective dysregulation.[36]

Subcortical structures

Few anatomic MRI studies of youths with BD have examined the thalamus. The thalamus is a key structure operating as a relay station between cortical and subcortical brain regions, and its role has been implicated in the pathophysiology of mood disorders.[37,38] However, in youths with BD, most ROI studies have been negative.[10,39–42] The one exception is an older study by Dasari and colleagues[40] who found smaller thalamic volumes in a sample of adolescents with BD when compared with those in HC. Interestingly, Frazier and colleagues[41] looked at a sample of youths with BD with and without psychosis and a group of youths with schizophrenia and found that only the schizophrenia group had smaller thalamic volumes compared with those of HC, suggesting that thalamic abnormalities may be specific to schizophrenia.

Collectively, cross-sectional ROI and studies of the amygdala in BD adolescents have found smaller[9,15,39] or a trend[43] toward smaller amygdala volumes compared with those of HC. In the only longitudinal study of youths with BD to look at the amygdala, Blumberg and associates[44] scanned adolescents and young adults on two separate occasions approximately 2 years apart and found that youths with BD had smaller amygdala volumes at both time periods compared with those of HC. A VBM followed by ROI analysis found left amygdala gray matter reductions but only after liberal statistics were applied.[45] Furthermore, another study of a younger population of youths with BD did not find abnormalities in amygdala volumes but instead found smaller hippocampi compared with those of HC.[10] Smaller total hippocampal volumes have also been reported in two other studies of adolescents with BD,[15,46] although there have also been negative studies in this population.[39,43,45] Interestingly, in a more recent VBM study, relative to HC, healthy bipolar offspring had significantly increased GM volumes in left parahippocampal/hippocampal gyrus following whole-brain analysis.[47] This finding in youths at genetic risk but who were without psychiatric illness suggests that increased gray matter volume in the parahippocampal/hippocampal gyrus may be a potential biomarker for risk for BD or, alternatively, a neuroprotective marker. In addition, in a recent study, Bearden and colleagues[46] used a novel 3-dimensional model of the hippocampus after manual tracing and found that adolescents with BD (n = 16) had smaller total hippocampus and localized deficits in the head and tail of the left hippocampal regions compared with those of HC (n = 20).

Overall, anatomic ROI MRI investigations in youths with BPD have not found abnormalities in the basal ganglia,[39,41,48,49] with the exception of two studies that reported enlarged striatal structures[9,17] compared with those of HC. Furthermore, Ahn and colleagues[48] found that prepubertal youths with BPD had larger right nucleus accumbens, and a VBM study reported smaller left nucleus accumbens volumes after liberal statistics was applied.[45]

Summary of structural neuroimaging findings

In summary, anatomic MRI studies to date in children and adolescents with BD report differences in a number of brain structures. For example, WM studies have reported increased WMH[12-14] and shape and fractional anisotropy abnormalities in regions of the CC in youths with BD compared with those in HC. In addition, fractional anisotropy abnormalities have been found in the superior longitudinal fasciculus I and the cingulate-paracingulate WM, which may be state and trait markers of BD illness, respectively.[27] These major WM tracts are important in interhemispheric and intrahemispheric communication between frontolimbic, frontoparietal, and temporoparietal regions. In addition, in a longitudinal VBM study, WM abnormalities were found over time in regions of the right posterior frontal/parietal cortex, left temporoparietal junction, right parietooccipital junction, left parietal lobe, and right cerebellum.

Other ROI structural findings in BD include abnormalities in regions of the parietal lobe (bilateral postcentral gyri), temporal lobe (STG and left fusiform gyrus, parahippocampal gyri) and frontal lobe (OFC, middle frontal gyrus, subgenual PFC), cingulate gyrus (left ACC, and bilateral posterior cingulate gyrus), and cerebellum.[10,16,28,30-33] Cross-sectionally, VBM studies are consistent with ROI studies and have also reported gray matter abnormalities in the frontal lobe (left DLPFC, OFC, right inferior frontal/precentral gyrus),[17,34] temporal lobe (inferior and middle temporal gyrus/uncus and left insula), and cingulate gyrus (anterior cingulated gyrus and left posterior cingulate gyrus).[35]

Longitudinally, a VBM study in youths and young adults with BD as compared with HC found decreased gray matter volumes over time in the anterior cingulated gyrus, bilaterally.[35] Furthermore, youths with BD were found to have smaller gray matter volumes in regions of the temporal lobe compared with those in schizophrenia youths who had reduced gray matter volumes in regions of the frontal lobe.[35] Furthermore, in a pre-post BD conversion longitudinal study, youths with BD were found to have cortical gray matter gains over the left OFC, VLPFC, and temporal lobe and losses over the right temporal lobe, OFC, left posterior cingulate cortex (PCC), and bilaterally in the ACC (and subgenual).[36] These findings were similar to those in MDI youths who had not converted to BD.

With the exception of one study,[40] thalamus abnormalities have not been found[10,39-42] and may be specific to schizophrenia.[41] Cross-sectional and longitudinal ROI studies of amygdala volumes in BD adolescents have found smaller[9,15,39,44] or a trend[43,45] toward smaller amygdala volumes compared with those of HC; however, a ROI study in a younger sample of youths with BD did not.[10] Smaller total hippocampal volumes, including localized deficits in the head and tail of the left hippocampal regions,[46] have also been reported in youths with BD,[10,15,41,46] although there have also been negative studies.[39,43,45] Interestingly, increased gray matter volumes in the left parahippocampal/hippocampal gyrus following whole-brain analysis[47] was found in HC at genetic risk for BD, suggesting its possible role as a biomarker for risk for BD or, alternatively, perhaps as a neuroprotective marker. The notion that increased parahippocampal gyri gray matter volume may be a biomarker for BD is further supported by the fact that youth affected by the illness have also been reported to have increased gray matter volume in that region.[29] Overall, anatomic ROI MRI investigations in youths with BD have not found abnormalities in the basal ganglia,[22,39,41,48,49] with the exception of two studies that reported enlarged striatal structures[9,17] compared with those of HC. Larger right nucleus accumbens[48] and smaller left nucleus accumbens[45] volumes have been reported in an ROI and VBM study, respectively.

Functional Imaging

Functional MRI uses the blood oxygenation level-dependent response to measure the hemodynamic consequences of neuronal activity. Some of the limitations of fMRI are its poor signal-to-noise ratio, sensitivity to state-dependent features, and the need for task modification for children and adolescents based on maturation levels and psychiatric impairment. Before January 2005, there had been only two studies that used fMRI in the study of youths with BD. One study incorporated a Stroop task,[50] and the other used an emotional processing task.[51] The findings of these studies along with newly published studies are described below in accordance with the type of task used.

Attention and mental flexibility tasks

Blumberg and colleagues[50] found increased activation in the left putamen and thalamus in adolescents with BD (n = 20; 10 with BD, 10 controls) during a Stroop activation paradigm task designed to measure directed attention. The authors also noted a lack of normal age-related signal increase in the rostroventral PFC and striatum. A study by Nelson and colleagues[52] used a response flexibility task to assess 25 youths with BD (five hypomanic, 20 euthymic) and 17 HC. The response flexibility task requires participants to both inhibit and replace a prepotent motor response with another motor response after the initial response has been cued.[52] The authors reported that those affected with BD had abnormal activation patterns in the left DLPFC, the primary motor cortex, and the precuneus, compared with those in HC. The authors speculated that executive functioning abnormalities in the DLPFC resulted in subjects with BD relying on the primary motor cortex to successfully complete the flexibility task. In a subgroup analysis of only youths with BD without comorbid ADHD (n = 10) compared with HC, the authors reported that the primary study findings were unchanged. Furthermore, a subgroup analysis of unmedicated youths with BD versus HC also demonstrated similar findings.

Adler and colleagues[53] used a simplified Continuous Performance Task (CPT) for children and adolescents to study youths with BD (mixed or manic) with comorbid ADHD (n = 11) and without (n = 15). The authors reported that compared with youths with BD alone, youths with BD+ADHD had reduced activation in the VLPFC and ACC and greater activation in the posterior parietal cortex and middle temporal gyrus. These findings support suggestions that adolescents diagnosed with BD+ADHD differ neurofunctionally from adolescents with BD alone. Unfortunately, the authors did not include a HC cohort to assess whether or not there was a continuum of dysfunction in these regions in the BD groups, with the BD and comorbid ADHD group expressing the most severe abnormalities.

Face-/emotion-processing studies

Several studies have been published using an fMRI test in which blocks of pictures of faces depicting different emotions were presented during scanning, and subjects were asked to rate how each picture made them feel. Investigators used variations of this method to examine changes in ROIs of the brain connected to emotional response and facial encoding. For instance, Dickstein and colleagues[54] performed a study of 23 youths with BD (seven hypomanic, five depressed, and 11 euthymic) and 22 HC, scanned while viewing emotional faces (happy, angry, fearful, and neutral) and given a surprise recognition memory test 30 minutes postscan. The authors found that youths with BD exhibited reduced memory for emotional faces, relative to HC, particularly on fearful faces.[54] Furthermore, youths with BD had increased neural activation in the striatum (caudate and putamen) and in regions of the PFC (ACC and OFC) when successfully encoding emotional faces (happy, angry, and all) compared with that in HC.[54] Post hoc analysis revealed that the findings were not dependent on mood state or presence of ADHD.[54]

Pavuluri and colleagues[55] examined 10 euthymic, unmedicated youths with BD and 10 HC and found that compared with HC, those with BD had reduced activation in the OFC and DLPFC, and there was greater bilateral parahippocampal gyrus activation in the BD group compared with that in HC for angry relative to neutral faces. For happy faces relative to neural faces, there was an attenuation of activation in the OFC, medial PFC (MPFC), and DLPFC, and greater activation in the right posterior parietal cortex and supplementary motor area, right amygdala, right medial parahippocampal gyrus and the tail region of the left hippocampus, and bilateral pregenual ACC in BD youths compared with that in HC.

Rich and colleagues[56] found that compared with HC (n = 21), youths with BD (n = 22, 12 euthymic, four depressed, six hypomanic) had greater activation in the left amygdala, left accumbens, left putamen, and left VLPFC when rating face hostility and greater activation in the left amygdala and bilateral accumbens when rating their fear of the face. In a later study performed by this same group, the authors used a similar face-processing task to assess the functional connectivity or temporal correlation of the amygdala to other brain structures in BD youths (n = 33; 18 euthymic, 11 hypomanic, three depressed, one mixed) and HC (n = 24).[57] The authors reported that youths with BD had significantly reduced connectivity between the left amygdala and the right posterior cingulate/precuneus and right fusiform gyrus/parahippocampal gyrus.[57] Both of these studies by Rich and colleagues included post hoc analyses of mood state and comorbidity status and found no difference in activation patterns between euthymic and noneuthymic youths or in youths with and without comorbidity (ADHD and anxiety disorders) compared with those in HC.

Other tasks

Chang and colleagues[51] studied a group of all male, euthymic youths with genetic BD (parent with BD) performing a visuospatial working memory task and an affective task of visualizing positive, negative, and neutral pictures while undergoing an fMRI study. The authors found that on the visuospatial task, youths with BD had greater activation in the bilateral ACC, left putamen, left thalamus, left DLPFC, left superior and inferior frontal gyrus, and left STG/insula. HC had greater activation in the cerebellar vermis. In viewing negatively valenced pictures, youths with BD had greater activation in bilateral DLPFC, left inferior frontal gyrus, left superior/middle temporal gyrus, and the right insula. HC had greater activation in the right PCC. For positively valenced pictures, BD had greater activation than that in HC in the bilateral caudate and thalamus, left middle superior frontal gyrus, left ACC, precentral gyrus, paracentral lobule, and precuneus. In a study by Pavuluri and colleagues,[58] 10 unmedicated, euthymic subjects with BD and 10 HC were asked to match the color of a word with one of two colored circles below where the words had a positive, negative, or neutral emotional valence to assess frontal lobe and amygdala responses. In the negative affect condition, relative to the neutral condition, youths with BD demonstrated greater activation of bilateral pregenual ACC and left amygdala and less activation in right rostral VLPFC and DLPFC. The authors proposed that the pattern of reduced activation of the VLPFC and greater amygdala activation in bipolar children in response to negative stimuli suggests both disinhibition of emotional reactivity in the limbic system and reduced regulatory functioning of the PFC.[58] Finally, in the first study to demonstrate neural changes after resolution of bipolar depression, Chang and colleagues[59] obtained a baseline fMRI and then a follow-up MRI after 8 weeks of lamotrigine treatment in eight adolescents with the illness. These authors found that adolescents with

BD treated with lamotrigine demonstrated less amygdalar activation when viewing negative pictures as depressive symptoms improved.

Summary of functional neuroimaging findings

In early onset BD, cognitive and emotion-based tasks have been used as probes in attempts to understand the frontolimbic circuit thought to be involved in the pathophysiology of mood dysregulation and executive dysfunction seen in this disorder. Four studies in youths with BD focused primarily on cognitive-based tasks including the Stoop, visuospatial, response flexibility, and CPT tasks. Overall, these studies found that youths with BD had activation abnormalities in regions of the PFC (ACC, DLPFC, and VLPFC), thalamus, and striatum (putamen) compared with those in HC.[51–53] Other regions that appear to be abnormal during these tasks include the primary motor cortex, regions of the parietal lobe (precuneus, posterior parietal cortex) and temporal lobe (middle temporal gyrus, left STG/insula).[51–53] In addition, one of these studies noted a lack of normal age-related signal increase in the rostroventral PFC and striatum, suggesting abnormal developmental maturation of these regions in BD.[50] Furthermore, a study using the CPT in youths with BD and comorbid ADHD compared with youths with BD without ADHD found different activation patterns between groups. Reduced activation in the VLPFC and ACC and greater activation in the posterior parietal cortex and middle temporal gyrus were seen in those with the comorbid presentation when compared with those of youths with BD alone.[53]

Emotion-based fMRI studies consistently reported abnormalities in the amygdala, striatum (caudate and putamen), and regions of the PFC (ACC, OFC, DLPFC, and VLPFC) in youths with BD.[51,54–56,58] Other regions that were found to be abnormal in youths with BD include the temporal lobe (parahippocampal gyrus, left superior/middle temporal gyrus, right insula), parietal lobe (PL) (right posterior parietal cortex, paracentral lobule, and precuneus), hippocampus, accumbens, the thalamus, and the precentral gyrus.[54–57] In a functional connectivity fMRI study of the amygdala, significantly reduced connectivity between the left amygdala and the right posterior cingulate/precuneus and right fusiform gyrus/parahippocampal gyrus was found in youths with BD.[57] Interestingly, four of the fMRI studies performed subgroup analyses and found that their results were independent of mood state,[54,56,57] medication status,[52] or comorbidity (ADHD and anxiety disorder).[52,54,56,57] Finally, one fMRI study demonstrated a reduction in amygdalar activation in depressed youths with BD after successful lamotrigine treatment.[59]

Magnetic Resonance Spectroscopy

MRS provides information about tissue biochemistry and metabolism. The most commonly used type of MRS used in psychiatric research is proton MRS (1H MRS), which is typically used to measure N-acetyl aspartate (NAA; considered a marker of neuronal integrity), creatine plus phosphocreatine (Cr-PCr; bioenergetics), myo-inositol-containing compounds (involved in phosphoinositide second-messenger cell-signaling pathway), glutamate/glutamine (Glx; marker of neurotransmission), and choline (biomarker for cell membrane phospholipid metabolism).[60]

Older MRS studies of BD have found biochemical abnormalities in regions of the FL (including the ACC and DLPFC) and BG in early onset BD. The FL has been the most extensively studied and abnormal levels of NAA, Glx, Cr, and myo-inositol, suggesting that neuronal integrity, neurotransmission, bioenergetic markers, and cell membrane metabolism are impaired in this region in youths with BD.[5] For example, medication-free youths with BD have shown elevated Glx ratios in the frontal lobe and basal ganglia,[61] and several studies have found decreased NAA in the frontal lobes.[62–66]

Cecil and colleagues[62] also found elevated levels of composite amino acids (aspartate, γ-aminobutyric acid, glutamate, and glutamine) in FL white matter. These same authors later studied children with a mood disorder and a family history of BD and found decreased NAA and Cr in the cerebellar vermis and increased myo-inositol in the FL,[63] suggesting that the biochemical differences found in their sample of youths at risk may represent early markers of BD.[63] In another study, youths with BD were found to have increased myo-inositol/Cr in the ACC, which decreased with lithium treatment.[67] Finally, Davanzo and colleagues[68] found that youths with BD had significantly higher myo-inositol/Cr-PCr and myo-inositol levels in the ACC than those in youths with intermittent explosive disorder and HC and concluded that these differences may differentiate the two clinical populations.

Over the past several years, two additional MRS studies have been performed, which considered the effect of medication and comorbidity on ACC metabolites. In the first study, Moore and colleagues[69] assessed a group of youths with BD, 10 who were unmedicated and eight who were taking risperidone, and found that children with BD exhibiting manic symptoms requiring treatment had lower Glx/Cr than that in children with BD being stably treated with the atypical antipsychotic risperidone. The authors proposed that mania might be associated with reduced Glx/Cr levels in the ACC, which is increased following successful treatment with risperidone.

In another study by Moore and colleagues,[70] 30 youths were evaluated using MRS in which, 15 youths had ADHD, eight had BD+ADHD, and seven were HC. The authors found that children with ADHD had a significantly higher ratio of Glx to myo-inositol-containing (Glx-to-Ino) compounds in the ACC than that of children with BD+ADHD and HC. These findings suggest that the Glx-to-Ino ratio may be able to differentiate between youths with ADHD and those with BPD+ADHD.[70]

MRS Summary

In summary, overall MRS studies of BD have found biochemical abnormalities in regions of the FL (including the ACC and DLPFC) and basal ganglia in early onset BD.[61–66] Findings of decreased NAA and Cr in the cerebellar vermis and increased myo-inositol in the frontal lobe of at-risk youths suggest that these biochemical abnormalities may represent early markers of BD.[63] Two wrap-around treatment studies in youths with BD found that abnormally high levels of myo-inositol/Cr decreased and reduced levels of Glx/Cr increased in response to lithium and risperidone treatment, respectively.[67,69] Furthermore, youths with BD had significantly higher myo-inositol/Cr-PCr and myo-inositol levels in the ACC than those in youths with intermittent explosive disorder and HC, and children with ADHD had a significantly higher ratio of Glx-to-Ino compounds in the ACC than that of children with BD+ADHD and HC.[70]

DISCUSSION

Taken together, the reviewed studies have found converging evidence for functional, anatomic, and biochemical abnormalities in structures involved in the neuroanatomic models of emotion processing and regulation: the limbic-thalamic-prefrontal circuit and the limbic-striatal-pallidal thalamic circuit.[38,71,72] Furthermore, the advances in neuroimaging methodologies provide additional support for older MRI data and have provided new insights into the pathophysiology of early onset BD. Specifically, older structural ROI neuroimaging studies found differences in total cerebral volume, STG, putamen, thalamic, amygdala, and hippocampal volumes, and WMH, whereas a VBM study found additional abnormalities in the basal ganglia, ACC, and OFC. More recent structural studies have found similar structural abnormalities and have provided new information regarding additional regions that may be involved in BD. For instance, prior imaging studies regarding WM abnormalities were limited to the evaluation of WMH. More recently, a longitudinal VBM study found that BD youths had reduced WM in the left frontal lobe and in the bilateral posterior parietotemporal junction at initial scanning and in the right posterior frontal/parietal cortex, left temporoparietal junction, right parietooccipital junction, left PL, and right cerebellum at follow-up.[35] In addition, DTI has found abnormalities in frontal WM tracts and specific fasiculi, including the CC, superior longitudinal fasciculus I, and the cingulate-paracingulate WM, in BD. These major WM tracts are important in interhemispheric and intrahemispheric communication between frontolimbic, frontoparietal, and parietal-temporal regions. Specifically, superior longitudinal fasciculus I contains WM of the superior parietal lobule, precuneus, postcentral gyrus, precentral gyrus, and the posterior part of the superior frontal gyrus as well as the supplementary motor area.[73] The cingulate-paracingulate WM contains tracts to/from the ACC and PCC and the paracingulate gyri and is the major WM tract connecting the limbic system to frontal and parietal cortices.[27,74] The CC is the major commissural tract providing interhemispheric communication of homologous regions of the cerebral hemisphere, and the body of the CC allows communication between motor, somatosensory, and parietotemporal regions.[75] Interestingly, these major WM tracts appear to connect cortical and subcortical regions thought to be involved in the pathophysiology of BD. Given the new findings of WM pathology in BD, further investigations are warranted. Specifically, multimodal techniques, including ROI studies on high-resolution anatomic images, VBM, and DTI, which will provide concurrent information regarding gray matter and WM pathology in the same sample, will aid in determining whether WM abnormalities are associated with corresponding cortical and subcortical gray matter abnormalities and whether they precede or coincide with aberrant gray matter development.

Recent advances in structural neuroimaging include higher-resolution scanning, larger sample sizes, longitudinal studies, automated and semiautomated cortical parcellation methods, and VBM. Overall, ROI studies have found abnormalities in cortical structures, such as regions of the frontal lobe (OFC, MFG), parietal lobe (bilateral post-central gyri), temporal lobe (STG and left fusiform gyrus, parahippocampal gyri), cingulate gyrus (left ACC and bilateral PCC), and cerebellum and subcortical structures, such as the amygdala and hippocampus. VBM studies are consistent with ROI studies and have reported gray matter abnormalities in the frontal lobe (left DLPFC, OFC, and right inferior frontal/precentral gyrus), temporal lobe (inferior and middle temporal gyrus/uncus and left insula), cingulate gyrus (ACC and left PCC), and in limbic structures. Longitudinally, the ACC has been found to be reduced over time in youths with BD. Furthermore, youths with BD pre-post manic conversion had cortical gray matter gains over the left frontal and temporal regions and gray matter loss over right frontal, temporal, and cingulate regions. These findings were similar to youths with MDI who had not converted to BD, suggesting that these findings are not specific to BD and may represent affect dysregulation more generally. Although abnormal structure does not necessarily imply abnormal function, the structural findings suggest impairments in more than one prefrontal-subcortical circuit. This is not surprising given the variability in symptom profile in mania and depression, the associated cognitive dysfunctions, and the heterogeneity within the diagnosis. For instance, the DLPFC, OFC/VLPFC, and the ACC are thought to be composed of separate closed-circuit connections whose corresponding simplistic functions include executive function, mood modulation, and motivation, respectively.[76] These closed-circuit connections also receive open-circuit information from somatosensory and heteromodal association areas from regions such as the parietal and temporal lobe, resulting in modulation of function. Abnormalities in any of these regions could result in the abnormal function of other regions, either directly or indirectly. Given the complexity of this disorder, it is unlikely that 1 or a few regions will be isolated as abnormal; thus, further evaluation of the anatomic networks involved in early onset BD is necessary. These types of studies should include longitudinal evaluation of both normal and abnormal maturation of anatomic networks with age, using a combination of whole-brain assessments and ROI analysis. Although VBM is rapid and fully automated, it is not a replacement for manual ROI-based analyses. VBM provides an unbiased tool, which is useful for whole-brain exploratory analyses but should be corroborated by more robust ROI analyses. Furthermore, since both methods provide different types of information, future studies should include both types of measurements. A newer method that holds promise in identifying cortical gray matter abnormalities includes whole-brain cortical thickness measurements, which may be more sensitive in detecting abnormalities in cortical gray matter, buried deep within sulci.[77]

A variety of tasks have been used as probes in attempts to understand the mood dysregulation and cognitive deficits seen in youths with BD. Attempts to consolidate the information provided by fMRI in youths with BD is difficult given the heterogeneity of the youths included in the studies. For example, youths with BD were studied in various mood states both within and between studies. In addition, the inclusion of medications and comorbidity is variable throughout the studies. However, overall, the fMRI studies in youths using both cognitive and affective tasks in BD have reported consistent abnormalities in regions of the frontal-striatal-thalamic-amygdala circuit. For instance, in 3 cognitive-based tasks (Stroop, flexibility task, and visuospatial task), youths with BD were found to have abnormal activation patterns in frontal (DLPFC, ACC, and inferior frontal gyrus), striatal, and thalamic circuits. Additionally, regions of the temporal lobe (STG) and parietal lobe (precuneus) were also found to have abnormal activation patterns. Emotion-based fMRI studies in which participants were asked to view emotionally valenced faces, pictures, or words also consistently reported abnormalities in the amygdala, striatum, and regions of the PFC (ACC, OFC, DLPFC, and VLPFC). Other regions that were found to be abnormal in more than one study include the temporal lobe (parahippocampal gyrus, hippocampus, left superior/middle temporal gyrus, and insula) and parietal lobe (posterior parietal cortex, paracentral lobule, and precuneus). In summary, despite the heterogeneity of the current fMRI studies, there appears to be a growing literature that supports the involvement of prefrontolimbic circuit(s) in the pathophysiology of BD.

MRS studies of BD have consistently found biochemical abnormalities in regions of the frontal lobe (including the ACC and DLPFC) and BG in early onset BD. The frontal lobe has been the most extensively studied, and abnormal levels of NAA, Glx, Cr, and myo-inositol have been reported, suggesting that neuronal integrity, neurotransmission, bioenergetic markers, and cell membrane metabolism are impaired in this region in youths with BD. Further biochemical evaluation of other regions such as the amygdala and hippocampus would provide further evidence that these areas are impaired in youths with BD. In addition, having information regarding specific biochemical abnormalities in these brain structures (such as abnormal neurotransmission) may provide a way to both target and monitor pharmacologic and potentially nonpharmacologic treatments.

Recent studies of BD in children and adolescents have also begun to uncover endophenotypic markers of illness in the brain. For example, in a DTI study that included a healthy, at-risk cohort of youths, the superior longitudinal fasciculus I was found to have reduced integrity compared with that of HC group, which suggests that it may be a trait marker of BD illness.[27] Furthermore, another study found increased gray matter volumes in the left parahippocampal/hippocampal gyrus[47] in healthy youths at genetic risk for BD, which also has the potential biomarker for risk for BD. In addition, findings of abnormal NAA and Cr in the cerebellar vermis and increased myo-inositol in the FL of at-risk youths suggest that these biochemical abnormalities may represent early makers of BD.[63] Establishing reliable markers could lead to improvements in early identification, prevention, and treatment of youths with BD; therefore, further study of healthy youths at genetic risk of BD is warranted.

New leads regarding the impact of confounding factors, such as comorbidity, mood state, and medication status on neuroimaging findings, in the study of BD have also begun to appear in the literature. For instance, several fMRI studies, including cognitive and emotion-based studies, found that mood state, comorbidity (ADHD and anxiety disorder), or medication status did not influence their findings after subgroup analysis.[52,54,56,57] The lack of findings in the subgroups in these studies may be due to small subgroup sizes; however, it may suggest that youths with BD have persistent neurocircuitry abnormalities that are detectable despite mood state, medication status, or comorbidity. In contrast to these findings, several studies have reported that both medication and comorbidities do have an impact on data. For example, a CPT study in youths with BD and comorbid ADHD reported reduced activation in the VLPFC and ACC and greater activation in the posterior parietal cortex and middle temporal gyrus compared with that in BD youths without comorbidity.[53] Unfortunately, this study did not include a HC cohort to determine if youths with BD without comorbidity had similar but less severely affected activation patterns or a completely different pattern of activation altogether. Furthermore, one MRS study in youths with BD did find distinct biochemical abnormalities in the ACC compared with those in youths with intermittent explosive disorder and HC. In another MRS study in children with ADHD, biochemical differences in the ACC were found in children compared with those with BD+ADHD and HC.[70] Furthermore, in a wrap-around medication study using fMRI, a reduction in amygdalar activation when viewing negative pictures was noted after successful lamotrigine treatment in depressed BD youths.[59] In addition, two MRS studies in youths with BD also found biochemical changes in the ACC in response to lithium and risperidone treatment.[67,69] Further investigations of the impact of confounding factors in neuroimaging studies are needed given the necessity of including youths in neuroimaging studies who have a high frequency of medication use, comorbidity, and rapidly fluctuating mood states.

Despite the recent advances in neuroimaging investigation in youths with BD, significant limitations still exist. For example, most studies to date are limited due to heterogeneous bipolar samples, and comparison of studies is complicated because samples may differ, both within and across centers, depending on how widely the inclusion net is cast. In addition, differences in MRI scanners (make and magnet strength) and imaging methodology may also contribute to inconsistent findings. Other clinical variables that are important to consider with regard to samples across studies include family history, medication exposure, psychosis, and history of rapid cycling. In addition, although the sample size of recent studies has increased, larger studies including more than 50 subjects per group have not been preformed in youths with BD, which makes subgroup analysis difficult. In addition, most samples of early onset BD include subjects who are being treated with medications, which may have a significant impact on the results regardless of the imaging modality used.[1,78–82] Finally, the study of the brain during a time when it is undergoing both progressive and regressive patterns of growth in different structures during the preteen to teenage years is a major challenge to the field. Therefore, it will be difficult to detect changes in brain structures across the life cycle with cross-sectional studies. To obtain a full sense of the developmental trajectory of these cortical and subcortical structures in the BD population, it is critical to pursue longitudinal imaging studies. These studies should have a sufficiently large sample size and a well-matched healthy comparison group, thereby allowing comparisons in relation to normal progressive and regressive brain changes.

The reviewed studies are finding converging evidence for functional, anatomic, and biochemical abnormalities in structures involved in the neuroanatomic models of emotion processing and regulation. Future multimodal neuroimaging studies using high-resolution structural scans, fMRI, MRS, and DTI will further delineate the under-lying anatomic, functional, and biochemical abnormalities involved in early onset BD. These studies should include both youth at risk and youths with current BD to evaluate both state and trait abnormalities. In addition, wrap-around medication studies will allow us to monitor the impact of medication regimens on the brains of those affected. Additionally, longitudinal studies with larger sample sizes are still needed.

REFERENCES

1. Grigoroiu-Serbanescu M, Martinez M, Nothen MM, et al. Different familial trans-mission patterns in bipolar I disorder with onset before and after age 25. Am J Med Genet 2001;105:765–73.
2. LaRoche C, Cheifetz P, Lester EP, et al. Psychopathology in the offspring of parents with bipolar affective disorders. Can J Psychiatry 1985;30:337–43.
3. Schulze TG, Muller DJ, Krauss H, et al. Further evidence for age of onset being an indicator for severity in bipolar disorder. J Affect Disord 2002;68:343–5.
4. Strober M, Morrell W, Burroughs J, et al. A family study of bipolar I disorder in adolescence. Early onset of symptoms linked to increased familial loading and lithium resistance. J Affect Disord 1988;15:255–68.
5. Frazier JA, Ahn MS, DeJong S, et al. Magnetic resonance imaging studies in early-onset bipolar disorder: a critical review. Harv Rev Psychiatry 2005;13:125–40.
6. Good CD, Johnsrude IS, Ashburner J, et al. A voxel-based morphometric study of ageing in 465 normal adult human brains. Neuroimage 2001;14:21–36.
7. Mechelli A, Price CJ, Froiston KJ, et al. Voxel-based morphometry of the human brain: methods and applications. Current Medical Imaging Reviews 2005;1:105.
8. Smith SM, Jenkinson M, Johansen-Berg H, et al. Tract-based spatial statistics: vox-elwise analysis of multi-subject diffusion data. Neuroimage 2006;31:1487–505.
9. DelBello MP, Zimmerman ME, Mills NP, et al. Magnetic resonance imaging anal-ysis of amygdala and other subcortical brain regions in adolescents with bipolar disorder. Bipolar Disord 2004;6:43–52.
10. Frazier JA, Chiu S, Breeze JL, et al. Structural brain magnetic resonance imaging of limbic and thalamic volumes in pediatric bipolar disorder. Am J Psychiatry 2005;162:1256–65.
11. Friedman L, Findling RL, Kenny JT, et al. An MRI study of adolescent patients with either schizophrenia or bipolar disorder as compared to healthy control subjects. Biol Psychiatry 1999;46:78–88.
12. Botteron KN, Vannier MW, Geller B, et al. Preliminary study of magnetic reso-nance imaging characteristics in 8- to 16-year-olds with mania. J Am Acad Child Adolesc Psychiatry 1995;34:742–9.
13. Lyoo IK, Lee HK, Jung JH, et al. White matter hyperintensities on magnetic resonance imaging of the brain in children with psychiatric disorders. Compr Psychiatry 2002;43:361–8.

14. Pillai JJ, Friedman L, Stuve TA, et al. Increased presence of white matter hyperintensities in adolescent patients with bipolar disorder. Psychiatry Res 2002;114:51–6.
15. Blumberg HP, Kaufman J, Martin A, et al. Amygdala and hippocampal volumes in adolescents and adults with bipolar disorder. Arch Gen Psychiatry 2003;60:1201–8.
16. Chen HH, Nicoletti MA, Hatch JP, et al. Abnormal left superior temporal gyrus volumes in children and adolescents with bipolar disorder: a magnetic resonance imaging study. Neurosci Lett 2004;363:65–8.
17. Wilke M, Kowatch RA, DelBello MP, et al. Voxel-based morphometry in adolescents with bipolar disorder: first results. Psychiatry Res 2004;131:57–69.
18. Breeze JL, Hesdorffer DC, Hong X, et al. Clinical significance of brain white matter hyperintensities in young adults with psychiatric illness. Harv Rev Psychiatry 2003;11:269–83.
19. Moore PB, El-Badri SM, Cousins D, et al. White matter lesions and season of birth of patients with bipolar affective disorder. Am J Psychiatry 2001;158:1521–4.
20. Norris SD, Krishnan KR, Ahearn E. Structural changes in the brain of patients with bipolar affective disorder by MRI: a review of the literature. Prog Neuropsychopharmacol Biol Psychiatry 1997;21:1323–37.
21. Stoll AL, Renshaw PF, Yurgelun-Todd DA, et al. Neuroimaging in bipolar disorder: what have we learned? Biol Psychiatry 2000;48:505–17.
22. Chang K, Barnea-Goraly N, Karchemskiy A, et al. Cortical magnetic resonance imaging findings in familial pediatric bipolar disorder. Biol Psychiatry 2005;58: 197–203.
23. McIntosh AM, Job DE, Moorhead TW, et al. White matter density in patients with schizophrenia, bipolar disorder and their unaffected relatives. Biol Psychiatry 2005;58:254–7.
24. Brambilla P, Nicoletti MA, Sassi RB, et al. Magnetic resonance imaging study of corpus callosum abnormalities in patients with bipolar disorder. Biol Psychiatry 2003;54:1294–7.
25. Yasar AS, Monkul ES, Sassi RB, et al. MRI study of corpus callosum in children and adolescents with bipolar disorder. Psychiatry Res 2006;146:83–5.
26. Adler CM, Adams J, DelBello MP, et al. Evidence of white matter pathology in bipolar disorder adolescents experiencing their first episode of mania: a diffusion tensor imaging study. Am J Psychiatry 2006;163:322–4.
27. Frazier JA, Breeze JL, Papadimitriou G, et al. White matter abnormalities in children with and at risk for bipolar disorder. Bipolar Disord 2007;9:799–809.
28. Sanches M, Sassi RB, Axelson D, et al. Subgenual prefrontal cortex of child and adolescent bipolar patients: a morphometric magnetic resonance imaging study. Psychiatry Res 2005;138:43–9.
29. Frazier JA, Breeze JL, Makris N, et al. Cortical gray matter differences identified by structural magnetic resonance imaging in pediatric bipolar disorder. Bipolar Disord 2005;7:555–69.
30. Chiu S, Widjaja F, Bates ME, et al. Anterior cingulate volume in pediatric bipolar disorder and autism. J Affect Disord 2008;105:93–9.
31. Kaur S, Sassi RB, Axelson D, et al. Cingulate cortex anatomical abnormalities in children and adolescents with bipolar disorder. Am J Psychiatry 2005;162:1637–43.
32. Najt P, Nicoletti M, Chen HH, et al. Anatomical measurements of the orbitofrontal cortex in child and adolescent patients with bipolar disorder. Neurosci Lett 2007; 413:183–6.
33. Monkul ES, Hatch JP, Sassi RB, et al. MRI study of the cerebellum in young bipolar patients. Prog Neuropsychopharmacol Biol Psychiatry 2008;32:613–9.

34. Dickstein DP, Milham MP, Nugent AC, et al. Frontotemporal alterations in pediatric bipolar disorder: results of a voxel-based morphometry study. Arch Gen Psychiatry 2005;62:734–41.
35. Farrow TF, Whitford TJ, Williams LM, et al. Diagnosis-related regional gray matter loss over two years in first episode schizophrenia and bipolar disorder. Biol Psychiatry 2005;58:713–23.
36. Gogtay N, Greenstein D, Lenane M, et al. Cortical brain development in nonpsychotic siblings of patients with childhood-onset schizophrenia. Arch Gen Psychiatry 2007;64:772–80.
37. Drevets WC. Neuroimaging studies of mood disorders. Biol Psychiatry 2000;48: 813–29.
38. Soares JC, Mann JJ. The anatomy of mood disorders: review of structural neuroimaging studies. Biol Psychiatry 1997;41:86–106.
39. Chang K, Karchemskiy A, Barnea-Goraly N, et al. Reduced amygdalar gray matter volume in familial pediatric bipolar disorder. J Am Acad Child Adolesc Psychiatry 2005;44:565–73.
40. Dasari M, Friedman L, Jesberger J, et al. A magnetic resonance imaging study of thalamic area in adolescent patients with either schizophrenia or bipolar disorder as compared to healthy controls. Psychiatry Res 1999;91:155–62.
41. Frazier JA, Hodge SM, Breeze JL, et al. Diagnostic and sex effects on limbic volumes in early-onset bipolar disorder and schizophrenia. Schizophr Bull 2008;34:37–46.
42. Monkul ES, Nicoletti MA, Spence D, et al. MRI study of thalamus volumes in juvenile patients with bipolar disorder. Depress Anxiety 2006;23:347–52.
43. Chen BK, Sassi R, Axelson D, et al. Cross-sectional study of abnormal amygdala development in adolescents and young adults with bipolar disorder. Biol Psychiatry 2004;56:399–405.
44. Blumberg HP, Fredericks C, Wang F, et al. Preliminary evidence for persistent abnormalities in amygdala volumes in adolescents and young adults with bipolar disorder. Bipolar Disord 2005;7:570–6.
45. Dickstein DP, Garvey M, Pradella AG, et al. Neurologic examination abnormalities in children with bipolar disorder or attention-deficit/hyperactivity disorder. Biol Psychiatry 2005;58:517–24.
46. Bearden CE, Soares JC, Klunder AD, et al. Three-dimensional mapping of hippocampal anatomy in adolescents with bipolar disorder. J Am Acad Child Adolesc Psychiatry 2008;47:515–25.
47. Ladouceur CD, Almeida JR, Birmaher B, et al. Subcortical gray matter volume abnormalities in healthy bipolar offspring: potential neuroanatomical risk marker for bipolar disorder? J Am Acad Child Adolesc Psychiatry 2008;47:532–9.
48. Ahn MS, Breeze JL, Makris N, et al. Anatomic brain magnetic resonance imaging of the basal ganglia in pediatric bipolar disorder. J Affect Disord 2007;104:147–54.
49. Sanches M, Roberts RL, Sassi RB, et al. Developmental abnormalities in striatum in young bipolar patients: a preliminary study. Bipolar Disord 2005;7:153–8.
50. Blumberg HP, Martin A, Kaufman J, et al. Frontostriatal abnormalities in adolescents with bipolar disorder: preliminary observations from functional MRI. Am J Psychiatry 2003;160:1345–7.
51. Chang K, Adleman NE, Dienes K, et al. Anomalous prefrontal-subcortical activation in familial pediatric bipolar disorder. Arch Gen Psychiatry 2004;61:781–92.
52. Nelson EE, Vinton DT, Berghorst L, et al. Brain systems underlying response flexibility in healthy and bipolar adolescents: an event-related fMRI study. Bipolar Disord 2007;9:810–9.

53. Adler CM, Delbello MP, Mills NP, et al. Comorbid ADHD is associated with altered patterns of neuronal activation in adolescents with bipolar disorder performing a simple attention task. Bipolar Disord 2005;7:577–88.

54. Dickstein DP, Rich BA, Roberson-Nay R, et al. Neural activation during encoding of emotional faces in pediatric bipolar disorder. Bipolar Disord 2007;9:679–92.

55. Pavuluri MN, O'Connor MM, Harral E, et al. Affective neural circuitry during facial emotion processing in pediatric bipolar disorder. Biol Psychiatry 2007;62:158–67.

56. Rich BA, Vinton DT, Roberson-Nay R, et al. Limbic hyperactivation during processing of neutral facial expressions in children with bipolar disorder. Proc Natl Acad Sci U S A 2006;103:8900–5.

57. Rich BA, Fromm SJ, Berghorst LH, et al. Neural connectivity in children with bipolar disorder: impairment in the face emotion processing circuit. J Child Psychol Psychiatry 2008;49:88–96.

58. Pavuluri MN, O'Connor MM, Harral EM, et al. An fMRI study of the interface between affective and cognitive neural circuitry in pediatric bipolar disorder. Psychiatry Res 2008;162:244–55.

59. Chang KD, Wagner C, Garrett A, et al. A preliminary functional magnetic resonance imaging study of prefrontal-amygdalar activation changes in adolescents with bipolar depression treated with lamotrigine. Bipolar Disord 2008;10:426–31.

60. Urenjak J, Williams SR, Gadian DG, et al. Proton nuclear magnetic resonance spectroscopy unambiguously identifies different neural cell types. J Neurosci 1993;13:981–9.

61. Castillo M, Kwock L, Courvoisie H, et al. Proton MR spectroscopy in children with bipolar affective disorder: preliminary observations. AJNR Am J Neuroradiol 2000;21:832–8.

62. Cecil KM, DelBello MP, Morey R, et al. Frontal lobe differences in bipolar disorder as determined by proton MR spectroscopy. Bipolar Disord 2002;4:357–65.

63. Cecil KM, DelBello MP, Sellars MC, et al. Proton magnetic resonance spectroscopy of the frontal lobe and cerebellar vermis in children with a mood disorder and a familial risk for bipolar disorder. J Child Adolesc Psychopharmacol 2003; 13:545–55.

64. Cecil KM, Jones BV. Magnetic resonance spectroscopy of the pediatric brain. Top Magn Reson Imaging 2001;12:435–52.

65. Chang K, Adleman N, Dienes K, et al. Decreased N-acetylaspartate in children with familial bipolar disorder. Biol Psychiatry 2003;53:1059–65.

66. Winsberg ME, Sachs N, Tate DL, et al. Decreased dorsolateral prefrontal N-acetyl aspartate in bipolar disorder. Biol Psychiatry 2000;47:475–81.

67. Davanzo P, Thomas MA, Yue K, et al. Decreased anterior cingulate myo-inositol/ creatine spectroscopy resonance with lithium treatment in children with bipolar disorder. Neuropsychopharmacology 2001;24:359–69.

68. Davanzo P, Yue K, Thomas MA, et al. Proton magnetic resonance spectroscopy of bipolar disorder versus intermittent explosive disorder in children and adolescents. Am J Psychiatry 2003;160:1442–52.

69. Moore CM, Biederman J, Wozniak J, et al. Mania, glutamate/glutamine and risperidone in pediatric bipolar disorder: a proton magnetic resonance spectroscopy study of the anterior cingulate cortex. J Affect Disord 2007;99:19–25.

70. Moore CM, Biederman J, Wozniak J, et al. Differences in brain chemistry in children and adolescents with attention deficit hyperactivity disorder with and without comorbid bipolar disorder: a proton magnetic resonance spectroscopy study. Am J Psychiatry 2006;163:316–8.

71. Phillips ML, Drevets WC, Rauch SL, et al. The neurobiology of emotion perception I: the neural basis of normal emotion perception. Biol Psychiatry 2003;54:504–14.

72. Phillips ML, Drevets WC, Rauch SL, et al. The neurobiology of emotion perception II: implications for major psychiatric disorders. Biol Psychiatry 2003;54:515–28.

73. Makris N, Kennedy DN, McInerney S, et al. Segmentation of subcomponents within the superior longitudinal fascicle in humans: a quantitative, in vivo, DT-MRI study. Cereb Cortex 2005;15:854–69.

74. Makris N, Pandya DN, Normandin JJ, et al. Quantitative DT-MRI investigations of the human cingulum bundle. CNS Spectr 2002;7:522–8.

75. Witelson SF. Hand and sex differences in the isthmus and genu of the human corpus callosum: a postmortem morphological study. Brain 1989;112:799–835.

76. Salloway S, Malloy P, Duffy JD. The frontal lobes and neuropsychiatric illness: American Psychiatric Pub, 2001 book.

77. Fischl B, Dale AM. Measuring the thickness of the human cerebral cortex from magnetic resonance images. Proc Natl Acad Sci U S A 2000;97:11050–5.

78. Buchsbaum MS, Hazlett EA, Haznedar MM, et al. Visualizing fronto-striatal circuitry and neuroleptic effects in schizophrenia. Acta Psychiatr Scand 1999; 99:129–37.

79. Holcomb HH, Cascella NG, Thaker GK, et al. Functional sites of neuroleptic drug action in the human brain: PET/FDG studies with and without haloperidol. Am J Psychiatry 1996;153:41–9.

80. Mayberg HS, Brannan SK, Tekell JL, et al. Regional metabolic effects of fluoxetine in major depression: serial changes and relationship to clinical response. Biol Psychiatry 2000;48:830–43.

81. Moore GJ, Bebchuk JM, Wilds IB, et al. Lithium-induced increase in human brain grey matter. Lancet 2000;356:1241–2.

82. Sassi RB, Nicoletti M, Brambilla P, et al. Increased gray matter volume in lithium-treated bipolar disorder patients. Neurosci Lett 2002;329:243–5.

Family and Genetic Association Studies of Bipolar Disorder in Children

Eric Mick, ScD[a],*, Stephen V. Faraone, PhD[b,c]

KEYWORDS

- Bipolar disorder • Childhood • Genetics
- Comorbidity • Age at onset

Pediatric bipolar disorder is associated with severe impairment, rapid cycling, early age at onset, and significant psychiatric comorbidity.[1–9] The presentation of bipolar disorder in children may not be unlike that described in adults as mixed mania by McElroy and colleagues,[10] a rapid-cycling and recurrent disorder with poor interepisode functioning, frequent onset in childhood and adolescence, high risk of suicide, high risk of substance use disorders, poor response to treatment, a history of poor school performance, and neuropsychological deficits suggestive of attention-deficit/hyperactivity disorder (ADHD). Whether pediatric bipolar disorder will be continuous with the disorder in adulthood can only be answered with follow-up studies of children, but Geller and colleagues[11,12] have conducted a 4-year longitudinal study of children with prepubertal-onset bipolar disorder that suggests that the rate of recovery from first episode in children with bipolar disorder is similar to that reported in adults.[13]

FAMILY STUDIES

Age at onset of bipolar disorder has been recognized for several decades as a potentially important marker of a more severe and more familial form of the disorder.[14] Tsuang and Faraone[14] reviewed family studies of mood disorders that dichotomized the age at onset into either early or mid-adulthood and found an elevated risk for

This work was supported in part by National Institutes of Health grant K01MH065523 and the support of members of the MGH Pediatric Psychopharmacology Council.

[a] Departments of Psychiatry, Massachusetts General Hospital and Harvard Medical School, 55 Fruit Street - Warren 705, Boston, MA 02114, USA
[b] Department of Psychiatry, SUNY Upstate Medical University, 750 East Adams Street, Syracuse, NY 13210, USA
[c] Department of Neuroscience & Physiology, SUNY Upstate Medical University, 750 East Adams Street, Syracuse, NY 13210, USA
* Corresponding author.
E-mail address: mick@helix.mgh.harvard.edu (E. Mick).

Child Adolesc Psychiatric Clin N Am 18 (2009) 441–453
doi:10.1016/j.chc.2008.11.008
1056-4993/08/$ – see front matter © 2009 Elsevier Inc. All rights reserved.

childpsych.theclinics.com

both bipolar disorder and unipolar depression among relatives of early onset probands versus relatives of later-onset probands. Subsequently, in a study of the old-order Amish, Pauls and colleagues[15] found increased lifetime rates of bipolar disorder among the first-degree relatives of patients who experienced their first affective symptoms before age 12 compared with relatives of those with onset at age 13 or later. Bellivier and colleagues[16] conducted an admixture analysis of 368 adult referrals with bipolar disorder and determined that the distribution of age at onset could be best described by three subgroups based on age at onset (at 17 years, 25 years, and 40 years) and that age at onset group definition was correlated in affected siblings. Thus, the age at onset of bipolar disorder may identify a subgroup of cases with specific familial vulnerability for the disorder. These findings suggest that samples of children with bipolar disorder may be highly enriched with familial cases of the disorder and therefore particularly informative for genetic research studies.

The first family study of child probands with bipolar disorder was published in 1985 (**Fig. 1**). In this uncontrolled study, Dwyer and colleagues[17] showed an excess of bipolar disorder and unipolar depression in the relatives of 20 outpatient children with bipolar disorder diagnosed per the criteria of the Diagnostic and Statistical Manual of Mental Disorders, 3rd edition (DSM-III). The point estimates of risk for mood disorders in relatives were replicated in subsequent controlled family studies of child probands with DSM-III bipolar disorder[18-20] as well as in our pilot family study of DSM-III text revision (R) bipolar disorder child probands.[21] Four recent family studies of DSM-IV bipolar disorder[4,6,8,9] also document a statistically significant excess risk of the disorder in relatives of bipolar disorder probands (see **Fig. 1**). The estimates of risk to first-degree relatives in families of child probands are consistently larger than the 8.7% estimate of recurrence risk of bipolar disorder in first-degree relatives of adult bipolar disorder cases.[22]

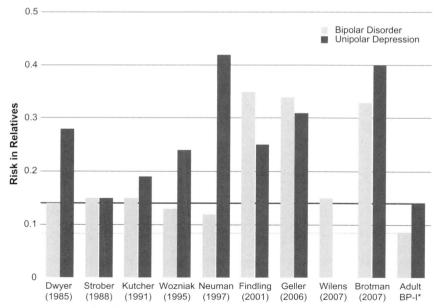

Fig. 1. Recurrence risk of bipolar disorder and unipolar depression in family studies of pediatric bipolar disorder*. Weighted estimate of recurrence risk in first-degree relatives in the data of Smoller and Finn (2003).[22]

LINKAGE STUDIES

There have been no family linkage studies of pediatric bipolar disorder conducted, but secondary analyses of linkage samples in which adults with bipolar disorder were stratified by age at onset are available. In the National Institute of Mental Health (NIMH) Genetics Initiative bipolar disorder sample,[23] age at onset of mania was significantly heritable and linked to loci on chromosomes 12p (marker D12S1292), 14q (marker GATA31B), and 15q (marker GATA50C) in 86 families multiply affected with bipolar disorder. A second study was conducted[23] in which suggestive logarithm of odds (LOD) scores (6q25, 9q34, and 20q11) found in the total sample were increased (ie, 9q34, between markers D9S290 and D9S915) when examined exclusively in the subset of families (N = 58) defined by onset of bipolar disorder before age 20. Lin and colleagues[24] reported two other areas of linkage to bipolar disorder, at 21q22.13 and 18p11.2, that were influenced by age at onset in a genome-wide scan of 874 individuals from 150 multiplex families. Estimates of linkage at 21q were increased in subjects with age at onset $\leq$21 years (LOD = 3.29; empiric chromosome-wide P value = .009), whereas linkage in the 18p region (LOD = 2.83; empiric chromosome-wide P value = .05) was increased in subjects with age at onset > 21 years. The European Collaborative Study of Early Onset Bipolar Affective Disorder (BPAD) (in France, Germany, Ireland, Scotland, Switzerland, England, and Slovenia) performed a genome scan and nonparametric linkage analysis using 384 microsatellite markers in 87 sib pairs ascertained through an early onset type I proband ($\leq$21 years).[25] This study suggests eight regions of linkage with P values <.01 (2p21, 2q14.3, 3p14, 5q33, 7q36, 10q23, 16q23, and 20p12), with the most significant linkage at the 3p14 region. Zandi and colleagues[26] examined age at onset ($\leq$21 years) as a covariate in a linkage scan of 98 bipolar disorder pedigrees and found that linkage to marker D3S2418 on chromosome 3q28 was greatest in early onset subjects; the LOD score was increased from 0.06 to 3.49 with the inclusion of age at onset as a covariate.

Although the region of linkage has not been consistently replicated with an early onset phenotype, the strength of association was consistently greater in the early onset subphenotype. This literature extends the results from family studies documenting increased familiality of pediatric bipolar disorder and suggests that the increased family risk may result from a greater genetic influence on pediatric bipolar disorder.

The Child Behavior Checklist Phenotype

We conducted a meta-analysis[27] of several studies employing the Child Behavior Checklist (CBCL) in samples of children with bipolar disorder and found a relatively homogenous profile of behavioral problems associated with the disorder defined by clinically significant elevations (ie, T-score $\geq$70) of the Anxious/Depressed, Attention Problems, and Aggression clinical subscales. This profile has been shown to be heritable in several large independent twin samples,[28–31] with additive genetic effects consistently explaining up to 67% of the variance in the profile score. The wide availability and simple administration of the CBCL, the reported association with pediatric bipolar disorder, and demonstrated heritability of a subset of clinical subscales suggest that this CBCL profile may be a valuable phenotype for genetic research of pediatric bipolar disorder.

Although it has been shown to discriminate ADHD from bipolar disorder in samples of children with ADHD,[32] this CBCL phenotype has not demonstrated good screening properties in samples with very low base rates of bipolar disorder[31,33] or in clinical settings with highly symptomatic referrals.[34] In a sample of 1,346 twins drawn from the general community, for example, Volk and colleagues[31] found that 0.6% of the sample (N = 9) met criteria for bipolar spectrum disorders while 2.5% (N = 33) met criteria for the CBCL phenotype (ie, T-score >70 on three suggested subscales). Similarly, McGough and colleagues[33] identified bipolar spectrum disorders in 1.9% (N = 10) of 540 children from affected ADHD sib-pair families but found that the CBCL phenotype criteria were met in 8% (N = 45). Thus, this associated behavioral phenotype is not a diagnostic proxy for pediatric bipolar disorder.

Focusing only on the lack of a specific relationship with bipolar disorder may be obscuring the potential utility of the CBCL phenotype in genetic studies of the disorder. If one of the goals of psychiatric genetics is to identify susceptibility genes for psychopathology, then a simple measure of an observable susceptibility for that psychopathology may be a more powerful phenotype to study. Conceivably, such a phenotype would be more proximal to the effect of susceptibility genes than an end-stage, categorical clinical diagnosis. For example, Volk and colleagues[31] found a nominally significant association with this CBCL phenotype and markers in the *DAT* gene (*SLC6A3*) consistent with associations observed in children and adults with bipolar disorder and this gene.[35–37] McGough and colleagues[33] found suggestive evidence of linkage near marker D2S151 at chromosome 2q23 with the CBCL phenotype consistent with findings, suggesting interaction between genes on chromosomes 2q22-2q24 and 6q23-6q24 in families of adult probands with bipolar disorder.[38] Too much should not be made of these potentially converging patterns of association in studies examining CBCL phenotype and clinical diagnosis of bipolar disorder, but it is interesting that the patterns emerged from samples in which the majority of children positive for the CBCL phenotype were not diagnosed with a bipolar spectrum disorder. Despite the obvious diagnostic limitations of the CBCL for bipolar disorder in children, it may still be a useful susceptibility phenotype for genetic studies of pediatric bipolar disorder.

CANDIDATE GENE ASSOCIATION STUDIES

Despite the evidence documenting that early onset bipolar disorder increases the familial recurrence rate of bipolar disorder and the strength of associations in linkage studies, there has been very little genetic research focused specifically on pediatric bipolar disorder. In this review, we focus exclusively on genes tested for association in samples of children with bipolar disorder, specifically excluding from the review studies of childhood-onset mood disorders that are not enriched with bipolar disorder. As shown in **Table 1**, four of the six reports come from a single sample of approximately 50 families.[35,39–43] Positive associations have been reported with markers in the *BDNF*, *DAT* (*SLC6A3*), and *GAD1* genes. In 2008, we attempted to independently replicate the findings of Geller and colleagues[39–41] in 170 affected offspring trios defined by a child (12.9 ± 5.3 years of age) with DSM-IV bipolar I disorder (Mick E, and colleagues, unpublished data, 2008).[43] For this review, we have pooled the number of transmitted and untransmitted alleles from family trios ascertained by our group at Harvard/Massachusetts General Hospital (MGH) with those reported by Geller and colleagues (see **Table 1**).

The Serotonin Transporter Gene (SLC6A4)

The serotonin transporter is a monoamine transporter protein that transports serotonin from synaptic spaces into presynaptic neurons. A 44-bp variable-number tandem-repeat (VNTR) polymorphism in the promoter region (HTTLPR) of the serotonin transporter gene (*SLC6A4*) influences the transcription and function of the transporter.[43] Meta-analysis of this polymorphism indicates that the short allele was associated with a small but statistically significant increased risk for bipolar disorder (odds ratio

Table 1
Association results of candidate genes for pediatric bipolar disorder

Gene	Marker	Allele*	WASH-U			Harvard/MGH			Pooled Results		
			T:U	OR (95% CI)	p	T:U	OR (95% CI)	p	T:U	OR (95% CI)	p
COMT	Val158Met	COMT-I	23:28	0.82 (0.47–1.42)	0.48	85:67	1.27 (0.92–1.75)	0.14	108:95	1.14 (0.86–1.50)	0.74
BDNF	Val66Met	Val66	21:9	2.3(1.09–4.98)	0.01	43:35	1.23 (0.79–1.92)	0.37	64:44	1.45 (0.99–2.13)	0.12
SLC6A4	HTTLPR	Short	26:25	1.04 (0.60–1.80)	0.89	73:84	0.87 (0.63–1.19)	0.38	99:109	0.91 (0.69–1.19)	0.85
SLC6A3	rs41084	T	—	—	—	103:68	1.51 (1.12–2.05)	0.03	—	—	—
GAD1	rs2241165	A	29:14	2.07 (1.11–3.87)	0.02	—	—	—	—	—	—

Abbreviations: MGH, Massachusetts General Hospital; OR (95% CI), odds ratio and 95% confidence interval from basic TDT; T:U, transmitted: untransmitted counts from basic TDT.
* Val66 (G allele at rs6265), COMT-L (Met158; A allele at rs4680), Short (14-repeat allele).

[OR] = 1.13, 95% confidence interval [CI] = 1.05–1.22).[44] In a study of 46 trios of affected offspring with pediatric bipolar disorder (11.1 ± 3.0 years of age with a mean onset of 8.1 ± 4.0 years), Geller and colleagues[39] found no evidence of association with *SLC6A4* at this HTTLPR locus. In addition, Mick and colleagues[43] found no evidence of association, and the pooled results presented in **Table 1** were also negative.

Catechol-O-Methyltransferase Gene

Catechol-O-methyltransferase (COMT) catalyzes the transfer of a methyl group from S-adenosylmethionine to catecholamines, including the neurotransmitters dopamine, epinephrine, and norepinephrine.[45] A variant caused by a G-to-A transition at codon 158 of the *COMT* gene results in a valine-to-methionine substitution.[46] Homozygosity for 158met leads to a three- to four-fold reduction in enzymatic activity, compared with homozygosity for 158val.[46] Meta-analysis[47] of 13 association studies found that the low-activity allele significantly increased the risk for bipolar disorder, but the OR was small: 1.18 (CI, 1.02–1.35). Lachman and colleagues[48] reported that in the population of patients with velo-cardio-facial syndrome (who are hemizygous for the region of chromosome 22 containing *COMT*), there was an association between the low-activity allele, 158met, and the development of rapid-cycling bipolar spectrum disorder. Geller and colleagues[40] reported no association with the val158met marker in 52 affected offspring trios (11.1 ± 3.0 years of age with a mean onset of 8.1 ± 4.0 years) or in a subsample of trios in which the affected offspring presented with ultradian rapid cycling (≥365 episodes per year), however. The lack of association between *COMT* and pediatric bipolar disorder was replicated in our pooled analyses (see **Table 1**).

Brain-derived Neurotrophic Factor Gene

BDNF supports survival of central nervous system neurons and stimulates growth and differentiation of developing neurons.[49] A polymorphism producing an amino acid substitution (valine to methionine) at codon 66 of the *BDNF* may affect intracellular trafficking and activity-dependent secretion of *BDNF*.[50] Large studies of adults with bipolar disorder suggest that the 66val allele[51,52] may be a susceptibility locus for the disorder. Furthermore, Muller and colleagues[53] reported that this *BDNF* variant predicted rapid cycling as defined by DSM-IV, and Strauss and colleagues[54,55] have reported evidence of association with childhood-onset mood disorder. Geller and colleagues[41] replicated this association and observed a significant overtransmission of the Val66 allele in 53 affected offspring trios of children with pediatric bipolar disorder (10.7 ± 2.7 years of age with a mean onset of 7.6 ± 3.6 years). We failed to replicate an association with *BDNF*[43] in a sample of 170 children with DSM-IV bipolar disorder. Although the estimate of association was considerably attenuated and not statistically significant in the pooled results (see **Table 1**), the *P* value was relatively small (*P* = .1) and the OR remained relatively large at 1.5.

Despite the lack of replication observed in our data, *BDNF* may continue to be an interesting candidate gene for pediatric bipolar disorder. Pandey and colleagues[56] observed significantly lower *BDNF* mRNA levels in lymphocytes of children with bipolar disorder compared with those in healthy control children. Furthermore, treatment with mood stabilizers normalized *BDNF* mRNA level at 8 weeks, and change in symptoms of bipolar disorder was correlated with change in *BDNF* mRNA levels.[56] In addition, Bulgin and colleagues[57] found evidence that the val66met polymorphism in *BDNF* affected theta electroencephalographic asymmetry in the parietal brain region of subjects with childhood-onset depression but not in that of normal controls. These results, and the magnitude of the association estimated from pooled analysis in **Table 1**, suggest that additional attempts at replicating an association with *BDNF* and pediatric bipolar disorder are warranted.

The Dopamine Transporter Gene (SLC6A3)

Because the DAT plays a central role in regulation of dopaminergic neurotransmission via reuptake of synaptic dopamine,[58,59] the *DAT* gene (*SLC6A3* located on chromosome 5p15.3) is a compelling candidate gene for several psychiatric disorders. In children, it has been most studied in relation to ADHD.[60–62] Because the comorbidity between ADHD and bipolar disorder in children may represent a developmentally[63] and etiologically distinct familial subtype of the disorder,[64,65] *SLC6A3* may also be an interesting candidate gene for pediatric bipolar disorder.

Early candidate gene studies of a 40-bp VNTR polymorphism in the 3' untranslated region failed to find consistent evidence of association with bipolar disorder.[66–68] Greenwood and colleagues[36,37] report that multiple variants in the 3' region of *SLC6A3* may increase susceptibility for bipolar disorder, whereas Stober and colleagues[69] failed to find an association with bipolar disorder and single-nucleotide polymorphisms (SNPs) located in the 5' region of *SLC6A3*. We conducted a family-based association study of *SLC6A3* in 170 affected offspring trios defined by a child (12.9 ± 5.3 years of age) with DSM-IV bipolar I disorder and found a positive association with 4 SNPs (rs40184, rs11133767, rs3776512, and rs464049), but only rs40184 survived correction for multiple statistical comparisons (P = .034).[35] Greenwood and colleagues[37] also identified an association with rs11133767. We did not replicate the direction of effect and did not sample comparable markers to test for other possible replications, however.

Glutamate Decarboxylase 1 Gene

The *GAD1* gene codes the GAD67 enzyme, which catalyzes the decarboxylation of glutamate to γ-aminobutyric acid and is expressed exclusively in the brain unlike *GAD2*, which encodes GAD65 and is expressed in both the brain and pancreas.[70,71] Geller and colleagues[42] examined the association with a SNP (rs2241165) that tags an overtransmitted haplotype of *GAD1* associated with childhood schizophrenia.[72] In 48 affected offspring trios, Geller and colleagues[42] found that the A allele was also significantly associated with pediatric bipolar disorder.

NOVEL CANDIDATE GENES

The scope of genes examined needs to be broadened considerably, and the recent publication of genome-wide association (GWA) studies of bipolar disorder suggest several new candidate genes to study in samples of children.[73–75] The Wellcome Trust Case Control Consortium (WTCCC) study of 2,000 cases and 3,000 controls reported a genome-wide significant association on chromosome 16p12 with a SNP (rs420259) of the partner and localizer of the *BRCA2* gene (*PALB2*). Baum and colleagues[74] pooled a sample of 1233 bipolar cases and 1439 controls from the NIMH and Germany and found one genome-wide significant association (rs1012053) on chromosome 13q14 in the diacylglycerol kinase eta (*DGKH*) gene. In a sample of 1461 bipolar cases (from the Systematic Treatment Enhancement Program for Bipolar Disorder [STEP-BD] and the University College London [UCL]) and 2008 controls (from UCL and the NIMH), Sklar and colleagues[75] found genome-wide statistical significance in myosin5B (MYO5B; rs4939921 on chromosome 18), tetraspanin-8 (TSPAN8, rs1705236 on chromosome 12), and epidermal growth factor (EGFR, rs17172438 and rs729969 on chromosome 7) genes.

Additional, and perhaps more persuasive, candidate genes have been identified in secondary or meta-analyses of these GWA studies. For example, Sklar and colleagues[51] highlight an association with a SNP in the alpha-subunit of the L-type voltage-gated calcium channel (CACNA1C) that was replicated in the WTCCC[73] (OR = 1.21 and 1.16), although pooled analysis of this marker fell short of genome-wide statistical significance ($P = 3.15 \times 10^{-6}$). A SNP in the deafness autosomal recessive 31 (DFNB31) gene was one of the most significant associations in Baum and colleagues' study,[74] and proximal SNPs were nominally significantly associated both in the WTCCC and in the primary and replication samples of Sklar and colleagues.[75] With meta-analysis, Baum and colleagues[76] identified a nearly genome-wide significant association (ie, pooled P values $< 5 \times 10^{-6}$) with solute carrier family 39 (zinc transporter), member 3 (SLC39A3) gene on chromosome 19, and the junctional adhesion molecule 3 (JAM3) gene on chromosome 11. Finally, Ferreira and colleagues[77] conducted a collaborative genome-wide association study with the data from Sklar and colleagues and the WTCCC and a new series of 1098 bipolar cases and 1267 controls (ED-DUB-STEP2) and found genome-wide significant association ($P = 9.1 \times 10^{-9}$) with a SNP (rs10994336) in a gene (ANK3) coding ankyrin 3 and further evidence in favor of association with CACNA1C ($P = 7.0 \times 10^{-8}$).

FUTURE DIRECTIONS

Although these interesting new candidates should certainly be tested for association with pediatric bipolar disorder, these results also highlight the need for GWA studies of children with bipolar disorder. Because genome-wide studies are atheoretical with respect to the underlying genetic architecture influencing a phenotype, they are not limited by prior knowledge or current etiologic hypotheses. The genome-wide significant associations with ANK3 and CACNA1C suggest a new etiologic hypothesis that bipolar disorder is in part an "ion channelopathy," for example.[77]

Clearly, the extant literature of genetic association studies in children with bipolar disorder is inadequate. The positive genetic associations reported have either not been replicated or have been contradicted when examined in independent samples of children. It is important to note, however, that the number of informative families examined in this literature is quite small, and the studies are vastly underpowered to detect small effects. In fact, the upper limits of the CIs for all genes assessed suggest that even statistically insignificant associations are consistent with relatively genetic effects (ie, OR = 1.2). Unfortunately, then, the current literature comprises largely uninformative negative studies.

An adequately powered sample (eg, 1850 trios are required at $P<.05$ for OR $\geq$ 1.2) will likely require collaborative ascertainment of cases from multiple sites using valid and accepted measures of pediatric bipolar disorder. In the absence of a diagnostic gold standard for pediatric bipolar disorder, a pragmatic solution has been offered to facilitate the execution of randomized clinical trials in children with the disorder.[78] This approach has met with some success, as large multicenter randomized clinical trials of second-generation antipsychotics have been conducted in patients 10 to 17 years of age, leading to FDA approval for this age group.[79–81] Combined, these three studies recruited and assessed 627 children with bipolar disorder (average onset at 11 years of age) across multiple sites, demonstrating that pediatric bipolar disorder is a psychiatric disorder amenable to large-scale systematic research efforts. The sample size required is large, but not insurmountable, and the development of an active pediatric bipolar disorder genetics consortium to develop such a sample is a priority.

FINANCIAL DISCLOSURES

Dr. Eric Mick receives research support from McNeil Pediatrics, Ortho-McNeil Janssen Scientific Affairs, Pfizer, Shire Pharmaceuticals, and the NIMH and has had an advisory or consulting relationship with Pfizer, Shire Pharmaceuticals, and Validus Pharmaceuticals. Dr. Stephen Faraone receives research support from and consults to Shire Pharmaceutical Development. He receives grant support from Eli Lilly and the National Institutes of Health.

REFERENCES

1. Biederman J, Mick E, Faraone SV, et al. A Prospective Follow-Up Study of Pediatric Bipolar Disorder in boys with attention deficit/hyperactivity disorder. J Affect Disord 2004;82S:S17–S23.
2. Geller B, Williams M, Zimerman B, et al. Prepubertal and early adolescent bipolarity differentiate from ADHD by manic symptoms, grandiose delusions, ultra-rapid or ultradian cycling. J Affect Disord 1998;51:81–91.
3. Geller B, Craney JL, Bolhofner K, et al. One-year recovery and relapse rates of children with a prepubertal and early adolescent bipolar disorder phenotype. Am J Psychiatry 2001;158:303–5.
4. Geller B, Tillman R, Bolhofner K, et al. Controlled, blindly rated, direct-interview family study of a prepubertal and early-adolescent bipolar I disorder phenotype: morbid risk, age at onset, and comorbidity. Arch Gen Psychiatry 2006;63:1130–8.
5. Birmaher B, Axelson D, Strober M, et al. Clinical course of children and adolescents with bipolar spectrum disorders. Arch Gen Psychiatry 2006;63:175–83.
6. Brotman MA, Kassem L, Reising MM, et al. Parental diagnoses in youth with narrow phenotype bipolar disorder or severe mood dysregulation. Am J Psychiatry 2007;164:1238–41.
7. Wozniak J, Biederman J, Kiely K, et al. Mania-like symptoms suggestive of childhood onset bipolar disorder in clinically referred children. J Am Acad Child Adolesc Psychiatry 1995;34:867–76.
8. Wilens TE, Biederman J, Adamson J, et al. Association of bipolar and substance use disorders in parents of adolescents with bipolar disorder. Biol Psychiatry 2007;62:129–34.
9. Findling RL, Gracious BL, McNamara NK, et al. Rapid, continuous cycling and psychiatric co-morbidity in pediatric bipolar I disorder. Bipolar Disord 2001;3: 202–10.
10. McElroy SL, Keck JPE, Pope JHG, et al. Clinical and research implications of the diagnosis of dysphoric or mixed mania or hypomania. Am J Psychiatry 1992;149: 1633–44.
11. Geller B, Craney JL, Bolhofner K, et al. Two-year prospective follow-up of children with a prepubertal and early adolescent bipolar disorder phenotype. Am J Psychiatry 2002;159:927–33.
12. Geller B, Tillman R, Craney JL, et al. Four-year prospective outcome and natural history of mania in children with a prepubertal and early adolescent bipolar disorder phenotype. Arch Gen Psychiatry 2004;61:459–67.
13. Tohen M, Zarate CA Jr, Hennen J, et al. The McLean-Harvard First-Episode Mania Study: prediction of recovery and first recurrence. Am J Psychiatry 2003;160: 2099–107.

14. Tsuang MT, Faraone SV. The Genetics of Mood Disorders. Baltimore (MD): Johns Hopkins University Press; 1990.
15. Pauls DL, Morton LA, Egeland JA. Risks of affective illness among first-degree relatives of bipolar I old-order Amish probands. Arch Gen Psychiatry 1992;49: 703–8.
16. Bellivier F, Golmard JL, Rietschel M, et al. Age at onset in bipolar I affective disorder: further evidence for three subgroups. Am J Psychiatry 2003;160: 999–1001.
17. Dwyer JT, DeLong GR. A family history study of twenty probands with child-hood manic-depressive illness. J Am Acad Child Adolesc Psychiatry 1987;26: 176–80.
18. Kutcher S, Marton P. Affective disorders in first-degree relatives of adolescent onset bipolars, unipolars, and normal controls. J Am Acad Child Adolesc Psychiatry 1991;30:75–8.
19. Neuman RJ, Geller B, Rice JP, et al. Increased prevalence and earlier onset of mood disorders among relatives of prepubertal versus adult probands. J Am Acad Child Adolesc Psychiatry 1997;36:466–73.
20. Strober M, Morrell W, Burroughs J, et al. A family study of bipolar I disorder in adolescence. Early onset of symptoms linked to increased familial loading and lithium resistance. J Affect Disord 1988;15:255–68.
21. Wozniak J, Biederman J, Mundy E, et al. A pilot family study of childhood-onset mania. J Am Acad Child Adolesc Psychiatry 1995;34:1577–83.
22. Smoller JW, Finn CT. Family, twin, and adoption studies of bipolar disorder. Am J Med Genet 2003;123C:48–58.
23. Faraone SV, Su J, Glatt SJ, et al. Early onset bipolar disorder: evidence for linkage to chromosome 9q34. Bipolar Disord 2006;8:144–51.
24. Lin PI, McInnis MG, Potash JB, et al. Assessment of the effect of age at onset on linkage to bipolar disorder: evidence on chromosomes 18p and 21q. Am J Hum Genet 2005;77:545–55.
25. Etain B, Mathieu F, Rietschel M, et al. Genome-wide scan for genes involved in bipolar affective disorder in 70 European families ascertained through a bipolar type I early-onset proband: supportive evidence for linkage at 3p14. Mol Psychiatry 2006;11:685–94.
26. Zandi PP, Badner JA, Steele J, et al. Genome-wide linkage scan of 98 bipolar pedigrees and analysis of clinical covariates. Mol Psychiatry 2007;12:630–9.
27. Mick E, Biederman J, Pandina G, et al. A preliminary meta-analysis of the Child Behavior Checklist in pediatric bipolar disorder. Biol Psychiatry 2003; 53:1021–7.
28. Althoff RR, Rettew DC, Faraone SV, et al. Latent class analysis shows strong heritability of the Child Behavior Checklist-juvenile bipolar phenotype. Biol Psychiatry 2006;60:903–11.
29. Hudziak JJ, Derks EM, Althoff RR, et al. The genetic and environmental contributions to attention deficit hyperactivity disorder as measured by the Conners' rating scales–revised. Am J Psychiatry 2005;162:1614–20.
30. Hudziak J, Althoff RR, Rettew DC, et al. The prevalence and genetic architecture of CBCL-juvenile bipolar disorder. Biol Psychiatry 2005;58:562–8.
31. Volk HE, Todd RD. Does the Child Behavior Checklist juvenile bipolar disorder phenotype identify bipolar disorder? Biol Psychiatry 2007;62:115–20.
32. Faraone SV, Althoff RR, Hudziak JJ, et al. The CBCL predicts DSM bipolar disorder in children: A receiver operating characteristic curve analysis. Bipolar Disord 2005;7:518–24.

33. McGough JJ, Loo SK, McCracken JT, et al. CBCL Pediatric Bipolar Disorder Profile and ADHD: Comorbidity and Quantitative Trait Loci Analysis. J Am Acad Child Adolesc Psychiatry 2008.

34. Youngstrom E, Youngstrom JK, Starr M. Bipolar diagnoses in community mental health: Achenbach Child Behavior Checklist profiles and patterns of comorbidity. Biol Psychiatry 2005;58:569–75.

35. Mick E, Kim JW, Biederman J, et al. Family based association study of pediatric bipolar disorder and the dopamine transporter gene (SLC6A3). Am J Med Genet B Neuropsychiatr Genet 2008;147B:1182–5.

36. Greenwood TA, Alexander M, Keck PE, et al. Evidence for linkage disequilibrium between the dopamine transporter and bipolar disorder. Am J Med Genet 2001; 105:145–51.

37. Greenwood TA, Schork NJ, Eskin E, et al. Identification of additional variants within the human dopamine transporter gene provides further evidence for an association with bipolar disorder in two independent samples. Mol Psychiatry 2006;11:125–33.

38. Abou Jamra R, Fuerst R, Kaneva R, et al. The first genome-wide interaction and locus-heterogeneity linkage scan in bipolar affective disorder: strong evidence of epistatic effects between loci on chromosomes 2q and 6q. Am J Hum Genet 2007;81:974–86.

39. Geller B, Cook E. Serotonin transporter gene (HTTLPR) is not in linkage disequilibrium with prepubertal and early adolescent bipolarity. Biol Psychiatry 1999;45: 1230–3.

40. Geller B, Cook EH Jr. Ultradian rapid cycling in prepubertal and early adolescent bipolarity is not in transmission disequilibrium with val/met COMT alleles. Biol Psychiatry 2000;47:605–9.

41. Geller B, Badner JA, Tillman R, et al. Linkage disequilibrium of the brain-derived neurotrophic factor Val66Met polymorphism in children with a prepubertal and early adolescent bipolar disorder phenotype. Am J Psychiatry 2004;161: 1698–770.

42. Geller B, Tillman R, Bolhofner K, et al. GAD1 single nucleotide polymorphism is in linkage disequilibrium with a child bipolar I disorder phenotype. J Child Adolesc Psychopharmacol 2008;18:25–9.

43. Lesch K, Bengel D, Heils A, et al. Association of anxiety-related traits with a polymorphism in the serotonin transporter gene regulatory region. Science 1996;274: 1527–32.

44. Lasky-Su JA, Faraone SV, Glatt SJ, et al. Meta-analysis of the association between two polymorphisms in the serotonin transporter gene and affective disorders. Am J Med Genet B Neuropsychiatr Genet 2005;133B:110–5.

45. Axelrod J, Tomchick R. Enzymatic O-methylation of epinephrine and other catechols. J Biol Chem 1958;233:702–5.

46. Lachman HM, Papolos DF, Saito T, et al. Human catechol-O-methyltransferase pharmacogenetics: description of a functional polymorphism and its potential application to neuropsychiatric disorders. Pharmacogenetics 1996;6:243–50.

47. Craddock N, Dave S, Greening J. Association studies of bipolar disorder. Bipolar Disord 2001;3:284–98.

48. Lachman HM, Morrow B, Shprintzen R, et al. Association of codon 108/158 catechol-O-methyltransferase gene polymorphism with the psychiatric manifestations of velo-cardio-facial syndrome. Am J Med Genet 1996;67:468–72.

49. Rylett RJ, Williams LR. Role of neurotrophins in cholinergic-neurone function in the adult and aged CNS. Trends Neurosci 1994;17:486–90.

50. Egan MF, Kojima M, Callicott JH, et al. The BDNF val66met polymorphism affects activity-dependent secretion of BDNF and human memory and hippocampal function. Cell 2003;112:257–69.

51. Sklar P, Gabriel SB, McInnis MG, et al. Family-based association study of 76 candidate genes in bipolar disorder: BDNF is a potential risk locus. Brain-derived neurotrophic factor. Mol Psychiatry 2002;7:579–93.

52. Neves-Pereira M, Mundo E, Muglia P, et al. The brain-derived neurotrophic factor gene confers susceptibility to bipolar disorder: evidence from a family-based association study. Am J Hum Genet 2002;71:651–5.

53. Muller DJ, de Luca V, Sicard T, et al. Brain-derived neurotrophic factor (BDNF) gene and rapid-cycling bipolar disorder: family-based association study. Br J Psychiatry 2006;189:317–23.

54. Strauss J, Barr CL, George CJ, et al. Association study of brain-derived neurotrophic factor in adults with a history of childhood onset mood disorder. Am J Med Genet B Neuropsychiatr Genet 2004;131:16–9.

55. Strauss J, Barr CL, George CJ, et al. Brain-derived neurotrophic factor variants are associated with childhood-onset mood disorder: confirmation in a Hungarian sample. Mol Psychiatry 2005;10:861–7.

56. Pandey GN, Rizavi HS, Dwivedi Y, et al. Brain-derived neurotrophic factor gene expression in pediatric bipolar disorder: effects of treatment and clinical response. J Am Acad Child Adolesc Psychiatry 2008;47:1077–85.

57. Bulgin NL, Strauss JS, King NA, et al. Association study of theta EEG asymmetry and brain-derived neurotrophic factor gene variants in childhood-onset mood disorder. Neuromolecular Med 2008, in press.

58. Madras BK, Miller GM, Fischman AJ. The dopamine transporter: relevance to attention deficit hyperactivity disorder (ADHD). Behav Brain Res 2002;130:57–63.

59. Madras BK, Miller GM, Fischman AJ. The dopamine transporter and attention-deficit/hyperactivity disorder. Biol Psychiatry 2005;57:1397–409.

60. Li D, Sham PC, Owen MJ, et al. Meta-analysis shows significant association between dopamine system genes and attention deficit hyperactivity disorder (ADHD). Hum Mol Genet 2006;2276–84.

61. Brookes K, Mill J, Guindalini C, et al. A common haplotype of the dopamine transporter gene associated with attention-deficit/hyperactivity disorder and interacting with maternal use of alcohol during pregnancy. Arch Gen Psychiatry 2006;63:74–81.

62. Brookes K, Xu X, Chen W, et al. The analysis of 51 genes in DSM-IV combined type attention deficit hyperactivity disorder: association signals in DRD4, DAT1 and 16 other genes. Mol Psychiatry 2006;11:934–53.

63. Faraone SV, Biederman J, Wozniak J, et al. Is comorbidity with ADHD a marker for juvenile onset mania? J Am Acad Child Adolesc Psychiatry 1997;36:1046–55.

64. Faraone SV, Biederman J, Monuteaux MC. Attention deficit hyperactivity disorder with bipolar disorder in girls: further evidence for a familial subtype? J Affect Disord 2001;64:19–26.

65. Faraone SV, Biederman J, Mennin D, et al. Attention-deficit hyperactivity disorder with bipolar disorder: a familial subtype? J Am Acad Child Adolesc Psychiatry 1997;36:1378–87.

66. Bocchetta A, Piccardi MP, Palmas MA, et al. Family-based association study between bipolar disorder and DRD2, DRD4, DAT, and SERT in Sardinia. Am J Med Genet 1999;88:522–6.

67. Gomez-Casero E, Perez de Castro I, Saiz-Ruiz J, et al. No association between particular DRD3 and DAT gene polymorphisms and manic-depressive illness in a Spanish sample. Psychiatr Genet 1996;6:209–12.

68. Waldman ID, Robinson BF, Feigon SA. Linkage disequilibrium between the dopamine transporter gene (DAT1) and bipolar disorder: extending the transmission disequilibrium test (TDT) to examine genetic heterogeneity. Genet Epidemiol 1997;14:699–704.
69. Stober G, Sprandel J, Schmidt F, et al. Association study of 5'-UTR polymorphisms of the human dopamine transporter gene with manic depression. Bipolar Disord 2006;8:490–5.
70. Erlander MG, Tillakaratne NJ, Feldblum S, et al. Two genes encode distinct glutamate decarboxylases. Neuron 1991;7:91–100.
71. Bu DF, Tobin AJ. The exon-intron organization of the genes (GAD1 and GAD2) encoding two human glutamate decarboxylases (GAD67 and GAD65) suggests that they derive from a common ancestral GAD. Genomics 1994;21:222–8.
72. Addington AM, Gornick M, Duckworth J, et al. GAD1 (2q31.1), which encodes glutamic acid decarboxylase (GAD67), is associated with childhood-onset schizophrenia and cortical gray matter volume loss. Mol Psychiatry 2005;10: 581–8.
73. WTCCC TWTCCC. Genome-wide association study of 14,000 cases of seven common diseases and 3,000 shared controls. Nature 2007;447:661–78.
74. Baum AE, Akula N, Cabanero M, et al. A genome-wide association study implicates diacylglycerol kinase eta (DGKH) and several other genes in the etiology of bipolar disorder. Mol Psychiatry 2008;13:197–207.
75. Sklar P, Smoller JW, Fan J, et al. Whole-genome association study of bipolar disorder. Mol Psychiatry 2008;13:558–69.
76. Baum AE, Hamshere M, Green E, et al. Meta-analysis of two genome-wide association studies of bipolar disorder reveals important points of agreement. Mol Psychiatry 2008;13:466–7.
77. Ferreira MA, O'Donovan MC, Meng YA, et al. Collaborative genome-wide association analysis supports a role for ANK3 and CACNA1C in bipolar disorder. Nat Genet 2008;40:1056–8.
78. Carlson GA, Jensen PS, Findling RL, et al. Methodological issues and controversies in clinical trials with child and adolescent patients with bipolar disorder: report of a consensus conference. J Child Adolesc Psychopharmacol 2003;13: 13–27.
79. Tohen M, Kryzhanovskaya L, Carlson G, et al. Olanzapine versus placebo in the treatment of adolescents with bipolar mania. Am J Psychiatry 2007;164:1547–56.
80. Pandina GJ, Delbello M, Kushner S, et al: Risperidone for the treatment of acute mania in bipolar youth. In 54th Annual Meeting of the American Academy of Child and Adolescent Psychiatry, Boston (MA): 2007. p. 246.
81. Forbes A, Chang KD, Nyilas M, et al: Acute efficacy and tolerability of aripiprazole for the treatment of bipolar-I disorder in pediatric patients. In 161st Annual Meeting of the American Psychiatric Association, Washington, DC; 2008. p. 296–7.

Pharmacologic Treatment of Pediatric Bipolar Disorder

Jayasree J. Nandagopal, MD[a],*, Melissa P. DelBello, MD, MS[a],
Robert Kowatch, MD, PhD[b]

KEYWORDS

- Bipolar disorder • Mania • Depression
- Pharmacologic treatment • Pediatric

Bipolar disorder is being diagnosed and treated with increasing frequency in the pediatric population. In one office-based practice sample, there was a 40-fold rise in the number of children and adolescents treated for bipolar disorder between 1994 and 2003.[1] However, the diagnosis and treatment of bipolar disorder are often challenging in youth. Bipolar disorder presents differently in children and adolescents compared with adults, perhaps due to developmental differences in symptom expression. Nonetheless, traditional mood stabilizers and atypical antipsychotic agents are being used to treat all phases of pediatric bipolar disorder. Evidence supporting the use of these medications in acute manic or mixed episodes in youth is accumulating rapidly. However, prospective studies for the treatment of acute bipolar depression and maintenance therapy in children and adolescents are few, possibly due to its atypical

Disclosures: Dr. Nandagopal has received travel fund from Somerset and Cognitive Research Corporation and research support from Lexicor Medical Technology, Abbott, AstraZeneca, Bristol-Myers Squibb/Otsuka, Eli Lilly, Janssen, GlaxoSmithKline, Pfizer, Shire, Martek, Somerset and Repligen.
Disclosures: Dr. DelBello is a consultant or advisor for AstraZeneca, Bristol-Myers Squibb, Eli Lilly, GlaxoSmithKline and Pfizer, is on the speaker's bureau for AstraZeneca, Bristol-Myers Squibb, Eli Lilly, and GlaxoSmithKline, and receives research support from Abbott, AstraZeneca, Bristol-Myers Squibb/Otsuka, Eli Lilly, Janssen, GlaxoSmithKline, Pfizer, Shire, Martek, Somerset and Repligen.
Disclosures: Dr. Kowatch is a consultant/advisor for the Child Adolescent Bipolar Foundation, GlaxoSmithKline, Medscape, and Physician's Postgraduate Press, is on the speaker's bureau for AstraZeneca, is the editor of Current Psychiatry, and receives research support from Bristol-Myers Squibb, Stanley Research Foundation, NIMH, and NICHD.

[a] Department of Psychiatry, University of Cincinnati, College of Medicine, 260 Stetson Street, Suite 3200, ML 559, Cincinnati, OH 45267, USA
[b] Cincinnati Children's Hospital Medical Center, 3333 Burnet Avenue, Cincinnati, OH 45232-3039, USA
* Corresponding author.
E-mail address: jayasree.nandagopal@uc.edu (J.J. Nandagopal).

Child Adolesc Psychiatric Clin N Am 18 (2009) 455–469
doi:10.1016/j.chc.2008.11.004
1056-4993/08/$ – see front matter © 2009 Elsevier Inc. All rights reserved.
childpsych.theclinics.com

presentation, high rates of comorbidity, and the dearth of long-term outcome data in this population. No medication has been approved by the United States Food and Drug Administration (FDA) for treating all phases of bipolar disorder in children and adolescents, but the literature is swiftly evolving, and new data on the treatment of pediatric bipolar disorder are constantly emerging. This article summarizes the extant literature of published pharmacologic studies of children and adolescents with bipolar disorder. A literature search using Medline/PubMed was conducted to identify published peer-reviewed papers.

DIAGNOSIS OF BIPOLAR DISORDER IN CHILDREN AND ADOLESCENTS

Making an accurate diagnosis of bipolar disorder in children is often a difficult clinical task. Adults with bipolar disorder exhibit distinct episodes of mania and depression, as described in the Diagnostic and Statistical Manual of Mental Disorders, 4th edition, whereas children and adolescents with bipolar disorder generally present in mixed or dysphoric states characterized by irritability, aggression, and frequent outbursts of intense mood lability,[2,3] which could be nonepisodic and chronic.[4] Rates of cycling also differ between adults and youth with bipolar disorder. In general, bipolar youth seem to exhibit higher rates of cycling with fewer distinct episodes, of longer duration.[2,4,5] Geller and colleagues[6] observed that cycling in pediatric bipolar disorder was more complex with the presence of short cycles embedded within a more prolonged episode. They defined this phenomenon as ultrarapid (5–364 cycles/y) and ultradian cycling (>365 cycles/y, mania occurs for ≥ 4 h/d, with at least one cycle daily for 2 weeks).

Bipolar disorder in youth is associated with very high rates of comorbidity. The most common comorbid condition among bipolar youth is ADHD, which occurs at a rate of approximately 90% in prepubertal children and 30%–40% in adolescents with bipolar disorder.[7] Differentiating between bipolar disorder and ADHD can sometimes be a challenge, due to the presence of overlapping symptoms. In fact, some researchers have raised the question whether these are actually two distinct disorders. However, studies of familial aggregation patterns and clinical correlates indicate that pediatric bipolar disorder is distinct from ADHD.[5,8–10] Euphoria, grandiosity, hypersexuality, decreased need for sleep, and racing thoughts, which are core symptoms of mania, are not seen in ADHD. Co-occurring ADHD and bipolar disorder may represent a distinct subtype of bipolar disorder with distinct neurobiological alterations.[10,11] Other conditions that are commonly seen in children and adolescents with bipolar disorder are conduct disorder (CD), oppositional defiant disorder (ODD), substance use disorders, and anxiety disorders.[7,8,12,13] Medications, such as antidepressants, stimulants, corticosteroids, aminophylline, certain antibiotics and sympathomimetic amines, and medical disorders, such as temporal lobe epilepsy, hyperthyroidism, traumatic brain injuries, multiple sclerosis, systemic lupus erythematosus, and Wilson's disease, may worsen or mimic bipolar symptoms.[14] Hence, ruling out these confounders before making a diagnosis or initiating treatment is essential.

PHARMACOTHERAPY OF PEDIATRIC BIPOLAR DISORDER
Treatment of Bipolar Mania

Pharmacologic agents that are typically used to treat mania in youth include lithium, the antiepileptic drugs divalproex and carbamazepine, and the atypical antipsychotic agents risperidone, olanzapine, quetiapine, ziprasidone, and aripiprazole, with other adjunctive medications used as indicated. The only medications that are approved by the US FDA to treat acute mania in youth are lithium for children aged 12 years or older and risperidone and aripiprazole for children aged 10 years or older. In the past, there was limited information available regarding the use of these medications in youth, and therapy was largely based on adult literature, but knowledge has now begun to emerge on the treatment of pediatric bipolar disorder. Nevertheless, a majority of the pharmacologic trials done in children and adolescents with bipolar disorder are for the treatment of mania.

Mood stabilizers

Lithium, one of the oldest mood stabilizers available, has been safely used to treat bipolar disorder in both adults and youth. In a double-blind, placebo-controlled study, Geller and colleagues assessed adolescents with bipolar disorder I or II, mania, or major depressive disorder with at least one predictor of future bipolar disorder and co-occurring substance dependence during a 6-week outpatient trial that included random weekly urine drug assays and random and weekly serum lithium levels.[15] The authors found that lithium was effective for improving overall outcome measures as measured by a global functioning score. The mean age at onset of bipolar disorder was 9.6 ± 3.9 years, and the mean serum lithium level of active responders was 0.9 mEq/L.

A large open-label trial found lithium to be effective in treating acute mania in adolescents with bipolar disorder I.[16] Of 100 acutely manic adolescents who were treated with lithium, 63 were considered responders after 4 weeks of treatment; however, only 26 were considered remitters. Notably, 46% of the sample was also taking concomitant antipsychotic medications. The investigators observed similar response rates in adolescents with and without psychotic features when adjunctive antipsychotic medication was used, with 65.7% of patients presenting with prominent delusions or hallucinations at baseline, achieving stabilization of both manic and psychotic symptoms using combination treatment. Additionally, a majority of the patients who discontinued their antipsychotic medication after 1 month of combination therapy of antipsychotic and lithium experienced a worsening of symptoms that resolved only when antipsychotic therapy was resumed, suggesting that combination therapy may be required in acutely manic bipolar adolescents with psychosis. Interestingly, the presence of comorbid ADHD, prominent depressive symptoms, and substance use disorders did not affect response to lithium; this finding is in contrast to two previous studies that reported bipolar adolescents with ADHD to be at risk for poorer response to lithium.[17,18]

An open-label study comparing lithium, divalproex, and carbamazepine monotherapy in the treatment of manic or mixed episodes showed large effect sizes (Cohen d ≥ 1) for each medication in 42 bipolar adolescents with response rates of 53%, 38%, and 38%, respectively.[19] The authors pointed out that more than half of the patients did not respond to each of the three mood stabilizers and that combination therapy may be necessary for symptom remission in these patients. They performed a 6-month continuation open-label treatment protocol, during which the subjects could have their acute-phase mood stabilizer switched or augmented with another mood stabilizer, a stimulant, an antidepressant, or an antipsychotic agent, if they were deemed to be nonresponders to monotherapy with their mood stabilizers.[20] Of the 35 subjects who elected to continue in the extension phase, 20 (58%) required treatment with one or two mood stabilizers and either a stimulant, an atypical antipsychotic, or an antidepressant agent; 16 of the 20 subjects (80%) responded to combination therapy with two mood stabilizers, after not responding to a single mood stabilizer in the acute phase of treatment, suggesting that combination pharmacotherapy may be necessary. Similarly, a large open-label study examining the efficacy of combination therapy with lithium and divalproex for treating adolescents with bipolar disorder I or II reported significant improvement in all outcome measures (Young Mania Rating Scale [YMRS], Children's Depression Rating Scale-Revised [CDRS-R], and Children's Global Assessment Scale).[21] Of the 90 subjects studied, 73 (81%) were in manic or mixed mood states at baseline.

Open-label trials, retrospective chart reviews, and case reports have demonstrated the effectiveness of divalproex[22–26] and carbamazepine[27,28] in treating bipolar mania in youth. Response rates have ranged from 60% to 100% in these reports. Forty bipolar adolescents in manic, mixed, or hypomanic states enrolled in a 2- to 8-week, open-label study of divalproex.[25] A significant improvement in all efficacy measures, including the Mania Rating Scale, Manic Syndrome Scale, Behavior and Ideation Scale, and Hamilton Rating Scale for Depression, was observed. However, 43% of the patients used other psychotropic medications, such as haloperidol, lithium, benzodiazepines, and stimulants. However, in a recent (2007) double-blind placebo-controlled study in manic adolescents, divalproex ER was no more effective than placebo.[29] A retrospective chart review of clinical changes in hospitalized bipolar adolescents treated with lithium, divalproex, or carbamazepine monotherapy found lithium and divalproex to be more efficacious than carbamazepine.[22] The combination of carbamazepine and lithium has been reported to be effective in treating mania in case series of bipolar adolescents.[27,30,31] In an open-label study, 30 (85%) out of 35 adolescents who received carbamazepine for 16 to 18 weeks were responders; of these only 13 (37%) were on monotherapy.[32] Of the 22 subjects who were on other psychotropic medications, the majority were receiving either a second mood stabilizer or stimulants.

Recently, Kowatch and colleagues[33] reported results from a study of 153 subjects, aged 7 to 17 years with bipolar disorder, manic or mixed, who were randomized to lithium, divalproex, or placebo. At the end of 8 weeks, 41% of patients in the lithium group, 56% in the divalproex group, and 30% in the placebo group experienced more than 50% reduction in their YMRS scores. The YMRS score change in the divalproex group was statistically significant, whereas the lithium group demonstrated a trend in the same direction.

There are limited data regarding the efficacy and safety of other antiepileptic agents in treating bipolar mania in youth. A controlled trial assessing the efficacy of topiramate monotherapy for acute mania in children and adolescents had to be discontinued early, when several adult trials of topiramate failed to show efficacy.[34] Although the results of this pilot study were inconclusive, a statistically significant difference between the slopes of the linear mean profiles of the YMRS scores of the two groups using a post hoc repeated measures regression revealed a significant group difference. Open studies suggest that topiramate may be useful as adjunctive treatment in pediatric bipolar disorder.[35,36]

A multicenter, double-blind, randomized, placebo-controlled trial examining the efficacy of oxcarbazepine in treating children and adolescents with bipolar I disorder, manic or mixed, did not find oxcarbazepine to be superior to placebo on any measures.[37] In this study, 42% of the oxcarbazepine group and 26% of the placebo group achieved at least a 50% reduction in the primary efficacy measure, the YMRS score, relative to baseline, but the difference between groups was not statistically significant. The 42% response rate noted in the oxcarbazepine group in this study is similar to that observed in the open trial comparing lithium, divalproex, and carbamazepine.[19]

Trials in adults with bipolar disorder have found that gabapentin is ineffective for treating acute mania, but there is some evidence in support of its role as adjunctive treatment for treating anxiety disorders, such as social phobia and panic disorder.[38,39] It may, therefore, prove to be useful in treating comorbid anxiety in youth with bipolar disorder, because selective serotonin reuptake inhibitors (SSRIs) may precipitate manic or hypomanic symptoms.[40]

Atypical antipsychotic agents

Atypical antipsychotic agents are increasingly used to treat children and adolescents with bipolar disorder, and there are emerging data supporting their utility. As previously mentioned, risperidone and aripiprazole have been approved by the FDA for use in the treatment of mania in bipolar youth. A recent 3-week, multicenter, randomized, double-blind, placebo-controlled study assessing the efficacy of risperidone for acute mania in children and adolescents with bipolar I disorder reported that risperidone was more effective than placebo for reducing manic symptoms in bipolar youth.[41] Specifically, in this study, participants were randomized to treatment with placebo, risperidone 0.5 to 2.5 mg/d, or risperidone 3 to 6 mg/d. Both risperidone groups had significantly more responders than placebo, and there was no difference in efficacy between the 2 dosage groups. However, the lower-dose group had fewer adverse events (AEs) and treatment discontinuations, suggesting that lower doses of risperidone may be more beneficial than higher doses.

Pavuluri and colleagues[42] conducted a 6-month, open-label prospective trial examining the efficacy and safety of two combination therapies, divalproex plus risperidone and lithium plus risperidone, for manic or mixed episodes, and reported significant improvements in all outcome measures with both combination therapies and no significant group differences in safety and tolerability. In another study, the same group performed an open-label risperidone augmentation study in youth with preschool-onset bipolar disorder who did not respond to lithium monotherapy.[43] Specifically, 38 children and adolescents aged 4 to 17 years, presenting in manic or mixed mood states, received lithium monotherapy for 8 weeks; of these, 17 responded and 21 required augmentation with risperidone. Response rates in subjects treated with combination therapy was 85.7%. The predictors of inadequate response to lithium monotherapy in this study were the presence of comorbid ADHD, severity at baseline, history of physical or sexual abuse, and preschool age.

In 2007, the efficacy of aripiprazole for the treatment of bipolar mania in youth was evaluated in a 4-week, double-blind, placebo-controlled trial.[44] This trial compared two fixed doses of aripiprazole (10 mg/d or 30 mg/d) to placebo and found that both doses were superior to placebo. Subjects who completed 4 weeks continued assigned double-blind treatments for an additional 26 weeks. The AEs were mild to moderate in severity, and the most prominent AEs in the combined aripiprazole treatment groups were somnolence and extrapyramidal symptoms (parkinsonism and akathisia), and tolerability appeared to be dose-related. An 8-week, open-label study and a retrospective chart review reported aripiprazole to be effective and well tolerated in children and adolescents with bipolar mania.[45,46]

A double-blind, 28-day pilot study comparing quetiapine and divalproex for treating adolescent mania suggested that quetiapine was as effective as divalproex and that quetiapine reduced mania symptoms more rapidly than divalproex.[47] Rates of response and remission were also greater in the quetiapine group than in the divalproex group. Another controlled study demonstrated that the combination of quetiapine and divalproex may be more effective than divalproex alone.[48]

In a 3-week, double-blind, placebo-controlled trial conducted in 2007 studying quetiapine, subjects, aged 10 to 17 years, were randomized to either quetiapine 400 or 600 mg/d or placebo.[49] Results of this study indicate that both quetiapine groups had significant improvement in acute mania symptoms and overall functioning, compared with that of the placebo group. The YMRS score change was significantly greater than that of placebo at day 4 in the 400 mg/d group and at day 7 in the 600 mg/d group. The medication was generally well tolerated, but in patients taking concomitant psychostimulants, the incidence of commonly seen AEs was higher in a dose-dependent manner compared with that of those taking quetiapine alone.

Several studies have reported the effectiveness of olanzapine as primary and adjunctive treatments for bipolar mania in youth. Specifically, in an 8-week, open-label study of olanzapine monotherapy, olanzapine treatment was associated with significant improvement in mean YMRS scores, with an overall response rate of 61%.[50] Although olanzapine was well tolerated, there was a considerable increase in body weight over the study period (5.0 ± 2.3 kg).

Recently, a 3-week, multicenter, double-blind, placebo-controlled trial of olanzapine reported statistically significant reduction in YMRS scores and higher response and remission rates when compared with those of placebo.[51] However, significantly greater weight gain was noted with olanzapine than with placebo (3.7 kg versus 0.3 kg). The mean increases in prolactin, fasting glucose, fasting total cholesterol, uric acid, and hepatic enzymes were significantly greater in the olanzapine group than in the placebo group.

An 8-week, open-label trial reported statistically significant reduction in YMRS scores in manic youth treated with ziprasidone.[52] No significant AEs were observed in this study. A case series describing four children, ages 7 to 16 years, who were switched to ziprasidone from mood stabilizers, antiepileptics, or other atypical antipsychotics, suggested that ziprasidone may be effective and safe in treating bipolar hypomania or depression in youth.[53]

Ziprasidone was shown to be more effective than placebo in treating bipolar mania in a 4-week, multicenter, double-blind study.[54] Subjects, ages 10 to 17 years, were randomized to flexible-dose ziprasidone (80–160 mg/d) or placebo, titrated over 1 to 2 weeks. At week 1, ziprasidone was found to be more effective than placebo at reducing manic symptoms. Weight gain of ≥7% was reported in 7% of the ziprasidone group and 4% of the placebo group. QT (Q and T waves) corrected interval prolongation was observed in one subject treated with ziprasidone compared with none in the placebo group.

Despite emerging evidence suggesting the onset of pediatric bipolar disorder in the preschool years and findings from pharmacoepidemiologic studies showing that psychotropic agents are widely used in this age group, limited data are available on the safety and effectiveness of these agents in preschoolers. An 8-week, open-label trial comparing the safety and efficacy of olanzapine with risperidone in children, ages 4 to 6 years, indicated rapid and significant improvement in manic symptoms with both olanzapine and risperidone.[55] There was a statistically significant increase in weight with both risperidone (2.2 ± 0.4 kg) and olanzapine (3.2 ± 0.7 kg). An increase in prolactin level was observed with risperidone but not with olanzapine.

The efficacy of clozapine in treating bipolar mania in children and adolescents has been described in case series and reports.[56–58]

Side effects

Although data regarding the use of traditional mood stabilizers and atypical antipsychotic agents in treating mania in youth continue to emerge, these medications are associated with adverse effects. Lithium may cause nausea, vomiting, diarrhea, hypothyroidism, renal function abnormalities, polyuria, polydipsia, leukocytosis, weight gain, tremors, acne, and serious drug interactions. Potential side effects of divalproex include weight gain, hepatic failure, pancreatitis, thrombocytopenia, hair loss, and, rarely, polycystic ovarian disease in girls. Side effects associated with carbamazepine are agranulocytosis, aplastic anemia, hepatotoxicity, and multiple drug interactions. Lamotrigine has been reported to cause the fatal necrotizing rash of Stevens-Johnson syndrome (0.8%).[59] Topiramate can cause word-finding difficulties, paresthesia, weight loss, metabolic acidosis, and glaucoma.[35] Atypical antipsychotic medications are associated with significant weight gain, resulting in metabolic abnormalities, such as diabetes mellitus, dyslipidemia, and transaminase elevations. Weight gain is reportedly highest with clozapine and olanzapine followed by risperidone, quetiapine, ziprasidone, and aripiprazole.[60] Extrapyramidal side effects and tardive dyskinesia, though rare with these medications, have been reported. Careful monitoring is essential while using these medications in children and adolescents.

Other agents
Considering the morbidity associated with the side effects of medications commonly used to treat pediatric bipolar disorder, there is a need to identify alternative treatments that may be safe and effective for these patients. There is some initial evidence to suggest the effectiveness of the omega-3 fatty acids eicosapentaenoic acid (EPA) and/or docosahexaenoic acid (DHA) in the treatment of pediatric bipolar mania. An 8-week, open-label study using combined EPA and DHA (1290–4300 mg) in bipolar youth showed a modest improvement in manic symptoms.[61] Only 35% of subjects met the response criteria of >50% decrease on the YMRS. These findings need to be validated with randomized, double-blind, controlled trials.

Treatment guidelines
The choice of medication(s) is usually based on the evidence of efficacy, safety profile, phase of illness, presence of psychosis or rapid cycling mood swings, patient's and family's preferences, and history of medication response.[62] According to the Child and Adolescent Bipolar Foundation (CABF) expert consensus guidelines, monotherapy with traditional mood stabilizers or atypical antipsychotics should be the first-line treatment for bipolar I disorder, manic or mixed, without psychosis.[40] Augmentation with a second mood stabilizer or atypical antipsychotic was recommended for patients exhibiting partial response to monotherapy. For patients presenting with psychosis, initial treatment with a combination of a mood stabilizer and an atypical antipsychotic was suggested, based on an open trial that demonstrated that adolescents with acute mania and psychosis had significant response to lithium plus an adjunctive antipsychotic.[63] A combination treatment with three medications, such as lithium, divalproex, or carbamazepine, and an atypical antipsychotic was recommended for patients who did not respond to combination treatment with two medications. Clozapine was recommended for patients who did not respond to or were unable to tolerate any of the treatments outlined in the algorithm. Many youth with bipolar disorder may require combination pharmacotherapy for adequate symptom control, but limited data are available to support such treatment. Atypical antipsychotic agents are increasingly being used as first-line agents for treating mania in youth, especially if psychotic symptoms are present as part of the mania, because they are generally effective.

TREATMENT OF BIPOLAR DEPRESSION

Depression is a major component of the clinical presentation of children and adolescents with bipolar disorder. Bipolar adolescents whose index episode is major depression have a more protracted recovery than those with an index manic or mixed episode.[64] This illness phase has also been associated with a high-risk of suicide in youth and adults. However, limited knowledge is available to guide therapeutic approaches to bipolar depression in adolescents. Treating bipolar depression is a complicated task, as treatment with combinations of medications with the potential for aggravating manic symptomatology is often necessary. SSRIs have been reported to cause or exacerbate mania in youth with bipolar disorder. A retrospective study of children and adolescents with bipolar disorder reported that SSRIs were efficacious in the treatment of bipolar depression and that concomitant use of SSRIs during the treatment of active manic symptoms with mood stabilizers did not inhibit the antimanic effects of these medications.[65] However, SSRIs were also associated with relapse of manic symptomatology in patients with depressive symptoms in the absence of active mania.

Studies of adults with bipolar disorder have reported the effectiveness of lithium, divalproex, lamotrigine, quetiapine, olanzapine, and olanzapine/fluoxetine combination in the treatment of bipolar depression. In contrast, there are relatively few pharmacologic studies in youth with bipolar depression. A 6-week, open-label study of lithium monotherapy in 27 adolescents with bipolar I disorder reported that lithium was effective and relatively well tolerated in the treatment of an acute depressive episode.[66] Response and remission rates were 48% and 30%, respectively.

Lamotrigine has also been evaluated for the treatment of bipolar depression in youngsters. A small case series reported that lamotrigine was effective in treating adolescents with bipolar depression.[67] In an 8-week, open-label trial of lamotrigine in 20 adolescents diagnosed with bipolar disorder I (BD-I), bipolar disorder II (BD-II), or bipolar disorder not otherwise specified (BD-NOS) who were experiencing a depressive episode, lamotrigine was found to be effective as monotherapy or adjunctive therapy.[68] Concomitant medications such as other mood stabilizers, antipsychotics, and ADHD medications were allowed, as long as no dose changes had been made within 1 month of the study. The response rate based on the primary response criteria of a "1" or "2" on the Clinical Global Impression Scale was 84%, and that based on the secondary response criteria of at least a 50% reduction in CDRS-R scores was 63%. Although lamotrigine was well tolerated in this study, the potential risk of developing Stevens-Johnson syndrome could limit its use in children and adolescents, as the rate of developing a rash is higher in the pediatric population (0.8%) compared with that in adults (0.3%). However, a gradual dose titration is thought to minimize the risk of serious rash.

The CABF expert consensus treatment guideline group did not develop any treatment algorithm for bipolar depression due to insufficient data in children and adolescents.[40] However, they recommended lithium as a treatment option, based on adult studies. Lamotrigine and divalproex were also suggested as treatment alternatives. The guidelines also recommended that SSRIs and bupropion may be used with caution and only as adjunctive treatment after adequate mood stabilization. Larger, controlled pharmacologic studies to develop safe and effective treatments for pediatric bipolar depression are greatly needed.

MAINTENANCE TREATMENT

Pediatric bipolar disorder is associated with high rates of relapse, chronicity, poor medication adherence, and fluctuating syndromal and subsyndromal mood symptoms. Prospective studies of children and adolescents with bipolar disorder have reported recurrence rates ranging from 35% to 70% during follow-up periods of 6 months to 4 years.[69] Increased risk of relapse has been observed after discontinuation of maintenance treatment with lithium in adults with bipolar disorder. An 18-month prospective study of 37 adolescents with bipolar disorder reported that >90% of patients who were noncompliant with their lithium treatment relapsed, whereas only 37.5% of those who were compliant relapsed.[70] However, a placebo-controlled discontinuation study of bipolar adolescents who were responders following 4 weeks of treatment with lithium monotherapy and were randomly assigned to lithium or placebo during a 2-week, double-blind, placebo-controlled phase reported high rates of symptom exacerbation in both groups, with no statistically significant differences between the groups.[71] Additionally, less than half of the lithium-treated group sustained their response during the 2-week, double-blind discontinuation phase of the study, thereby questioning the ongoing efficacy of lithium. Findling and colleagues undertook an 18-month, double-blind trial to determine whether divalproex was superior to lithium in the maintenance treatment of bipolar disorder in youth who had been previously stabilized on a combination of lithium and divalproex.[72] In this study, subjects were treated with a combination of lithium and divalproex for up to 20 weeks, and those who achieved remission were then randomized in a double-blind fashion to monotherapy with either lithium or divalproex for up to 76 weeks. Divalproex and lithium were equally effective as maintenance treatment for bipolar youth who achieved syndromal remission with a combination of lithium and divalproex. Specifically, both treatment groups had a rapid median time to relapse (114 days for lithium-treated patients and 112 days for divalproex-treated patients) and did not differ in time until study discontinuation for any reason.

There is insufficient information available regarding the duration of maintenance treatment for young bipolar patients. According to the CABF guidelines[40] and the American Academy of Child and Adolescent Psychiatry (AACAP) practice parameters[62] for pediatric bipolar disorder, the medications used for acute stabilization should be maintained for 12 to 24 months. It was recognized that some patients may require lifelong treatment when the benefits of continued treatment outweigh the risks associated with it. The guideline recommends gradual taper, rather than abrupt discontinuation of medications, with careful monitoring to detect early symptoms of relapse. Educating patients and families about the early signs and symptoms of mood episodes is imperative, so that treatment can be reinstated as soon as possible.

TREATMENT OF COMORBID CONDITIONS

The majority of youth with bipolar disorder have co-occurring psychiatric illnesses, particularly ADHD, ODD, CD, anxiety disorders, and substance use disorders. ADHD is, by far, the most common comorbidity with pediatric bipolar disorder. The presence of comorbidities often worsens the prognosis of these patients and complicates their treatment. For bipolar youth with co-occurring ADHD, mood stabilization with a traditional mood stabilizer or an atypical antipsychotic medication is necessary before initiating stimulant therapy.[73]

The only double-blind, placebo-controlled trial of pediatric patients with co-occurring bipolar disorder and ADHD, whose manic symptoms were stabilized with divalproex, reported that adjunctive treatment with mixed amphetamine salts was safe and effective for treatment of ADHD symptoms.[74] Sustained-release psychostimulants may be preferable to short-acting stimulants, because rebound symptoms may be reduced with longer-acting agents. Psychosocial therapies may be employed to treat other comorbidities, such as anxiety disorders, ODD, CD, and substance use disorders. Lithium and topiramate have been shown to be effective in treating co-occurring substance abuse in adolescents with bipolar disorder.[15,35,75]

EARLY INTERVENTION STRATEGIES

Early intervention studies of psychotropic medications in high-risk offspring of bipolar parents seem promising. Chang and colleagues[76] found that high-risk offspring of bipolar parents with mood or behavioral disorders and at least mild affective symptoms, but not BD-I or BD-II, responded to 12-week, open-label, divalproex monotherapy. DelBello and colleagues[77] performed a 12-week, open-label trial of quetiapine in treating adolescents with a familial risk for developing BD-I and reported that quetiapine may be effective in treating mood symptoms in this population. However, Findling and colleagues[78] failed to observe any differences in mood symptom ratings, psychosocial functioning, or time to discontinuation of medication due to new mood episodes, over a 5-year period, between symptomatic at-risk youth (with BD-NOS or cyclothymia and a parent with BD) treated with divalproex versus placebo, although both groups showed improvement in mood and psychosocial functioning over time.

SUMMARY

Early identification and treatment of bipolar disorder in children and adolescents are important, albeit challenging. Delay in diagnosis and treatment could lead to greater psychosocial dysfunction and poorer outcome. Some psychotropic agents have been shown to have potential neuroprotective properties in bipolar youth,[79] indicating that these medications might be able to correct some of the neurobiological alterations associated with bipolar disorder. Future studies examining the safety, efficacy, tolerability, and neurobiological effects of psychotropic medications in children and adolescents with and at familial risk for developing bipolar disorder are needed, so that safe and effective early intervention and preventative strategies may be developed.

Recent research supports the use of several of the traditional mood stabilizers and atypical antipsychotic medications for the treatment of bipolar disorder in youth. However, the majority of the pharmacologic studies have focused on the treatment of bipolar mania, and very few data are available regarding the treatment of bipolar depression and, more importantly, maintenance (ie, prevention of recurrent mood episodes) therapy. Prospective, controlled studies evaluating the long-term safety and efficacy of psychotropic medications and the treatment of comorbid conditions in pediatric bipolar disorder are also needed to guide the treatment of these complex children and adolescents.

REFERENCES

1. Moreno C, Laje G, Blanco C, et al. National trends in the outpatient diagnosis and treatment of bipolar disorder in youth. Arch Gen Psychiatry 2007;64:1032–9.
2. Geller B, Tillman R, Craney JL, et al. Four-year prospective outcome and natural history of mania in children with a prepubertal and early adolescent bipolar disorder phenotype. Arch Gen Psychiatry 2004;61:459–67.
3. Geller B, Zimerman B, Williams M, et al. Diagnostic characteristics of 93 cases of a prepubertal and early adolescent bipolar disorder phenotype by gender, puberty and comorbid attention deficit hyperactivity disorder. J Child Adolesc Psychopharmacol 2000;10:157–64.

4. Tillman R, Geller B. Definitions of rapid, ultrarapid, and ultradian cycling and of episode duration in pediatric and adult bipolar disorders: a proposal to distinguish episodes from cycles. J Child Adolesc Psychopharmacol 2003;13:267–71.
5. Birmaher B, Axelson D, Strober M, et al. Clinical course of children and adolescents with bipolar spectrum disorders. Arch Gen Psychiatry 2006;63:175–83.
6. Geller B, Luby J. Child and adolescent bipolar disorder: a review of the past 10 years. J Am Acad Child Adolesc Psychiatry 1997;36:1168–76.
7. Kowatch RA, Youngstrom EA, Daielyan A, et al. Review and meta-analysis of the phenomenology and clinical characteristics of mania in children and adolescents. Bipolar Disord 2005;7:483–96.
8. Wozniak J, Biederman J, Kiely K, et al. Mania-like symptoms suggestive of childhood-onset bipolar disorder in clinically referred children. J Am Acad Child Adolesc Psychiatry 1995;34:867–76.
9. Findling RL, Youngstrom EA, McNamara NK, et al. Early symptoms of mania and the role of parental risk. Bipolar Disord 2005;7:623–34.
10. Faraone SV, Biederman J, Mennin D, et al. Attention-deficit hyperactivity disorder with bipolar disorder: a familial subtype? J Am Acad Child Adolesc Psychiatry 1997;36:1378–87.
11. Faraone SV, Biederman J, Monuteaux MC. Attention deficit hyperactivity disorder with bipolar disorder in girls: further evidence for a familial subtype? J Affect Disord 2001;64:19–26.
12. Youngstrom EA, Youngstrom JK, Starr M. Bipolar diagnoses in community mental health: Achenbach CBCL profiles and patterns of comorbidity. Biol Psychiatry 2005;58:569–75.
13. Axelson DA, Birmaher B, Strober M, et al. Phenomenology of children and adolescents with bipolar spectrum disorders. Arch Gen Psychiatry 2006;63:1139–48.
14. Kowatch RA, DelBello MP. Pharmacotherapy of children and adolescents with bipolar disorder. Psychiatr Clin North Am 2005;28:385–97.
15. Geller B, Cooper TB, Sun K, et al. Double-blind and placebo-controlled study of lithium for adolescent bipolar disorders with secondary substance dependency. J Am Acad Child Adolesc Psychiatry 1998;37:171–8.
16. Kafantaris V, Coletti DJ, Dicker R, et al. Lithium treatment of acute mania in adolescents: a large open trial. J Am Acad Child Adolesc Psychiatry 2003;42:1038–45.
17. Strober M, De Antonio M, Schmidt-Lackner S, et al. Early childhood attention deficit hyperactivity disorder predicts poorer response to acute lithium therapy in adolescent mania. J Affect Disord 1998;51:145–51.
18. Strober M, Morrell W, Burroughs J, et al. A family study of bipolar I disorder in adolescence: early onset of symptoms linked to increased familial loading and lithium resistance. J Affect Disord 1988;15:255–68.
19. Kowatch RA, Suppes T, Carmody TJ, et al. Effect size of lithium, divalproex sodium, and carbamazepine in children and adolescents with bipolar disorder. J Am Acad Child Adolesc Psychiatry 2000;39:713–20.
20. Kowatch RA, Sethuraman G, Hume JH, et al. Combination pharmacotherapy in children and adolescents with bipolar disorder. Biol Psychiatry 2003;53:978–84.
21. Findling RL, McNamara NK, Gracious BL, et al. Combination lithium and divalproex sodium in pediatric bipolarity. J Am Acad Child Adolesc Psychiatry 2003;42:895–901.
22. Davanzo P, Gunderson B, Belin T, et al. Mood stabilizers in hospitalized children with bipolar disorder: a retrospective review. Psychiatry Clin Neurosci 2003;57:504–10.

23. Papatheodorou G, Kutcher SP, Katic M, et al. The efficacy and safety of divalproex sodium in the treatment of acute mania in adolescents and young adults: an open clinical trial. J Clin Psychopharmacol 1995;15:110–6.

24. State RC, Frye MA, Altshuler LL, et al. Chart review of the impact of attention-deficit/hyperactivity disorder comorbidity on response to lithium or divalproex sodium in adolescent mania. J Clin Psychiatry 2004;65:1057–63.

25. Wagner KD, Weller EB, Carlson GA, et al. An open-label trial of divalproex in children and adolescents with bipolar disorder. J Am Acad Child Adolesc Psychiatry 2002;41:1224–30.

26. West SA, Keck PE Jr, McElroy SL, et al. Open trial of valproate in the treatment of adolescent mania. J Child Adolesc Psychopharmacol 1994;4:263–7.

27. Hsu LK. Lithium-resistant adolescent mania. J Am Acad Child Adolesc Psychiatry 1986;25:280–3.

28. Woolston JL. Case study: carbamazepine treatment of juvenile-onset bipolar disorder. J Am Acad Child Adolesc Psychiatry 1999;38:335–8.

29. Wagner KD, Redden L, Kowatch RA, et al. Safety and efficacy of Divalproex ER in youth with mania. Poster presented at the national meeting of the American Academy of Child and Adolescent Psychiatry. October 2007, Boston (MA), USA.

30. Hsu LK, Starzynski JM. Mania in adolescence. J Clin Psychiatry 1986;47:596–9.

31. Himmelhock JM, Garfinkel ME. Sources of lithium resistance in mixed mania. Psychopharmacol Bull 1986;22:613–20.

32. Kowatch RA, Carmody TJ, Suppes T, et al. Acute and continuation pharmacological treatment of children and adolescents with bipolar disorders: a summary of two previous studies. Acta Neuropsychiatrica 2000;12:145–9.

33. Kowatch RA, Findling RL, Scheffer RE, et al. Placebo controlled trial of divalproex versus lithium for bipolar disorder. Poster presented at the national meeting of the American Academy of Child and Adolescent Psychiatry. October 2007, Boston (MA), USA.

34. DelBello MP, Findling RL, Kushner S, et al. A pilot controlled trial of topiramate for mania in children and adolescents with bipolar disorder. J Am Acad Child Adolesc Psychiatry 2005;44:539–47.

35. DelBello MP, Kowatch RA, Warner J, et al. Adjunctive topiramate treatment for pediatric BPD: a retrospective chart review. J Child Adolesc Psychopharmacol 2000;12:323–30.

36. Yatham LN, Kusumakar V, Calabrese JR, et al. Third generation anticonvulsants in bipolar disorder: a review of efficacy and summary of clinical recommendations. J Clin Psychiatry 2002;63:275–83.

37. Wagner KD, Kowatch RA, Emslie GJ, et al. A double-blind, randomized, placebo-controlled trial of oxcarbazepine in the treatment of bipolar disorder in children and adolescents. Am J Psychiatry 2006;163:1179–86.

38. Pande AC, Davidson JR, Jefferson JW, et al. Treatment of social phobia with gabapentin: a placebo-controlled study. J Clin Psychopharmacol 1999;19:341–8.

39. Pande AC, Crockatt JG, Janney CA, et al. Gabapentin in bipolar disorder: a placebo-controlled trial of adjunctive therapy. Bipolar Disord 2000;2:249–55.

40. Kowatch RA, Fristad M, Birmaher B, et al. The Child Psychiatric Workgroup on Bipolar Disorder. Treatment guidelines for children and adolescents with bipolar disorder. J Am Acad Child Adolesc Psychiatry 2005;44:213–35.

41. Pandina GJ, DelBello MP, Kushner S, et al. Risperidone for the treatment of acute mania in bipolar youth. Poster presented at the national meeting of the American Academy of Child and Adolescent Psychiatry. Boston; October 2007.

42. Pavuluri MN, Henry DB, Carbray JA, et al. Open-label prospective trial of risperidone in combination with lithium or divalproex sodium in pediatric mania. J Affect Disord 2004;82(Suppl 1):S103–11.
43. Pavuluri MN, Henry DB, Carbray JA, et al. A one-year open-label trial of risperidone augmentation in lithium nonresponder youth with preschool-onset bipolar disorder. J Child Adolesc Psychopharmacol 2006;16:336–50.
44. Chang K, Nyilas M, Aurang C, et al. Efficacy of aripiprazole in children (10–17 years old) with mania. Poster presented at the national meeting of the American Academy of Child and Adolescent Psychiatry. Boston; October 2007.
45. Biederman J, Mick E, Spencer T, et al. An open-label trial of aripiprazole monotherapy in children and adolescents with bipolar disorder. CNC Spectr 2007; 12:683–9.
46. Barzman DH, DelBello MP, Kowatch RA, et al. The effectiveness and tolerability of aripiprazole for pediatric bipolar disorders: a retrospective chart review. J Child Adolesc Psychopharmacol 2004;14:593–600.
47. DelBello MP, Kowatch RA, Adler CM, et al. A double-blind randomized pilot study comparing quetiapine and divalproex for adolescent mania. J Am Acad Child Adolesc Psychiatry 2006;45:305–13.
48. DelBello MP, Schwiers M, Rosenberg H, et al. Quetiapine as adjunctive treatment for adolescent mania associated with bipolar disorder. J Am Acad Child Adolesc Psychiatry 2002;41:1216–23.
49. DelBello MP, Findling RL, Earley WR, et al. Efficacy of quetiapine in children and adolescents with bipolar mania: a 3-week, double-blind, randomized, placebo-controlled trial. Poster presented at the national meeting of the American Academy of Child and Adolescent Psychiatry. Boston; October 2007.
50. Frazier JA, Biederman J, Tohen M, et al. A prospective open-label treatment trial of olanzapine monotherapy in children and adolescents with bipolar disorder. J Child Adolesc Psychopharmacol 2001;11:239–50.
51. Tohen M, Kryzhanovskaya L, Carlson G, et al. Olanzapine versus placebo in the treatment of adolescents with bipolar mania. Am J Psychiatry 2007;164:1547–56.
52. Biederman J. An open-label trial of ziprasidone in children and adolescents with bipolar disorder. Presented at the annual meeting of the American and Canadian Academy of Child and Adolescent Psychiatry. October 2005, Toronto, Canada.
53. Barnett MS. Ziprasidone monotherapy in pediatric bipolar disorder. J Child Adolesc Psychopharmacol 2004;14:471–7.
54. DelBello MP, Findling RL, Wang PP, et al. Efficacy and safety of ziprasidone in pediatric bipolar disorder. Poster presented at the annual New Clinical Drug Evaluation Unit meeting. May 2008. Phoenix (AZ), USA.
55. Biederman J, Mick E, Hammerness P, et al. Open-label, 8-week trial of olanzapine and risperidone for the treatment of bipolar disorder in preschool-age children. Biol Psychiatry 2005;58:589–94.
56. Kovacs M, Pollock M. Bipolar disorder and comorbid conduct disorder in childhood and adolescence. J Am Acad Child Adolesc Psychiatry 1995;34:715–23.
57. Masi G, Mucci M, Millepiedi S. Clozapine in adolescent inpatients with acute mania. J Child Adolesc Psychopharmacol 2002;12:93–9.
58. Kowatch RA, Suppes T, Gilfillan SK, et al. Clozapine treatment of children and adolescents with bipolar disorder and schizophrenia: a clinical case series. J Child Adolesc Psychopharmacol 1995;5:241–53.
59. Calabrese JR, Sullivan JR, Bowden CL, et al. Rash in multicenter trials of lamotrigine in mood disorders: clinical relevance and management. J Clin Psychiatry 2002;63:1010–1.

60. Newcomer JW. Second-generation (atypical) antipsychotics and metabolic effects: a comprehensive literature review. CNS Drugs 2005;19:1–93.
61. Wozniak J, Biederman J, Mick E, et al. Omega-3 fatty acid monotherapy for pediatric bipolar disorder: a prospective open-label trial. Eur Neuropsychopharmacol 2007;17:440–7.
62. McClellan J, Kowatch R, Findling RL, Work Group on Quality Issues. Practice parameter for the assessment and treatment of children and adolescents with bipolar disorder. J Am Acad Child Adolesc Psychiatry 2007;46:107–25.
63. Kafantaris V, Coletti DJ, Dicker R, et al. Adjunctive antipsychotic treatment of adolescents with bipolar psychosis. J Am Acad Child Adolesc Psychiatry 2001;40:1448–56.
64. Strober M, Schmidt-Lackner S, Freeman R, et al. Recovery and relapse in adolescents with bipolar affective illness: a five-year naturalistic, prospective follow-up. J Am Acad Child Adolesc Psychiatry 1995;34:724–31.
65. Biederman J, Mick E, Spencer TJ, et al. Therapeutic dilemmas in the pharmacotherapy of bipolar depression in the young. J Child Adolesc Psychopharmacol 2000;10:185–92.
66. Patel NC, DelBello MP, Bryan HS, et al. Open-label lithium for the treatment of adolescents with bipolar depression. J Am Acad Child Adolesc Psychiatry 2006;45:289–97.
67. Carandang CG, Maxwell DJ, Robbins DR, et al. Lamotrigine in adolescent mood disorders. J Am Acad Child Adolesc Psychiatry 2003;42:750–1.
68. Chang K, Saxena K, Howe M. An open-label study of lamotrigine adjunct or monotherapy for the treatment of adolescents with bipolar depression. J Am Acad Child Adolesc Psychiatry 2006;45:298–304.
69. DelBello MP, Hanseman D, Adler CM, et al. Twelve-month outcome of adolescents with bipolar disorder following first hospitalization for a manic or mixed episode. Am J Psychiatry 2007;164:582–90.
70. Strober M, Morrell W, Lampert C, et al. Relapse following discontinuation of lithium maintenance therapy in adolescents with bipolar I illness: a naturalistic study. Am J Psychiatry 1990;147:457–61.
71. Kafantaris V, Coletti DJ, Dicker R, et al. Lithium treatment of acute mania in adolescents: a placebo controlled discontinuation study. J Am Acad Child Adolesc Psychiatry 2004;43:984–93.
72. Findling RL, McNamara NK, Youngstrom EA, et al. Double-blind 18-month trial of lithium versus divalproex maintenance treatment in pediatric bipolar disorder. J Am Acad Child Adolesc Psychiatry 2005;44:409–17.
73. DelBello MP, Soutullo CA, Hendricks W, et al. Prior stimulant treatment in adolescents with bipolar disorder: association with age at onset. Bipolar Disord 2001;3:53–7.
74. Scheffer R, Kowatch R, Carmody T, et al. A randomized placebo-controlled trial of mixed amphetamine salts for symptoms of comorbid ADHD in pediatric bipolar disorder following mood stabilization with divalproex sodium. Am J Psychiatry 2005;162:58–64.
75. Chengappa KN, Gershon S, Levine J. The evolving role of topiramate among other mood stabilizers in the management of bipolar disorder. Bipolar Disord 2001;3:215–32.
76. Chang KD, Dienes K, Blasey C, et al. Divalproex monotherapy in the treatment of bipolar offspring with mood and behavioral disorders and at least mild affective symptoms. J Clin Psychiatry 2003;64:936–42.

77. DelBello MP, Adler CM, Whitsel RM, et al. A 12-week single-blind trial of quetiapine for the treatment of mood symptoms in adolescents at high risk for developing bipolar I disorder. J Clin Psychiatry 2007;68:789–95.
78. Findling RL, Frazier TW, Youngstrom EA, et al. Double-blind, placebo-controlled trial of divalproex monotherapy in the treatment of symptomatic youth at high risk for developing bipolar disorder. J Clin Psychiatry 2007;68:781–8.
79. DelBello MP, Cecil KM, Adler CM, et al. Neurochemical effects of olanzapine in first-hospitalization manic adolescents: a proton magnetic resonance spectroscopy study. Neuropsychopharmacology 2006;31:1264–73.

Psychosocial Treatments for Childhood and Adolescent Bipolar Disorder

Amy E. West, PhD[a],*, Mani N. Pavuluri, MD, PhD[b]

KEYWORDS

- Pediatric bipolar disorder • Adolescent
- Psychosocial therapy • Family treatment
- Psychoeducation • Cognitive-behavioral therapy
- Group treatment

Pediatric bipolar disorder (PBD) is a serious disorder, is of early onset, and is associated with debilitating symptoms, including significant mood disturbance (eg, elated or irritable mood), episodes of rage, grandiosity or inflated self-esteem, hypersexual behavior, a decreased need for sleep, and poor judgment. Research on the characterization and accurate diagnosis of PBD has been plagued by uncertainty in the past, primarily due to high overlap with symptoms of attention-deficit hyperactivity disorder (ADHD), which causes confusion about whether PBD is a distinct disorder.[1] However, research to date has led to a general recognition that PBD represents a discrete cluster of symptoms that can be validated by reliable assessment with stability over time.[2]

The NIMH Research Roundtable of prepubertal bipolar disorder (BD) (2001) reached consensus that PBD can present as "narrow" or "broad" phenotypes.[3] Children and adolescents with the "narrow" phenotype have recurrent periods of major depression and mania or hypomania fitting the classical definitions of BD type I or BD type II described in the Diagnostic and Statistical Manual of Mental Disorders, 4th edition (DSM-IV).[4] However, compared with those with adult-onset BD, most of these children experience multiple episodes with rapid cycling and mixed mood states.[1,5] Children and adolescents with the "broad" phenotype have chronic, severe mood dysregulation (SMD) and hyperarousal[6] that is episodic in nature, but episodes may not meet intensity or duration criteria for BD I or II as defined by the DSM-IV.[3] These children

---

[a] University of Illinois at Chicago, 1747 West Roosevelt Road, MC 747, Chicago, IL 60608, USA
[b] University of Illinois at Chicago, 912 South Wood Street, MC 912, Chicago, IL 60612, USA
* Corresponding author.
E-mail address: awest@psych.uic.edu (A.E. West).

Child Adolesc Psychiatric Clin N Am 18 (2009) 471–482
doi:10.1016/j.chc.2008.11.009
1056-4993/08/$ – see front matter © 2009 Elsevier Inc. All rights reserved.

have complicated mood symptoms with significant comorbidity and associated impairment. There is still some debate in the literature as to whether children with the "broad" phenotype of BD are best characterized as part of the bipolar spectrum (eg, bipolar disorder not otherwise specified [BD NOS]) or as a distinct diagnostic category (eg, SMD;[7]). Despite continuing discussion about accurate characterization, it is widely recognized that children with both the narrow and broad phenotypes suffer from significant mood dysregulation and accompanying psychosocial deficits and would benefit from psychosocial intervention targeting their impairments.

Unfortunately, there are no authoritative data on the prevalence of PBD.[8] One community study evaluating rates of BDs in adolescents[9] showed a lifetime prevalence of 1% in youths 14–18 years old. In addition, Brotman and colleagues (2006) found the lifetime prevalence of SMD to be 3.3% in children aged 9–19 years, indicating that a larger percentage of the population may experience symptoms consistent with the broad phenotype of PBD.[6] Retrospective studies of adults with BD have reported that as many as 60% experienced symptoms before age 20, and 10%–20% reported symptoms before 10 years of age.[10–12] It remains unclear, however, whether there is continuity between the childhood-onset presentation and the more "classic" presentation of adult bipolar. Longitudinal studies will help clarify the progression of symptoms over the lifespan.

Despite the lack of knowledge on exact prevalence and the continuity/overlap between childhood-onset and adult-onset presentations, and regardless of whether they fall into broad or narrow phenotypic categories, it is well understood that the impact of symptoms of PBD on youth and their families is devastating. The unique symptom profile in PBD is associated with significant disruption in normative development, which manifests in impairments in social, emotional, and academic functioning.[9] For example, children with PBD have demonstrated academic underperformance and behavioral problems in school;[1] marked social impairments, including few or no friends, frequent teasing, and poor social skills;[1,13] and deficient family functioning, including poor sibling relationships, parent–child relationships characterized by frequent hostility and conflict, poor family problem solving, and poor agreement on parenting strategies.[1] These psychosocial impairments comprise a constellation of risks that may contribute to compounded psychological and psychosocial dysfunction throughout development. Indeed, by adolescence, children with BD exhibit low self-esteem, hopelessness, external locus of control, and poor coping;[14] high expressed emotion in family relationships;[14,15] more negative life events and chronic life stress, especially in the context of family relationships and school;[14,16] and poorer social skills performance.[17]

The accumulation of risk throughout childhood and adolescence makes PBD a significant public health concern, placing an enormous burden on educational and health care systems and on families of affected children. Children with PBD evidence increased behavioral problems, family stress, and academic underachievement, as well as an alarmingly high rate of repeated hospitalizations and suicide attempts.[18] As adults, they are likely to demonstrate impaired functioning, greater mental health care use, and lower rates of school graduation.[9] Given the significant psychosocial risk conferred on children with this disorder, and the poor long-term prognosis, it is no surprise that psychosocial intervention is increasingly recognized as an essential adjuvant intervention to pharmacotherapy in comprehensive treatment for PBD.[19]

ADJUNCTIVE PSYCHOSOCIAL TREATMENT FOR CHILDHOOD AND ADOLESCENT BD

Despite its recognition as an important aspect of multimodal treatment, the development and study of psychosocial interventions for childhood BD are in their relative infancy. However, there are several adjunctive psychosocial treatments that are being developed or tested for children and/or adolescents with bipolar spectrum disorders.

Multi-Family Psychoeducation Groups

Fristad and colleagues (2002) developed the multi-family psychoeducation groups (MFPG) adjunctive group treatment for parents and school-aged children with bipolar and depressive spectrum disorders.[20] MFPG consists of eight 90-minute sessions for parents, with concurrent sessions for children.[21] The goals of MFPG include teaching parents and children about the child's illness and its treatment, symptom management, and improving problem-solving and communications skills; and providing support, both from other group members and from professionals who understand the disorder. Important components of the treatment include direct education to parents in how to become more involved with their child's treatment and serve as an effective advocate, and the instruction of coping skills for children via the use of a "toolbox" approach, which has children identify pleasant and relaxing activities in 4 categories (creative, physical, social, and relaxing) that can be used to combat negative emotional states. The initial randomized clinical trial of 35 children indicated that families demonstrated increased knowledge about mood disorders, improved family interactions, improved ability to access services, and increased perceived social support from parents, compared with those of a wait-list control group.[21] Children's mood symptom severity did not decrease significantly following treatment. A larger-scale randomized controlled trial (RCT) was recently completed, but results have not yet been published.

Fristad and colleagues[22] have also developed an individual form of MFPG called individual family psychoeducation (IFP), incorporating similar concepts, but delivered across 24 child, parent, and family sessions. The IFP protocol delivers content similar to that of MFPG, with the addition of a "healthy habits" component to address sleep hygiene, nutrition, and exercise. An initial RCT of 20 children suggested that the IFP intervention had a positive impact on children's mood symptoms, family climate, and treatment use.[23]

Family-Focused Treatment for Adolescents

Miklowitz and colleagues[24] adapted their family-focused therapy (FFT)—that was originally developed for adults with BD—for adolescents. Family-focused treatment for adolescents (FFT-A) has the goal of reducing symptoms through increased awareness of how to cope with the disorder, decreased levels of expressed emotion from caregivers, and improvement in family problem-solving and communication skills. FFT seeks to accomplish these goals through the delivery of 3 treatment components, which include psychoeducation, communication enhancement training, and problem-solving skills training. The psychoeducation component involves developing an understanding of the symptoms, etiology, and course of the disorder, as well as the importance of pharmacotherapy adherence and relapse prevention. The communication-enhancement training component is focused on using role-playing and rehearsal to develop skills for active listening, offering positive feedback or constructive criticism, or requesting changes in others' behavior. The problem-solving component involves helping participants to identify problems, generate solutions, and implement those solutions in everyday life. These components are delivered across 21 50-minute sessions (12 weekly, 6 biweekly, and 3 monthly) for 9 months and include the patient, parents, and available siblings. A recently completed 2-year randomized clinical trial of FFT-A in adolescents with BD demonstrated that compared with adolescents who received the control treatment (psychopharmacology plus three sessions of psychoeducation), adolescents who received the FFT-A intervention had shorter times to recovery from depression, less time in depressive episodes, and lower depression severity scores for 2 years.[25]

Interpersonal and Social Rhythm Therapy for Adolescents

Hlastala and colleagues[26] are currently developing an adapted version of interpersonal and social rhythm therapy for adolescents (IPSRT) for adolescents with BD. IPSRT[27] is a manual-based psychotherapy founded on the theory that one aspect of vulnerability to BD is instability in circadian rhythms and neurotransmitter systems involved in regulation. In this model, psychosocial stressors are hypothesized to precipitate and/or exacerbate bipolar episodes through their ability to disrupt social and sleep routines. The IPSRT interventions seek to stabilize social and sleep routines and address interpersonal precipitants of dysregulation such as interpersonal disputes, role transitions, and interpersonal function deficits. IPSRT is primarily an individual treatment, but this adaptation will also incorporate brief family psychotherapy. A pilot study of this adapted IPSRT model is underway, but no results have been published yet.[26]

Dialectical Behavior Therapy for Adolescents

Goldstein and colleagues[28] are adapting dialectical behavior therapy (DBT) for adolescents with BD. DBT[29] is a psychotherapy developed for adults with borderline personality disorder, the main target of which is emotion dysregulation, including high sensitivity to emotional stimuli and extreme emotional intensity. This adapted intervention is delivered over the course of 1 year, and is composed of two modalities: family skills training (delivered to the family unit) and individual psychotherapy with the adolescent patient. The acute treatment period is 6 months and includes 24 weekly sessions that alternate between individual and family therapy. Continuation treatment consists of 12 additional sessions tapering in frequency over the rest of the 1 year. A small, preliminary open trial of DBT in 10 adolescents with BD found decreases in suicidality, nonsuicidal self-injurious behavior, emotional dysregulation, and depression symptoms after the intervention.[28]

Child- and Family-Focused Cognitive-Behavioral Therapy

Child- and family-focused cognitive-behavioral therapy (CFF-CBT) was adapted from FFT[24] and developed as an adjunctive psychosocial intervention for children 8–12 years old with bipolar spectrum disorders and their families.[30] CFF-CBT was designed to meet the specific developmental needs of children 8–12 years old with a bipolar spectrum disorder. We believe that CFF-CBT comprises four innovative aspects in the treatment of PBD in that it: (1) is designed to be developmentally specific to children aged 8–12 years; (2) is driven by the distinct needs of these children with PBD and their families (eg, affect modulation); (3) involves intensive work with parents parallel to the work with children to directly address parents' own therapeutic needs as well as to help them develop an effective parenting style for their child with BD; and (4) integrates psychoeducation, CBT, and interpersonal therapy techniques, tailored to the unique needs of these children, to augment the effects of pharmacotherapy. Diverse therapeutic techniques are employed across multiple domains, including individual, peer, family, and school to address the impact of PBD in the child's broader psychosocial context.

Empirical Foundation for CFF-CBT

As shown in **Fig. 1**, the psychotherapeutic methods used in CFF-CBT are driven by three areas of research evidence: (1) affective circuitry brain dysfunction in PBD; (2)

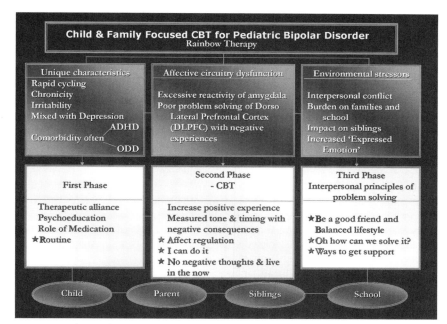

Fig. 1. CFF-CBT for pediatric bipolar disorder.

developmentally specific symptoms of PBD; and (3) impact of PBD on psychosocial and interpersonal functioning. First, studies of biological dysfunction in PBD implicate the brain structures involved in affective circuitry and may include the dorsolateral prefrontal cortex (DLPFC), ventrolateral prefrontal cortex (VLPFC), and amygdala.[31,32] The DLPFC is implicated in problem solving,[33] whereas the VLPFC and amygdala work in concert to regulate affective responses.[31,32] Functional neuroimaging studies have demonstrated reduced activation in the DLPFC and VLPFC, possibly contributing to problem-solving difficulties during excessive emotional reactivity, and increased activation of the amygdala.[34]

Second, children with BD evidence many unique symptom patterns that require tailored intervention. For example, they are more likely than their adult counterparts to exhibit ultrarapid or ultradian cycling and to present in mixed states, with manic symptoms coinciding with depressive symptoms.[1,5,35] This continuous and mixed pattern of cycling likely contributes to a clinical presentation as chronically and significantly irritable, which is typical of children and young adolescents with BD, compared with that of older adolescents and adults.[1,5,36] In addition, parents are likely to report that their children's irritability will often escalate into rage attacks and explosive outbursts, sometimes with little provocation.[37] The complex symptom picture in children with PBD is often made even more complicated by the presence of comorbid disorders, such as ADHD and oppositional defiant disorder.[1,36] Finally, there is some preliminary evidence suggestive of trait-level neurocognitive dysfunction in PBD in the key domains of attention, working memory, executive function, and verbal learning, which may severely impede learning and academic function.[38]

Third, due to the rapid mood changes and recalcitrant nature of the disorder – from irritable, excitable, impulsive, intrusive, and loud, to sullen, withdrawn and weepy – these children often have significant interpersonal problems with peers and family members.[1] Peer rejection and family conflict may erode the child's sense of self and contribute to feelings of worthlessness.[30] Conflict and expressed emotion often result from the exhaustion and strain endured by parents.[24]

Organization and Essential Components of CFF-CBT

Based on the scientific understanding of affective circuitry, developmentally specific symptoms, and psychosocial and interpersonal functioning in PBD, the core concepts and initial CFF-CBT curricula were developed. CFF-CBT is a 12-session protocol-driven treatment program meant to be delivered weekly over the course of 3 months (**Table 1**). Each session is approximately 1 hour. The majority of sessions are for the parent and child together, but some for the parent only, and some for the child only. Recently, CFF-CBT has also been adapted to a group format, which consists of parallel parent and child groups that run for 1.5 hours each week for 12 weeks. Although there is established content for each session and an ideal sequence to the delivery of this content, the treatment protocol can be implemented in a flexible manner as long as the essential ingredients are included. The acronym "RAINBOW" was formed to help parents and children remember the key components of CFF-CBT. The essential components of CFF-CBT "RAINBOW" covered throughout the treatment sessions are as follows:

R: Routine

The goal of this component is to increase affect regulation and decrease symptom exacerbation by establishing a predictable, simplified routine that will reduce excessive reactivity and tense negotiations in response to changes in the patient's schedule. Parents are encouraged to establish routines around sleep, diet, medication, and making transitions. Parents are also urged to integrate soothing and pleasurable activities into their own and their child's routine.

Table 1
CFF-CBT treatment overview

Session	Participants	Topics Covered
1	Child and parents together	Orientation to treatment Diagnosis and symptoms of PBD
2	Child and parents together	Psychoeducation about PBD Establishing a routine
3	Parents only	Affect regulation Parental efficacy boosting
4	Child only	Affect regulation skills Mood monitoring
5	Child only	Combating negative cognitions Behavioral control
6	Child only	Positive mantras
7	Child only	Social skills and interpersonal problem solving
8	Parents only	Effective communication and problem solving
9	Parents (and siblings, if applicable)	Coping skills for siblings
10	Child and parents together	Managing life stressors
11	Child and parents together	Social support
12	Child and parents together	Review and maintenance plan

A: Affect regulation

The goal of this component is to provide psychoeducation about symptoms of PBD and neurochemical underpinnings, teach behavioral management and coping strategies, and provide affective education to the children. Parents are educated about the biological basis of their child's illness and the nature of bipolar symptoms. Parents are instructed in various behavioral management techniques borrowed from Barkley[39] and Greene[40] to establish appropriate systems for negotiation and creating consistent consequences. Children are educated about recognizing and responding to affective states and consistently self-monitoring moods. They are given a system to monitor their moods several times throughout each day.

I: I can do it!

The goal of this component is to increase parents' and children's beliefs in their ability to cope with the disorder and to solve issues that arise. CFF-CBT employs techniques designed to increase a sense of self-efficacy in children and parents, including having children and parents generate a list of positive self-statements, encouraging parents to focus on the child's positive qualities, and helping parents to give consistent positive reinforcement for good behavior. Parents are encouraged to approach interactions with their children using a mixture of quiet confidence, firm limit setting, calming tones, empathy, and a focus on positive reframing, which we believe to be an effective combination for children who are highly sensitive to criticism and whose negative mood states are easily triggered. This style of interaction is likely to be more effective than shouting, threatening, and/or swift punishment in regulating the child's response and instilling a sense of confidence in both the child and parent that the particular situation will resolve positively.

N: No negative thoughts and live in the now!

The goals of this component are two-fold. The first goal is to decrease negativistic thinking and thought distortions associated with depression. Children and families are taught how to differentiate between helpful and unhelpful thoughts and to reframe unhelpful thoughts into helpful ones that increase their sense of hope, beliefs in efficacy around coping, and ability to solve problems. The second goal of this component is to encourage children and parents to focus on the present moment and to avoid becoming overwhelmed by thoughts of what might happen in the future. Based on evidence from the emerging literature on the use of mindfulness techniques in cognitive-behavioral therapy for depression,[41] children and parents are encouraged to focus on coping in the present moment, rather than dwelling on past failures or anticipating future failures. Mindfulness techniques, such as the use of positive mantras, are incorporated.

B: Be a good friend and a balanced lifestyle for parents

The goals of this component are, again, two-fold. The first is to improve social functioning in children. Children with PBD often have significant difficulties in peer relationships. Thus, a major goal of this component is to help children establish and maintain friendships. Children are taught the skills necessary to be a good friend and are provided opportunities within the therapy session to practice the skills. Parents are also encouraged to seek opportunities for children to practice newly developed skills and develop friendships (such as sleepovers, play dates, and supervised group activities). The second goal of this component is to increase parents' sense of well-being and ability to cope through achieving a balanced lifestyle. Parents of children with BD often suffer from physical and emotional exhaustion, frustration, guilt, and feelings of isolation.[42] Therefore, we encourage parents to develop a more balanced lifestyle that involves finding ways to rest, replenish their energy, and enjoy life. As an initial strategy related to this goal, parents draw a pie diagram that depicts the amount of time they invest in "recharging their own batteries" versus being a spouse, worker, or parent. Then, the therapist and the parent together discuss how to "carve the pie" so that parents strike a healthier balance between the demands of caring for a child with PBD and taking care of themselves.

O: Oh, how can we solve the problem?

The goal of this component is to engage parents and children in a collaborative and effective problem-solving process. As part of this treatment component, parents are encouraged to view their children as partners in the problem-solving process and to explain the pros and cons of potential solutions in an empathic way. Parents and children are encouraged to try creative ways to approach problem solving to minimize reactivity and the exacerbation of negative emotion.

W: Ways to get support

The goal of this component is to increase social support. Isolation, shame, and lack of access may prevent parents of children with BD from finding friends or family members who can provide respite and support. Therefore, the techniques used in this component emphasize the identification and active seeking out of people who can help the child and the parents through difficult situations. School advocacy is also a part of this component. Teachers are provided with a portfolio of CFF-CBT materials, information about the diagnosis, and information about ways in which the disorder may interfere with a child's performance in school. Parents are encouraged to engage the child's individual therapist or school counselor in further advocating for the child's needs at school.

Evidence Supporting CFF-CBT

The preliminary open trial of CFF-CBT[30] was conducted to assess its feasibility, patient adherence to the treatment (including dropouts), therapist adherence to the treatment protocol, and parent satisfaction with the treatment experience. In addition, outcome measures were administered to explore the effect of the treatment on symptom severity and overall functioning. Thirty-four children and young adolescents were assessed for bipolar symptoms and global functioning pre- and post-treatment. Results indicated that the CFF-CBT intervention was feasible to deliver and that patients were very satisfied with their experience. In addition, preliminary evidence demonstrated a reduction in symptoms of attention problems, aggression, mania, psychosis, depression, and sleep disturbance, and increased global functioning after the intervention.

Despite these encouraging initial gains, our clinical experience has taught us that these improvements are unlikely to be sustained without continued maintenance treatment. Therefore, we conducted a study of a maintenance model of CFF-CBT, comprising psychosocial booster sessions and optimized pharmacotherapy.[43] The 34 patients who underwent the initial 12-session treatment were followed up over a 3-year period and assessed for symptom experience and global functioning at years 1, 2, and 3 during the maintenance phase. During these 3 years, maintenance treatment consisted of ongoing medication management with psychosocial booster sessions using the CFF-CBT ingredients. Results indicated that patients were able to maintain the initial positive effects of the treatment over the 3-year follow-up period with continued booster treatment. These findings suggest that maintenance treatment models may help facilitate the long-term management of symptoms and represent an important step in addressing the low recovery and high relapse rates associated with PBD.

The results of both these studies must be interpreted with caution as the designs were open trials with no control group, and raters were not blinded to patient's participation in CFF-CBT. The initial improvements and maintenance of improvements over time could have been due to expectancy effects, the natural course of the disorder, continued stabilization on medication, or the continuation of additional attention and structure, rather than to the specific intervention. A RCT is in development.

Finally, CFF-CBT has also been adapted to group format, comprising 12 weeks of parallel parent and child groups. The group treatment is manual-based and delivers the same content as that in the individual treatment format. However, parent support and skill building are enhanced through the interchange that occurs when multiple parents are present in a single group session. A preliminary open trial of the CFF-CBT group treatment was completed to test feasibility. Results indicated that the group adaptation is feasible to deliver and resulted in a significant increase in parents' report of their child's coping skills, a decrease in parenting stress, an increase in parents' knowledge and self-efficacy in coping with the disorder, and a decrease in parent-reported symptoms of mania after treatment (West A, unpublished data, 2008).

SUMMARY

PBD is a devastating illness that is associated with psychosocial impairments in social, emotional, and academic functioning.[9] Despite what we know about the suffering endured by children and families afflicted by PBD, there is little research on how psychosocial treatment used in conjunction with medication might enhance treatment, prevent poor outcomes, and improve the quality of life for these families. In the 2007 American Academy of Child and Adolescent Psychiatry Practice Parameters for the Treatment of Childhood BD, McClellan and colleagues stated that, "a comprehensive multimodal treatment approach combining psychopharmacology with adjunctive psychosocial therapies is almost always indicated for early-onset BD."[19] Yet, to date, there are few empirically supported psychosocial treatments for PBD. The psychosocial treatments discussed above represent the entirety of burgeoning evidence-based psychotherapeutic approaches to treating BD in children and adolescents. Although they may have different populations of interest (eg, school-aged versus adolescents) and different theoretical orientations (eg, psychoeducation vs. cognitive-behavioral vs. interpersonal) driving their targeted interventions, they share many ingredients in common. Components of treatment emphasized in all these approaches include psychoeducation about the disorder, the importance of effective communication and problem solving, and the development of healthy coping skills, for example.

It remains to be determined how exactly psychosocial intervention may enhance medication treatment and contribute to sustained remission and improved quality of life for children and adolescents with BD. Most of these interventions are in the early stages of development, and even those that have been tested through more rigorous designs (eg, MFPG and FFT) had smaller sample sizes that limit the interpretability of their results. However, the results of all of the preliminary studies of these interventions suggest that they are feasible and may add utility beyond medication or treatment as usual in addressing specific aspects of the disorder. Certainly, few would challenge the notion that we have a long way to go in developing treatments that are effective in the long-term management of childhood and adolescent BD. These psychosocial interventions, as further developed, may provide important insight, knowledge, and skills to families that prove integral to treatment success and are not addressed with medication alone or generic psychotherapy approaches. Therefore, the testing of such interventions is an important step in the development of effective evidence-based practices.

However, there are both scientific and practical challenges to developing and testing psychosocial interventions for PBD. First, the spectrum of BDs encompasses diverse symptom profiles, and each child may experience the disorder in a slightly different way, which makes flexibility and adaptability imperative, even in "packaged" treatment approaches. Unfortunately, this phenomenon presents obvious challenges in a climate of RCTs that emphasize control, rigor, and strict treatment fidelity. Second, PBD is a refractory and episodic illness, which can make teasing out the results of an actual intervention from the natural course of the disorder complicated. Patients with PBD naturally fluctuate in their mood states, which can cloud the effects of treatment and make it difficult to determine whether the intervention is working or the patient is just cycling in and out of different mood states. Third, medication is the first-line treatment for PBD, and the medication regimens for these children are often quite complicated and need to be adjusted frequently to address recurring symptoms and side effects. The constant flux of medication treatment can present a challenge when trying to clarify the unique effects of psychotherapy beyond medication's stabilization of symptoms. Finally, PBD is a chronic disorder and few would argue that an initial injection of any psychosocial treatment approach will sustain improvements over the long term. Even with rapidly advancing medical technology, the current profile of successful treatment is likely to include lifelong medication management enhanced by psychosocial intervention, ongoing therapy booster sessions, crisis management and case management as needed, social support, and advocacy throughout childhood, adolescence, and adulthood, as patients navigate different life systems.

These challenges point to the need for rigorously designed, large-sample, and longitudinal research, which unfortunately often clashes with what is feasible in clinical practice settings, where low base rates, diagnostic confusion, comorbidity, high dropout rates, lack of resources, and severe symptoms requiring ongoing crisis management often impede a researcher's ability to carry out these kinds of studies. However, the potential benefits of these kinds of interventions in increasing treatment engagement and adherence, improving important domains of psychosocial functioning that optimize quality of life, and ultimately enabling patients to manage the symptoms of the disorder long term certainly merit the investment of resources into their investigation. The ultimate goal of the study of psychosocial treatments for BD in childhood is to identify important psychosocial treatment targets (eg, psychoeducation, affect regulation skills, cognitive restructuring, family communication) and incorporate them into practical and cost-efficient treatment models. Ideally, these models will be easy to train, transport, and implement, yet represent comprehensive and efficacious approaches to improving patient outcomes in the short- and long term. Such treatments will offer providers an organized framework for implementing evidence-based approaches, thus optimizing both the individual patient's experience as well as reducing the public health burden of childhood and adolescent BD.

REFERENCES

1. Geller B, Craney J, Bolhofner K, et al. Two-year prospective follow-up of children with a prepubertal and early-adolescent bipolar disorder phenotype. Am J Psychiatry 2002;159(6):927–33.

2. Geller B, Craney J, Bolhofner K, et al. One-year recovery and relapse rates of children with a prepubertal and early adolescent bipolar disorder phenotype. Am J Psychiatry 2001;158:303–5.
3. National Institutes of Mental Health. Roundtable on prepubertal bipolar disorder. J Am Acad Child Adolesc Psychiatry 2001;40(8):871–8.
4. American Psychiatric Association. Diagnostic and statistical manual of mental disorders. (4th edition). Washington, DC: Author; 1994.
5. Findling R, Gracious B, McNamara N, et al. Rapid continuous cycling and psychiatric comorbidity in pediatric bipolar I disorder. Bipolar Disord 2001;3:202–10.
6. Brotman M, Schmajuk M, Rich B, et al. Prevalence, clinical correlates, and longitudinal course of severe mood dysregulation in children. Biol Psychiatry 2006; 60(9):991–7.
7. Leibenluft E, Charney D, Towbin K, et al. Defining clinical phenotypes of juvenile mania. Am J Psychiatry 2003;160:430–7.
8. Pavuluri M, Birmaher B, Naylor M. Pediatric bipolar disorder: a review of the past 10 years. J Am Acad Child Adolesc Psychiatry 2005;44(9):846–71.
9. Lewinsohn P, Klein D, Seeley J. Bipolar disorders in a community sample of older adolescents: prevalence, phenomenology, comorbidity, and course. J Am Acad Child Adolesc Psychiatry 1995;34:454–63.
10. Egeland J, Hostetter A, Pauls D, et al. Prodromal symptoms before onset in manic-depressive disorder suggested by first hospital admission histories. J Am Acad Child Adolesc Psychiatry 2000;39:1245–52.
11. Lish J, Dime-Meenan S, Whybrow P, et al. The national depressive and manic-depressive association (DMDA) survey of bipolar members. J Affect Disord 1994;31:281–94.
12. Loranger A, Levine P. Age at onset of bipolar affective illness. Arch Gen Psychiatry 1978;35:1345–8.
13. Wilens T, Biederman J, Forkner P, et al. Patterns of comorbidity and dysfunction in clinically referred preschool and school-age children with bipolar disorder. J Child Adolesc Psychopharmacol 2003;13(4):495–505.
14. Rucklidge J. Psychosocial functioning of adolescents with and without pediatric bipolar disorder. J Affect Disord 2006;91(2–3):181–8.
15. Miklowitz D, Biukians A, Richards J. Early-onset bipolar disorder: a family treatment perspective. Dev Psychopathol 2006;18:1247–65.
16. Kim E, Miklowitz D, Biukians A, et al. Life stress and the course of early-onset bipolar disorder. J Affect Disord 2007;99(1–3):37–44.
17. Goldstein T, Mullen K, Miklowitz D. Social skills knowledge and performance among adolescents with bipolar disorder. Bipolar Disord 2006;8:350–61.
18. Lewinsohn P, Olino T, Klein D. Psychosocial impairment in offspring of depressed parents. Psychol Med 2005;35(10):1493–503.
19. McClellan J, Kowatch R, Findling R, et al. Practice parameter for the assessment and treatment of children and adolescents with bipolar disorder. J Am Acad Child Adolesc Psychiatry 2007;46(1):107–25.
20. Fristad M, Goldberg-Arnold J, Gavazzi S. Multi-family psychoeducation groups (MFPG) for parents of children with bipolar disorder. Bipolar Disord 2002;4: 254–62.
21. Fristad M, Gavazzi S, Mackinaw-Koons B. Family psychoeducation: An adjunctive intervention for children with bipolar disorder. Biol Psychiatry 2003;53: 1000–8.
22. Young M, Fristad M. Evidence based treatments for bipolar disorder in children and adolescents. J Contemp Psychother 2007;37:157–64.

23. Fristad M. Psychoeducational treatment for school-aged children with bipolar disorder. Dev Psychopathol 2006;18:1289–306.
24. Miklowitz D, George E, Axelson D, et al. Family-focused treatment for adolescents with bipolar disorder. J Affect Disord 2004;82(Suppl 1):113–28.
25. Miklowitz D, Axelson D, Birmaher B, et al. Family-focused treatment for adolescents with bipolar disorder. Arch Gen Psychiatry 2008;65(9):1053–61.
26. Hlastala S, Frank E. Adapting interpersonal and social rhythm therapy to the developmental needs of adolescents with bipolar disorder. Dev Psychopathol 2006;18:1267–88.
27. Frank E. Treating bipolar disorder: a clinician's guide to interpersonal and social rhythm therapy. New York: Guilford Press; 2005.
28. Goldstein T, Axelson D, Birmaher B, et al. Dialectical behavior therapy for adolescents with bipolar disorder: a 1-year open trial. J Am Acad Child Adolesc Psychiatry 2007;46(7):820–30.
29. Linehan M. Cognitive-behavioral treatment of borderline personality disorder. New York: Guildford Press; 1993.
30. Pavuluri M, Graczyk P, Henry D, et al. Child- and family-focused cognitive-behavioral therapy for pediatric bipolar disorder: development and preliminary results. J Am Acad Child Adolesc Psychiatry 2004;43:528–37.
31. Pavuluri M, Henry D, Nadimpalli S, et al. Biological risk factors in pediatric bipolar disorder. Biol Psychiatry 2006;60:936–41.
32. Rich B, Vinton D, Roberson-Nay R, et al. Limbic hyperactivation during processing of neutral facial expressions in children with bipolar disorder. Proc Natl Acad Sci USA 2006;103(23):8900–5.
33. Perlstein W, Elbert T, Stenger V. Dissociation in human prefrontal cortex of affective influences on working memory-related activity. Proc Natl Acad Sci USA 2002; 99:1736–41.
34. Pavuluri M, O'Connor M, Harral E, et al. Affective neural circuitry during facial emotion processing in pediatric bipolar disorder. Biol Psychiatry 2007;62(2):158–67.
35. Pavuluri M, Naylor M, Janicak P. Recognition and treatment of pediatric bipolar disorder. Contemporary Psychiatry 2002;1:1–10.
36. Wozniak J, Biederman J, Kiely K, et al. Mania-like symptoms suggestive of childhood-onset bipolar disorder in clinically-referred children. J Am Acad Child Adolesc Psychiatry 1995;34:867–76.
37. Biederman J, Faraone S, Milberger S, et al. A prospective 4-year follow-up study of attention-deficit hyperactivity and related disorders. Arch Gen Psychiatry 1996; 53:437–46.
38. Pavuluri M, Schenkel L, Aryal S, et al. Neurocognitive functioning in unmedicated manic and medicated euthymic pediatric bipolar patients. Am J Psychiatry 2006; 163:286–93.
39. Barkley RA. Defiant children: a clinician's manual for parenting training. New York: Guilford Press; 1987.
40. Greene R. The explosive child. New York: Harper Collins; 2001.
41. Segal Z, Williams J, Teasdale J. Mindfulness-based cognitive therapy for depression: a new approach to preventing relapse. New York: Guilford Press; 2002.
42. Fristad M, Goldberg-Arnold J. Family interventions for early-onset bipolar disorder. In: Geller B, DelBello M, editors. Bipolar disorder in childhood and early adolescence. New York: Guilford Press; 2003. p. 295–313.
43. West A, Pavuluri M. Maintenance model of integrated psychosocial treatment in pediatric bipolar disorder. J Am Acad Child Adolesc Psychiatry 2007;46(2): 205–12.

Alternative Treatments in Pediatric Bipolar Disorder

Mona Potter, MD[a], Alana Moses, BA[b], Janet Wozniak, MD[a],*

KEYWORDS

- Complementary and alternative treatments
- Pediatric bipolar disorder • Omega-3-fatty acid • Inositol
- St. John's wort • SAMe • Melatonin • Acupuncture

Part of the controversy surrounding the diagnosis of bipolar disorder in youth is the concern that children given the diagnosis may be subjected to treatments that are fraught with potentially impairing and serious side effects. The standard treatments for pediatric-onset bipolar disorder include the mood stabilizers comprising lithium, anticonvulsants, and atypical antipsychotics. All of these medications are associated with both serious and annoying side effects. None of these medications offers a guarantee of recovery. In the naturalistic setting when used for children with bipolar disorder, although they are more useful in the treatment of bipolar symptoms than antidepressants or stimulants, lithium and the anticonvulsants divalproex and carbamazepine are associated with slow onset of action and frequent relapse.[1] In a placebo-controlled trial by Kowatch and colleagues[2] of the traditional mood stabilizers lithium, divalproex, and carbamazepine, treatment of pediatric mania was marked by frequent adverse events, noncompliance, and treatment dropouts, as well as discouraging effect sizes, demonstrating effectiveness in less than 50% of youth studied. In another double-blind, placebo-controlled trial of lithium in adolescents with bipolar disorder and substance abuse, lithium was moderately effective; however, the benefit was limited to substance abuse symptoms only, not the core symptoms of bipolar disorder.[3] In a multisite study with divalproex sodium, Wagner[4] reported that of the 40 subjects enrolled, only 17 completed the open trial due to side effects and ineffectiveness, and only three entered the double-blind follow-up phase. An open-label trial of Depakote ER (divalproex sodium) resulted in a high dropout rate and only partial efficacy for bipolar symptoms.

[a] Department of Child and Adolescent Psychiatry, Massachusetts General Hospital and McLean Hospital, Yawkey Center for Outpatient Care, Yawkey 6A, 55 Fruit Street, Boston, MA 02114, USA
[b] Department of Pediatric Psychopharmacology, Massachusetts General Hospital, 185 Alewife Brook Parkway, Suite 2000, Cambridge, MA 02138, USA
* Corresponding author.
E-mail address: jwozniak@partners.org (J. Wozniak).

Child Adolesc Psychiatric Clin N Am 18 (2009) 483–514
doi:10.1016/j.chc.2008.11.001
1056-4993/08/$ – see front matter © 2009 Elsevier Inc. All rights reserved.

childpsych.theclinics.com

Although more encouraging results have emerged with the use of atypical antipsychotics,[5–8] these treatments have been associated with severe weight gain and an increased risk for the development of diabetes as well as tardive dyskinesia. In addition, there is resistance among families and clinicians to the use of "antipsychotic" medication in youth, because these medications are perceived as "powerful," and there is a lack of information regarding the effects of these medications on developing brains. Because monotherapy use of mood stabilizing medications in pediatric bipolar disorder has shown only modest effects for many youth, researchers have looked to the practice of combining mood stabilizing medications. For example, Findling and colleagues[9–11] reported that symptoms of bipolar disorder in youth may be safely treated with a combination of lithium and divalproex sodium with greater efficacy than either agent could provide if used solo. Finding safe and effective combinations or new treatments with minimal side effects has become a priority for clinicians given the morbidity associated with bipolar disorder and the relapsing nature of the illness.

Adding to the concerns regarding the use of these conventional treatments, adverse effects and noncompliance may be more significant problems in the management of children and adolescents than in that of adults. Youth, especially adolescents, may be particularly self-conscious and intolerant of side effects such as weight gain, acne, or sedation. Parents of children and adolescents express particular concerns regarding the possibility of cognitive impairments in youth whose main developmental task is learning. When combined pharmacotherapy is used, the risk for adverse events is compounded by the possibility of drug–drug interactions and the need for routine blood collection for drug monitoring. Poor adherence to treatment can further compromise clinical outcome.

In summary, pediatric-onset bipolar disorder is associated with high levels of morbidity and documented disability, yet there is no gold standard of treatment, and none of the conventional treatments can claim a high level of efficacy combined with a low level of adverse events.[12] Taken together, this state of affairs indicates the need for more safe and effective treatments for the management of pediatric bipolar disorder. Increasingly, clinicians, researchers, and patients and their families are turning to an array of natural products considered complementary and alternative treatments. Although these agents have little evidence of efficacy, the fact that they appear to be safe and even healthful make them attractive options as monotherapy or in combination with each other or with conventional treatments. Although studies of these agents generally report disappointing efficacy rates, the fact that complementary treatments are usually part of a normal diet and likely to have no or minimal downside in terms of side effects leaves many individuals wondering, "Why not try them?"

Alternative treatments should be thoughtfully considered for children with bipolar disorder, as youngsters, especially, may be vulnerable to the morbid side effects of known pharmaceutical agents due to the demands of growth and development. Furthermore, as bipolar disorder may be a lifelong condition, the exigencies of early and aggressive treatment need to be balanced by the side effects of early and lengthy exposure to agents with serious side effects. Alternative treatments offer a healthy option for treating developing youth with psychiatric disturbance. As bipolar disorder in children is severely impairing, lack of intervention is usually not an option. In this article, we review some of the agents that have been noted to have mood stabilizing or antidepressant action and, therefore, have the potential to be most useful in the treatment of pediatric bipolar disorder. We review the agent's role in biological mechanisms, its purported mechanism of action, the agent's use in psychiatry, studies addressing efficacy and safety in adults, and when available, studies addressing safety and efficacy in youth.

OMEGA-3 FATTY ACIDS

Fatty acids fall into the family called lipids. Lipids make up over half the mass of the brain, and they are especially important in the structure and function of cell membranes. Cell membrane functioning is critical for cell-to-cell communication, as receptor proteins and ion channels are found in the cell membrane. Omega-3 fatty acids and other polyunsaturated fatty acids are a component of the human diet, are important components of cell membranes, and act as precursors for prostaglandins and eicosanoids (second messengers) in normal cell physiology. The two omega-3 fatty acids most implicated in psychiatric functioning are eicosapentaenoic acid (EPA) (20:5n-3) and its metabolic product docosahexaenoic acid (DHA) (22:6n-3).

Unsaturated fatty acids, especially the omega-3s, are known primarily for their healthy effect on the cardiovascular system and their anti-inflammatory properties (vs the unhealthy saturated fats, which contribute to coronary artery disease, and the omega-6s, which have a pro-inflammatory effect). A fatty acid is "highly unsaturated" or "polyunsaturated" if it contains more than four double bonds in its long chain (ie, at multiple locations, there are double bonds that are not "saturated" with hydrogen atoms). Double bonds result in greater flexibility of the fatty acid, leading to greater cell membrane fluidity and better effects on health. The term "omega-3" is a chemistry term that refers to the position of the first of these double bonds. That is, for omega-3s, the first double bond is located three carbons from the end (or "omega") carbon atom of the molecule.

Our bodies require fuel (from carbohydrates, proteins, and fats, which are rich in energy) and carbon skeletons to construct the materials needed to function. Certain nutrient fuels are considered "essential" if they must be ingested and cannot be constructed from other molecules. Essential nutrients include eight of the 20 amino acids, vitamins (organic molecules), minerals (inorganic molecules), and essential fatty acids. EPA is an essential fatty acid, and our bodies can make DHA from EPA. EPA is a component of the human diet if fish, especially salmon, cod, mackerel, and tuna, is consumed. Our bodies do, in fact, have a process for manufacturing EPA, via another essential fatty acid, alpha linolenic acid (ALA), but it is not very efficient. ALA is fairly common in our diet, found in vegetable sources such as flaxseed, walnuts, and canola oil. Less than 10% of the ALA consumed is converted to EPA and DHA, making supplementation with flaxseed oil a possible but poor way of increasing the body's EPA and DHA stores.

In an influential and intriguing letter to the editor in Lancet, Hibbeln linked fish consumption (rich in omega-3 fatty acids) to worldwide rates of depression.[13] Countries with high fish consumption have the lowest rates of depression, including Japan. The shift in the fatty acid profile of the Western diet is a result of the industrial revolution, with the advent of the vegetable oil industry, the increased use of cereal grains for livestock feed (as opposed to grass grazing cattle), and the reduced consumption of wild plants, animals, and fish.[13–16] Epidemiologic data have linked the national prevalence of depression worldwide, including postpartum depression, as well as bipolar disorder, to reduced dietary intake of omega-3 fatty acids in the form of fish consumption.[13,17]

In addition to the importance of omega-3 levels, the ratio of omega-6 fatty acids to omega-3 acids has been implicated in increasing rates of depression. Although omega-3 is low in our Western diet, omega-6 fatty acids are fairly common in our diet, primarily from vegetable oils and in particular from corn, safflower, and soybean.[18–20] Arachidonic acid is a common omega-6 fatty acid. In the absence of omega-3 fatty acids, our bodies will use omega-6 fatty acids in our cell membranes. These omega-6 fatty acids, due to the configuration of the double bonds, are less flexible than the omega-3 fatty acids and speculatively result in less efficient cell membrane performance. In addition, arachidonic acid plays a central role in the production of inflammatory eicosanoids, and increase in inflammation from the products of the arachidonic acid pathway has been implicated in disease: cardiovascular disease, joint disease, and mental illness.

Various studies have suggested that omega-3 fatty acids may have beneficial effects on health in general by lowering serum lipids, decreasing platelet aggregation, preventing diabetes, and maintaining arterial elasticity.[21–26] As omega-3 fatty acids have been shown to be both protective against coronary heart disease[27] and implicated in mood disorders, a relative deficiency of omega-3 fatty acids may help explain the observed link between heart disease, cardiac mortality, and depression. Converging evidence thus suggests that omega-3 fatty acids may be protective for both heart disease and mood disorder, which has important clinical implications, especially given the increased risk for diabetes associated with the atypical antipsychotics commonly used in the treatment of bipolar disorder and treatment-resistant depression.

Abnormalities in fatty acid composition of phospholipids in cell membranes have been described in psychiatric disorders in general and in bipolar disorder in particular.[18,28–34] These studies use red blood cell (RBC) membranes as a proxy for brain cell membranes. Patients with depression have increased plasma and RBC membrane arachidonic acid (omega-6) to EPA (omega-3) ratios.[35] Another study showed a significant depletion of RBC fatty acids, particularly DHA, in depressed subjects relative to healthy control subjects.[19] Also, greater severity of depression has been associated with lower RBC membrane levels and low dietary intake of omega-3 fatty acids.[19]

The phospholipid hypothesis of mental illness proposes that neurotransmitter receptor functioning is affected by the fatty acid composition of the phospholipids of the cell membrane.[32–34] With reduced omega-3 fatty acids, the fatty acid composition of the cell membrane phospholipids would be altered, possibly leading to altered neurotransmitter binding and psychopathology. Several studies have shown reduced levels of omega-3 fatty acids in the RBC membranes,[29] fibroblasts,[36] and even in the postmortem brain tissue of schizophrenic patients.[37] Other studies demonstrate increased uptake of omega-3 fatty acids into the RBC membranes of treated subjects, raising the question as to whether subjects have a dietary deficiency in omega-3 fatty acids, which can be corrected by supplementation.[38] Another possibility is that some affected individuals are unable to take up omega-3 adequately into cell membranes. No clear guidelines exist on normal blood levels of omega-3 fatty acids, but the increase in blood levels and RBC cell membranes with supplementation argues for the idea that individuals who are depleted can benefit from supplementation.

Clinical trial evidence is mixed as to whether supplementation with the omega-3 fatty acids EPA and/or DHA may play a therapeutic role in the management of mood disorders. There have been a handful of studies, with overall equivocal findings, addressing the use of omega-3 fatty acids for the treatment of bipolar disorder.[28,33,39,40] The first study of omega-3 fatty acids for bipolar disorder was a 4-month, double-blind, placebo-controlled study in which the authors added EPA+DHA, a total of 9.6 g (6.2 and 3.4 g, respectively), to ongoing treatment in 30 adults with bipolar disorder.[28] These authors reported a significantly longer period of remission for those supplemented with omega-3s. Furthermore, these omega-3 supplemented subjects performed better on the Clinical Global Impression (CGI) Scale, Global Assessment Scale (GAS), and Hamilton Depression Scale (HAM-D) than the placebo group (there was no difference in the Young Mania Rating Scale [YMRS]). On the other hand, a discouraging outcome was reported by authors associated with The Stanley Foundation Bipolar Network, which conducted a 4-month, double-blind, randomized controlled study of EPA monotherapy in 116 bipolar adults. This long-term monotherapy large-scale study failed to show efficacy. A dose of 6 g/d of EPA used as monotherapy was compared with placebo for 4 months in the treatment of either acute depression or rapid-cycling illness.[40] The authors note that this dose may have been too large for demonstrating efficacy. Dose-ranging studies in depression and schizophrenia found efficacy at lower dose levels, 1 to 3 g, but not for higher doses. For example, Frangou and colleagues[41] studied 1 g versus 2 g in a 12-week, double-blind, placebo-controlled trial of bipolar I and II depression. These authors report improved clinical outcomes compared with those of placebo on the Hamilton Depression Rating Scale (HDRS) and the CGI, but not on the YMRS, with no difference between the treatment groups. Peet and colleagues[42] studied 1 g, 2 g, and 4 g of EPA in a randomized, double-blind, placebo-controlled trial of depression and found that the 1 g/d group (but not the 2 or 4 g/d group) performed better than placebo on all three depression rating scales used. Also, this study, unlike that of Stoll and colleagues,[29] used EPA only, without DHA. A dose-finding study of DHA in 35 depressed outpatients used three dosing arms with double-blind assessment of 1 g, 2 g, and 4 g DHA per day and found response rates of 83%, 40%, and 0% respectively. Taken together, these studies suggest that omega-3 fatty acids may be most effective in a lower dosing range and that higher doses may be ineffective. Pediatric studies, in particular, could benefit from a study on dosing of omega-3 fatty acids for mood disorders. In the one study in youth with bipolar disorder, effectiveness was noted in individuals receiving 2 g or greater, but doses beyond 2 g were not associated with greater improvement.[43]

In the only study addressing omega-3 fatty acids in pediatric bipolar disorder, a modest improvement in YMRS scores was reported in an 8-week open-label trial for bipolar disorder. Twenty subjects, aged 6 to 17 years, were administered 1290 to 4300 mg combined EPA and DHA. The subjects experienced a statistically significant decrease in the YMRS scores measuring the core symptoms of mania, from a mean score of 28.9 at baseline to an endpoint score of 19.1, with an attendant increase in RBC membrane and plasma EPA and DHA levels. The findings of the one open-label pediatric trial of omega-3 fatty acids showing improvement in manic symptoms should be considered in light of some methodological limitations. Because it was an open study, assessments were not blind to treatment status. These findings await validation via randomized, double-blind controlled clinical trials. Furthermore, the sample was heterogeneous and included subjects meeting criteria for bipolar II disorder and bipolar disorder not otherwise specified and with comorbid attention-deficit/hyperactivity disorder, conduct disorders, and generalized anxiety disorder but in insufficient numbers to make comparisons regarding response or tolerability in these subgroups. Finally, the effect was modest for an open-label trial and indicates that double-blind conditions would result in even lower efficacy rates. However, this modest positive effect, which would be discouraging for a pharmaceutical agent, appears attractive considering the healthful effects of the treatment. Because of the documented efficacy of omega-3 fatty acids in the treatment of adult depression,[42] and since depression is a prominent feature of the mixed presentation of pediatric bipolar disorder, more work is needed to explore the effectiveness of these compounds in the treatment of pediatric bipolar disorder. Negative studies in adults need not rule out the possibility that used in developing brains, and proximal to the onset of the illness, omega-3 fatty acids could play a therapeutic role. Notably, studies supplementing infant formula with omega-3 fatty acids find positive effects on development and cognition.[44]

Because omega-3 fatty acids are part of normal metabolism, the likelihood of unwanted side effects is low. Thus far, the only adverse effects reported with omega-3 fatty acids are the following minor issues. Mild gastrointestinal disturbance (loose stool) can be minimized by taking omega-3 fatty acids with food. A "fishy" taste or fishy burps decrease compliance, but these can be mitigated by taking omega-3 fatty acids with food or switching brands. Decrease in platelet aggregation, although beneficial in the prevention of atherosclerotic plaques, can lead to increase in bleeding time, but no study has suggested that this is a clinically significant adverse effect.

INOSITOL

Inositol is a structural isomer of glucose. *Myo*-inositol comprises 95% of the total free inositol in the human body.[45,46] Inositol is present in numerous foods in low amounts; it is present in higher amounts in beans, grains, nuts, and many fruits.[47] The average adult human consumes about 1 g of inositol in the daily diet.[48,49] Inositol, located primarily within cell membranes, is ubiquitous in biological organisms; it is a precursor to, as well as a product of, the phosphatidylinositol (PI) cycle.[48,49] The PI cycle is the second messenger system for numerous neurotransmitter receptors, including cholinergic muscarinic, alpha 1 noradrenergic, serotonin (5-hydroxytryptamine (5-HT$_{2A}$ and 5-HT$_{2C}$), and dopaminergic D$_1$ receptors. Inositol has been referred to as vitamin B$_8$.

The initial rationale for recent attempts to treat depression by dietary supplementation with inositol came from the finding that inositol was shown to be decreased in the cerebrospinal fluid (CSF) of patients with depression[50] although others did not replicate this finding.[51] Atack and colleagues[52,53] studied CSF inositol in patients treated with inositol for depression. Baseline CSF inositol did not predict response to inositol treatment. Increased levels of the monophosphatase enzyme that breaks down inositol have been reported in patients with depression and schizophrenia. Inositol is also decreased in the frontal cortex of postmortem brains of patients with bipolar disorder and suicide victims compared with that in normal controls.[53,54]

Silverstone and colleagues[55] showed that chronic treatment with either lithium or sodium valproate in bipolar patients may normalize PI cycle functioning. Lithium may exert its clinical mood stabilizing effects due to its actions on the phosphoinositol second messenger system (PI cycle).[55] Berridge and colleagues[56] suggested that lithium acts in bipolar disorder by affecting the enzyme inositol 1-monophosphatase and causing a relative inositol deficiency. A possible excess of inositol in mania suggested its possible deficit in depression. In addition, in animal models of depression, inositol has been shown to reduce depressive behaviors.[48,57] Positive studies of inositol in humans have been reported in the treatment of depression, panic disorder, obsessive-compulsive disorder, and bulimia.[48,58] In Europe, over-the-counter inositol has long been used as a folk remedy for depression.[48,59]

Although scientific evidence suggests that inositol and the PI cycle are affected in depression and impacted by lithium treatment, the mechanism of action of inositol remains unclear. Indirectly from the available evidence, we presume that subjects with mood disorders experience a decrease in brain *myo*-inositol, which adversely affects the functioning of the PI second messenger system, which in turn results in mood changes. Dietary supplement with inositol, therefore, improves the functioning of the PI system, thereby treating the depressive symptoms.[45,46] Lithium may operate conversely by lowering or blocking *myo*-inositol, the so-called inositol depletion hypothesis: that is, lithium produces a lowering of *myo*-inositol in the brain, via inositol monophosphatase, bringing about a mood stabilizing effect.[60,61]

Mood stabilizer medications may be better thought of as producing an action that stabilizes inositol and its actions. Lithium, valproate, and carbamazepine in human astrocyte cells decreased inositol uptake at high inositol concentrations and increased inositol uptake at low inositol concentrations, suggesting a much more complicated mode of action.[53,62–64] Kaya and colleagues[65] found that erythrocyte inositol 1-mono-phosphatase activity was higher in lithium-treated euthymic patients than that in non–lithium-treated patients; increased inositol 1-monophosphatase activity by chronic lithium use suggests paradoxically, over time, an upregulation of the enzyme activity.

In response to the seemingly contradictory findings, Belmaker evolved the inositol polyphosphate signal suppression hypothesis and hypothesized that inositol's effect in the brain was much more complex than simply being a matter of too much or too little.[59] He writes, "Inositol has been shown to regulate the function of the PI cycle in a complex manner. Complex regulation of a cycle can lead to "pendulum" effects where a push from either direction causes an identical effect." Belmaker notes that inositol supplementation with lithium reverses the effects of lithium. On the other hand, inositol supplementation as monotherapy had effects similar to those of lithium. This author writes, "This apparent paradox may hint at a solution to the mystery of how lithium administration benefits both mania and depression." Further, because the PI cycle serves as a second messenger for several balancing and mutually interactive neurotransmitters, Belmaker and colleagues[59] hypothesizes that exogenous inositol could hypothetically alleviate inositol deficiency in one system without increasing inositol above normal levels in another.

Trials with inositol in pediatric bipolar disorder are limited to measuring brain levels and ratios in neurochemical spectroscopic studies of treated and untreated youth; there are no clinical trials examining the efficacy of inositol in the treatment of pediatric bipolar disorder or any pediatric psychiatric condition. Davanzo and colleagues[66] measured changes in *myo*-inositol levels in the anterior cingulate cortex of 11 children (mean age, 11.4 years) diagnosed with bipolar disorder, currently manic, hypomanic, or mixed, before and after lithium therapy (mean serum level, 0.64 mEq/L) and in 11 case-matched controls at baseline and on day 7 using proton magnetic resonance spectroscopy (^{1}H MRS). There was a significant decrease in anterior cingulate *myo*-inositol/creatinine (Cr) ratio following 7 days of lithium therapy in children and adolescents with bipolar disorder. When responders and nonresponders were compared at week 1, *myo*-inositol/Cr was decreased at 1 week versus baseline in the lithium-responder group, but not in the lithium nonresponder group, consistent with[45,46] and contrasting with[67] previous studies. These same authors compared *myo*-inositol levels in the anterior cingulate of 10 youth with bipolar I disorder on various medications (most recent episode, manic or mixed), 10 youth with intermittent explosive disorder, and 13 normal comparison youth using ^{1}H MRS.[68] The patients with bipolar disorder had significantly higher mean anterior cingulate *myo*-inositol and *myo*-inositol/Cr-phosphocreatine measures than those of patients with intermittent explosive disorder and normal comparison subjects. There were no significant differences in levels between youth with intermittent explosive disorder and normal comparison subjects. There was no significant difference in levels between groups in the occipital cortex.

Patel and colleagues[69] reported on an open-label study of 28 inpatient adolescents (12–18 years; mean age, 15.5 years) who met the Diagnostic and Statistical Manual of Mental Disorders, fourth edition (DSM-IV) criteria for diagnosis of bipolar I disorder, were currently depressed, and were given lithium doses adjusted to serum levels of 1.0 to 1.2 mEq/L. *Myo*-inositol concentrations in the medial as well as the left and right lateral prefrontal cortices were measured using ^{1}H MRS scan at baseline, day 7, and day 42 of treatment. Lithium administration did not result in significant changes from baseline in *myo*-inositol concentrations in the medial as well as the left and right lateral prefrontal cortices. Consistent with previous studies,[45,46,70] these authors suggested, based on their findings, that the inositol-depletion hypothesis may not be the mechanism of action of lithium in patients with bipolar depression.

MRS studies have also been completed on adult subjects, some supplemented with inositol. Frey and colleagues[71] studied 22 unmedicated, depressed bipolar and unipolar patients and found reduced *myo*-inositol concentrations in the frontal lobes compared with those in 22 healthy controls, although this finding was significant only when the groups were paired by age (<40 y). Moore and colleagues[45,46] found an initial significant increase in *myo*-inositol/Cr levels in the occipital cortex gray matter and parietal white matter of 17 healthy subjects taking a dietary supplement of 12 g/d *myo*-inositol, but this level returned to baseline by day 8. Moore and colleagues[46] also investigated lithium's effects on in vivo brain *myo*-inositol levels in 12 adults (mean age, 36.6 years) diagnosed with DSM-IV diagnosis of bipolar disorder, most recently depressed. Patients underwent a drug washout period of at least 14 days and then underwent baseline MRS scan before initiation of treatment with lithium. Brain *myo*-inositol levels were measured by ^{1}H MRS after acute (5–7 days) and chronic (3–4 weeks) lithium treatment. In the right frontal lobe, the *myo*-inositol concentrations during both acute and chronic treatment were significantly lower than those at baseline before correction for multiple comparisons, but not after correction. Lowering of *myo*-inositol levels per se did not appear to be associated with therapeutic efficacy. Authors hypothesized that the initial reduction of *myo*-inositol initiates a cascade of secondary changes in the protein kinase C signaling pathway and gene expression in the central nervous system, effects that may ultimately be responsible for lithium's therapeutic efficacy. No significant differences were found in the temporal, occipital, and parietal lobes.

Taken together, these neuroimaging studies suggest that inositol is implicated in the pathophysiology of bipolar disorder, and that treatment with exogenous inositol or with medications that affect brain inositol levels (eg, lithium) results in brain chemistry changes associated with clinical improvement. The conflicting results lend credence to Belmaker's statements highlighting the complexity of the role of inositol.

Double-blind, controlled trials of inositol treatment of depression in adults offer conflicting evidence regarding the use of inositol in clinical practice. Levine and colleagues[72] conducted a 4-week study of 27 adults with DSM-III-R diagnosis of major depression or bipolar disorder who were depressed and had failed antidepressant treatment or had dropped out due to side effects. Subjects were given either inositol 12 g/d or placebo. Treatment with inositol resulted in significantly greater improvement in HDRS score than that for placebo in females (but not in males) with unipolar depression at 4 weeks (no difference at 2 weeks). In a follow-up study,[73] half of the patients who had responded well to inositol relapsed rapidly after inositol discontinuation, whereas none of those who responded to placebo relapsed rapidly after placebo cessation.

Several studies in adults have addressed the utility of inositol as an adjunctive treatment to selective serotonin reuptake inhibitors (SSRIs) or other treatment. Adding inositol to SSRI treatment under double-blind conditions in 27 adults with DSM-IV diagnosis of major depression resulted in no improvement in effect and no side effects.[74] Forty-two depressed adults who were failing a 3- to 4-week trial of SSRI were randomized to receive as an adjunct either inositol 12 g/d or placebo. Inositol was found to have no effect in augmenting the response to SSRI therapy in depression.[75]

Three studies of inositol as an adjunctive treatment in bipolar adults have suggested at best a modest clinical effect of inositol. Twenty-two adults diagnosed with DSM-IV bipolar depression were given either inositol 12 g/d or placebo as add-on treatment to current medication. There was a nonsignificant but encouraging difference between the two groups, with 50% of inositol subjects improving versus 30% of placebo subjects.[76] The authors concluded that a controlled study with an adequate sample size may demonstrate efficacy for inositol in bipolar depression. In another study, 66 bipolar adults, currently depressed, were randomized to receive lamotrigine, risperidone, or inositol (target dose 10–25 mg) added on to regular treatment for 8 weeks.[77] There were no significant between-group differences; however, post hoc analysis suggested that lamotrigine may be superior to inositol and risperidone in improving treatment-resistant bipolar depression, and inositol outperformed risperidone, but not reaching statistical significance. Recovery rate with lamotrigine was 23.8%, that with risperidone 4.6%, and that with inositol 17.4%. A similar study by Evins and colleagues[56] randomized 17 depressed bipolar adults on therapeutic levels of lithium or valproate to receive either inositol 5 to 20 g/d or placebo as adjunctive treatment. Although 44% on inositol versus 0% on placebo met response criteria for symptoms of depression, this finding was not statistically significant.

There is no established recommended daily allowance (RDA) for inositol. Studies of adults have used dosages ranging from 6 to 25 g/d of inositol or *myo*-inositol given in divided doses. One study suggested that 12 g/d of inositol has been shown to raise CSF inositol levels by 70%.[78]

Regarding safety, like many nutraceutical agents, inositol has been found to be generally well tolerated in adult randomized controlled trials. Side effects reported in available studies include mild increases in glucose, flatus, nausea, sleepiness and insomnia, dizziness, and headache. Inositol has been studied as an adjunctive agent, and no drug interactions have been reported to date. There have been case reports of inositol-induced mania.[51]

ST. JOHN'S WORT

St. John's wort (*Hypericum perforatum*), a 5-petal perennial flowering plant that grows in many areas of the world, is one of the most extensively studied of medicinal plants.[79,80] Studied in psychiatric disorders, including depression, seasonal affective disorder, anxiety, obsessive-compulsive disorder, and social phobia, it has been used for depression in Europe for centuries and is approved for treatment of depression in Germany. In fact, St. John's wort products and tricyclic antidepressants (TCAs) have been reported to account for more than 80% of antidepressant use in Germany's children and adolescents.[81]

Although a number of biologically active constituents of St. John's wort have been identified, hypericin and hyperforin have been most often related to St. John's wort's antidepressant effects.[82–85] The exact antidepressant mechanism of action of St. John's wort is not fully understood. It has been reported to modulate neurotransmitter levels and receptors, including serotonin, norepinephrine, and dopamine,[82–84] as well as γ-aminobutyric acid and glutamate amino acid neurotransmitters.[82,84,85] Although there have been reports that St. John's wort inhibits monoamine oxidase (MAO), subsequent investigations have reported only a weak potency as a MAO inhibitor (MAOI) that is not strong enough to significantly contribute to the antidepressant effect of St. John's wort.[80,86] Additional proposed mechanisms of action include modification of inflammatory cytokines, inhibition of cortisol production, modulation of neuronal ionic conductance, elevation of intracellular sodium concentration, and induction of neurogenesis and neuroprotection.[82]

Although many studies (mostly conducted in Europe) have supported the antidepressant effects of St. John's wort, several key adult studies in the United States have been negative.[82,87] Linde and Berner[88] 2005 conducted a meta-analysis of randomized controlled trials in which they investigated 23 trials involving placebo-controlled groups and 13 trials comparing Hypericum extracts with standard antidepressants. They reported that in adults with mild to moderate depression, Hypericum perforatum extracts improved symptoms more than placebo and similarly to standard antidepressants. They reported, however, that pooled analysis of six large, more recent, and more precise trials restricted to patients with major depression showed only minimal benefits of Hypericum extract compared with those of placebo. This meta-analysis found that Hypericum extracts caused fewer adverse effects than older antidepressants and might have caused slightly fewer adverse effects than SSRIs. Since the 2005 meta-analysis, there have been at least six positive studies and at least two large negative studies regarding the antidepressant effect of St. John's wort.

St. John's wort has been studied for treatment of pediatric depression. In 2005, Simeon and colleagues[89] published an 8-week open-label pilot study of 26 adolescents (12 to 17 years old) diagnosed with major depressive disorder who were given St. John's wort 300 mg 3 times daily. Of the 11 patients who completed the study, nine (82%) showed significant clinical improvement at week 8. Statistically significant clinical improvements appeared during the first week and continued to be noted until week 8. Mild and transient side effects were noted and included restlessness, dry mouth, nightmares, confusion, loss of attentiveness, nausea, and fatigue. There were no significant changes in blood tests, urinalysis, weight, blood pressure, and electro-cardiogram. It is worth noting that 15 patients withdrew from the study due to persisting or worsening depression or noncompliance. In 2003, Findling and colleagues[79] published results of an 8-week open-label pilot study of 30 youth (6 to 16 years old) diagnosed with major depressive disorder, at least moderate severity, given St. John's wort 150 to 300 mg three times daily. Twenty-four percent met response criteria at the end of week 4 and 83% at the end of the study. Of the patients who completed 8 weeks, 93% chose to continue their treatment with St. John's wort after their participation in the study ended. The most common side effects were generally mild and transient and included dizziness, increased appetite, and loose stools. No clinically significant changes in weight, vital signs, laboratory parameters, or electrocardiogram were noted. In addition, to investigate the pharmacodynamics of St. John's wort in vivo, fasting predose morning 5-HT levels were obtained at baseline, at week 4, and at the end of the study. End of week 4 or 85-HT levels did not significantly differ from those at baseline. In 2001, Hubner and Tilman[90] reported on a multicenter postmarketing surveillance study. One hundred and one children younger than 12 years of age with symptoms of depression and psychovegetative disturbances were treated for 4 to 6 weeks with St. John's wort 300 to 900 mg/d (one coated tablet containing 300 mg Hypericum perforatum extract was standardized to contain 900 μg hypericin). Compliance, tolerability, and efficacy were assessed every 2 weeks by physicians and parents. Physicians' rating of effectiveness as "good" or "excellent" was 72% after 2 weeks, 97% after 4 weeks, and 100% after 6 weeks, although the amount of missing data also increased with time, with results based on 94% of the initial sample at 2 weeks, 89% at 4 weeks, and 76% at the final assessment. No adverse events were reported. Dropouts were due to achievement of therapeutic goal, inadequate therapeutic effect, difficulty swallowing tablets, and going on holiday.

Doses of 300 to 900 mg/d have been studied in children and 900 to 1800 mg/d in adults. Capsules are generally standardized to contain 0.3% to 0.5% hypericin and/ or 3% to 5% hyperforin per dose. Given that hyperforin and hypericin content can vary between commercially available St. John's wort products, users are encouraged to use the same brand on a regular basis, to help ensure consistency in response.[91]

The most commonly reported side effects of St. John's wort include dry mouth, gastrointestinal symptoms (such as constipation), dizziness/confusion, tiredness/ sedation, urinary frequency, anorgasmia, and swelling.[82,92] In addition, St. John's wort can cause photosensitivity.[93] A review of data from 35 double-blind randomized trials showed that dropout and adverse effect rates in patients receiving hypericum extracts were similar to those with placebo, lower than those with older antidepressants, and slightly lower than those with SSRI.[92]

Caution should be used in patients with personal or family history of bipolar disorder, because St. John's wort has been reported to induce mania[94,95] and worsen anxiety. In addition, St. John's wort has been theorized to cause an increase in thyroid-stimulating hormone (TSH), though a clear link has not been established.[96,97] Finally, in 2008, Karalapillai and Bellomo[98] reported the case of a 16-year-old girl who presented with a seizure due to an overdose of St. John's wort. She reportedly took up to 15 300 μg tablets a day in the 2 weeks leading to her seizure plus an additional 50 tablets just before presentation.

St. John's wort has been shown to significantly induce the activity of the cytochrome P-450 system, mostly CYP3A4 (but also CYP2C9 and CYP1A2) and the drug transporter P-glycoprotein, which may result in diminished clinical effectiveness or increased dosage requirements for substrates.[99–101] In addition, combination with SSRIs, MAOIs, and other antidepressants may result in serotonin syndrome.[82]

S-ADENOSYL-L-METHIONINE

S-Adenosyl-L-Methionine (SAMe) has been routinely prescribed in Europe as treatment for depression since the 1970s and has gained popularity in the United States since its release as an over the-counter dietary supplement in 1999. It is one of the better-studied natural agents used to treat depression.

SAMe is produced in mammals from the essential amino acid L-methionine and adenosine triphosphate (ATP). Adequate concentrations of folate and vitamin B_{12} are required for its production. SAMe is found throughout the human body, although particularly high concentrations have been measured in the liver, adrenal glands, and the pineal gland.[102,103] Concentrations are highest in childhood and decrease with age.[104]

SAMe serves as a crucial intermediate of three major pathways in all biological systems: methylation, transsulfuration, and aminopropylation. These pathways are known to be involved in the synthesis of nucleic acids, proteins, phospholipids, hormones, neurotransmitters, antioxidants, polyamines, catecholamines, and other biogenic amines;[105] it is required for the synthesis of norepinephrine, dopamine, and serotonin.[103]

In 1990, Bottiglieri and colleagues[106] demonstrated that CSF SAMe was significantly lower in severely depressed patients compared with that in neurological control groups and increased significantly following intravenous SAMe 200 mg/d or oral SAMe 1200 mg/d. In 1994, Bell and colleagues[107] conducted a double-blind randomized study comparing oral SAMe 1600 mg/d with oral desipramine 250 mg/d in 26 depressed adults for 4 weeks. Sixty-two percent of the patients treated with SAMe and 50% of the patients treated with desipramine significantly improved. Responders (defined by 50% decrease in their HAM-D score), regardless of type of treatment, showed a significant increase in plasma SAMe concentration with treatment.

Because SAMe takes part in many metabolic pathways, defining the mechanisms of action of SAMe's antidepressant effect is difficult. Possible direct or indirect metabolic or receptor effects on monoamine neurotransmission (eg, norepinephrine, dopamine, and serotonin) or on neuronal membrane structure and function in the brain have been theorized to play a role in SAMe's antidepressant effects.[102,105] In addition, Williams and colleagues[108] discussed the potential role SAMe plays in reversing regional brain volume loss in depressive rat models.

There are a number of studies evaluating the antidepressant effectiveness of SAMe in adults. In 2002, the Agency for Healthcare Research and Quality published a meta-analysis of placebo-controlled SAMe trials for the treatment of depression, osteoarthritis, and liver disease.[109] This meta-analysis noted that the majority of the 28 depression studies they evaluated enrolled small numbers of patients and varied greatly in their quality. The authors determined that, compared with placebo, treatment with SAMe was associated with an improvement of approximately six points in the score of the HDRS measured at 3 weeks. This was a statistically as well as clinically significant, albeit partial, response. When compared with treatment with TCAs, treatment with SAMe was not associated with a statistically significant difference in outcomes (though not all of these trials were adequately powered to discern a difference between SAMe and the tricyclics, some used only low to moderate doses of tricyclics, and a majority involved parenteral formulations of SAMe). Some studies have suggested a faster onset of action for SAMe than for conventional antidepressants and report that it may even accelerate the effect of conventional antidepressants.[103] More recently, Alpert and colleagues[102] conducted a 6-week open trial of 30 adults (23 completed the trial) with major depression to evaluate the safety, tolerability, and efficacy of oral SAMe when used as an adjunct among partial or nonresponders to SSRI antidepressants or venlafaxine. Subjects started with SAMe 400 mg twice a day to augment current treatment and then increased to 800 mg twice a day after 2 weeks. There was a significant decrease in depression severity from baseline to end point. No patient experienced serious adverse events, including serotonin syndrome. There was a significant but modest (4.9%) decrease in pretreatment to post-treatment homocysteine levels. The mean levels of folate, B_{12}, or homocysteine differ between responders and nonresponders.

Very limited data exist on the use of SAMe for treatment of pediatric depression. In 2004, Schaller and colleagues[110] described three case reports of the use of SAMe for pediatric major depression. Case 1 discussed an 11-year-old girl (34 kg) diagnosed with DSM-IV-TR major depression who was placed on 200 mg SAMe enteric-coated tablet each morning for 1 week and then increased to 400 mg every morning. Improvement began 4 days after increasing the dose, with modest improvement over 3 weeks. At 3 weeks, the dose was increased to 600 mg every morning, which resulted in complete resolution of depressive symptoms 2 days after the dose increase. She had no signs of mania or anxiety. Her Children's Depression Inventory (CDI) fell from 34 to 4. She had been on this dose for 6 months at the time of the report without complications and with continued efficacy. Case 2 described an 8-year-old girl (24 kg) with DSM-IV-TR major depression and CDI score of 29 who was treated with 200 mg of SAMe. She started showing improvement by day 2, and was at baseline by day 11. She had increased sadness at 3 months, and the dose was increased to 200 mg twice daily, with resultant decrease of CDI score to six. She had been on this dose for 6 months at the time of the report without complications and with continued efficacy. Case 3 described a 16-year-old boy diagnosed with DSM-IV-TR major depression and oppositional defiant disorder who refused traditional antidepressants but agreed to a trial of SAMe. He was started on 200 mg and the dose increased to 1800 mg/d over 10 days. He experienced slight tremor and anxiety on 1800 mg/d, but after decrease to 1400 mg/d the side effects abated. His mood and function improved to baseline over 1 to 2 weeks, though he continued to have residual oppositional behavior. After 2 to 3 months, he stopped taking SAMe, which resulted in relapse over the next 3 weeks. Restarting a dose of 800 mg every morning and 400 mg every afternoon restored him to baseline in 5 to 8 days.

The recommended adult dose of SAMe ranges from 400 to 1600 mg/d, although some individuals may require doses >3000 mg/d to alleviate depression;[102,103] there is no established dose range for children and adolescents. SAMe is available in capsule and powder form. Enteric-coated formulations have helped address the chemical instability of older formulations.[111,112]

As it is a dietary supplement, SAMe has not undergone the rigorous safety testing required for prescription drugs, and although short-term trials have suggested that SAMe is safe, no long-term data exist.[111] Potential adverse effects include gastrointestinal side effects (primarily flatulence and diarrhea), headache, dizziness, dry mouth, nausea, and cold or flu-like symptoms.[111] In addition, mild nausea, restlessness, and moderate increase in anxiety have been observed in some patients.[107]

SAMe should be avoided in patients with personal or family history of bipolar disorder unless patients are also taking a mood stabilizer, as there are several reports of SAMe-induced mania.[111,113] In addition, Iruela and colleagues[114] published a case report describing altered mentation, fever, hyperreflexia, and elevated Cr phosphokinase when SAMe (100 mg intramuscular) was combined with clomipramine 75 mg in a 71-year-old woman. Similar symptoms suggesting serotonin syndrome have not been described in controlled studies evaluating the efficacy and safety of SAMe administered in conjugation with older antidepressants.[102,112]

SAMe may affect homocysteine, prolactin, and thyroid hormones. Since SAMe is ultimately metabolized to homocysteine, it is theoretically possible that SAMe administration could lead to increased homocysteine levels.[102,111] In contrast, due to SAMe-associated elevations in 5-methyltetrahydrofolate, a cofactor of homocysteine metabolism, SAMe has been postulated to be effective in treating elevated homocysteine.[111] Thomas and colleagues[115] performed a double-blind, placebo-controlled trial in which 20 subjects with depression were given SAMe; they found a highly significant fall in prolactin concentrations in the SAMe-treated group after 14 days of treatment. Fava and colleagues[116] investigated the effects of treatment with SAMe on prolactin and TSH response to thyrotropin-releasing hormone (TRH) stimulation in seven depressed outpatient women (without childbearing potential) and 10 depressed outpatient men in a 6-week open study of oral SAMe (maximum dose, 1600 mg/d). There was a significant reduction after treatment with SAMe in the response of both prolactin and TSH to TRH stimulation in the group of depressed men, but not in the women.

Interactions with other drugs are not well known. Theoretically, SAMe may potentiate the activity and/or toxicities of MAOIs, TCAs, or SSRIs, although this has not been documented.

MELATONIN

Melatonin (N-acetyl-5-methoxytryptamine or 5-Methoxy, N-Acetyltryptamine), a hormone secreted from the pineal gland, is the principal hormone of the circadian system.[117] The amino acid L–tryptophan is converted to serotonin (5-HT) and then eventually to melatonin. Melatonin secretion starts between the third to sixth months of life. It then increases rapidly, with a peak in nocturnal melatonin concentrations between ages 3 to 7 years.[118–120]

In addition to effects on sleep and circadian body rhythm, melatonin has been proposed to affect mood (it has been studied in bipolar disorder, depression, and seasonal affective disorder), regulate the secretion of growth hormone and gonadotropic hormones, and have antioxidant activity. It is currently sold in the United States labeled as a "dietary supplement," though food does not supply meaningful amounts of melatonin.

Rapid-cycling bipolar disorder has been proposed to be associated with unstable circadian rhythms.[121] Patients with bipolar disorder have been reported to have lower baseline levels of melatonin and increased sensitivity to dim light (with dim light causing increased melatonin suppression in bipolar patients compared with that in healthy controls),[122–124] though other reports do not support these data.[125,126]

There is conflicting evidence regarding the efficacy of melatonin in the treatment of adults with bipolar disorder. In 2000, Bersani and Garavini[127] published an open-label trial in which 11 outpatients aged 22 to 43 years diagnosed with bipolar disorder, manic type, who experienced insomnia that did not respond to usual hypnotic therapies were given melatonin 3 mg nightly at 10:30 PM for 30 days. By the end of the treatment, all patients showed a longer sleep duration compared with that at baseline (mean hours of sleep increased from 2.43 ± 0.76 to 5.24 ± 1.51 per night) and a significant decrease in severity of mania (Brief Psychiatric Rating Scale total scores decreased from 22.72 ± 4.45 to 14.09 ± 4.43). In contrast, Leibenluft and colleagues[121] reported a double-blind, placebo-controlled evaluation in which five outpatients diagnosed with rapid-cycling DSM-III-R bipolar disorder were treated with melatonin 10 mg daily at 10:00 PM for 12 weeks (added on to a stable medication regimen). These authors found that administration of melatonin in these patients had no significant effects on mood or sleep. They noted that the administration of exogenous melatonin may have caused partial suppression of endogenous melatonin secretion in two of the patients, and melatonin withdrawal led to marked instability in the sleep–wake cycle of one of the patients. They hypothesized that bipolar patients may be more sensitive than controls to suppressive effects of exogenous melatonin on endogenous melatonin secretion.

Although there are no studies available evaluating the use of melatonin for treatment of pediatric bipolar disorder, Robertson and Tanguay[128] described the clinical course of a 10-year-old boy diagnosed with bipolar disorder who was nonresponsive to combinations of lithium (levels up to 1.5 mEq/L), thioridazine up to 80 mg/d, and valproic acid up to 750 mg/d. Although this child did respond to a combination of lithium and carbamazepine, he developed an adverse reaction that required discontinuation of carbamazepine. He required numerous inpatient psychiatric hospitalizations due to manic symptoms and aggression. His insomnia and manic episodes responded rapidly to a trial of melatonin 3 mg nightly, with recurrence of symptoms when efforts to stop the melatonin were made 1 month after starting it. Subsequent recurrence of symptoms responded to a dose increase to 9 mg/d and then to 12 mg/d augmented by alprazolam 0.375 mg/d. At the time of the publication of the study, the boy had been stable for 15 months without recurrence of full-blown manic episodes on melatonin 12 mg/d plus alprazolam 0.375 mg/d.

There is no established dose range for melatonin in the treatment of bipolar disorder. Usual doses of melatonin range from 0.1 to 5 mg/d, though staying in the range of 0.1 to 0.3 mg/d has been recommended.[118] Dose ranges are separated by "physiological" and "pharmacological" doses; dose timing is determined by whether melatonin is used for circadian regulation or for acute sleep-promoting effects.

Typical physiological nocturnal peak serum concentrations of melatonin are around 60 to 200 pg/mL, whereas daytime levels are as low as 3 to 10 pg/mL. Taking 0.1 to 0.3 mg of oral melatonin typically induces physiological serum melatonin levels.[117,118] Ingestion of 10 mg of melatonin can result in a 1000-fold increase in plasma melatonin level when compared with peak melatonin levels normally occurring at night in a young healthy adult.[117] Physiological doses of melatonin have been reported not to cause substantial changes in sleep architecture, though this is not the case with doses greater than 5 mg/d.[117]

The circadian effect largely depends on the time of melatonin administration and can produce opposite effects: morning administration may delay the onset of evening sleepiness by delaying the phase of the circadian rhythms, whereas evening ingestion can advance the circadian rhythms and sleep onset.[117] Rather than producing a rapid increase in subjective sleepiness or drowsiness, at physiological doses, melatonin has been reported to induce a behavioral state that resembles quiet wakefulness, which usually enables sleep initiation; it leads to minimal alterations in performance ability. Therefore, sleep results if the environmental conditions are appropriate for sleep, and an individual can override melatonin's effects on promoting sleep with stimuli such as turning lights on or sitting.[117]

Melatonin is generally well tolerated. The most common side effects that have been noted include drowsiness, headache, dizziness, and nausea.[129,130] Additional reported side effects include transient depressive symptoms, mild tremor, mild anxiety, abdominal cramps, irritability, reduced alertness, confusion, vomiting, and hypotension.[131]

Long-term clinical and experimental studies are needed to address questions regarding adverse effects of melatonin. Concerns have been raised that taking pharmacological doses of melatonin could induce a circadian rhythm disorder by disrupting the body's natural circadian body rhythms.[118,121] There is some evidence to suggest that altered melatonin levels may lead to disorders of prolactin and the hypothalamic-pituitary-gonadal axis (delayed puberty, precocious puberty, hypothalamic amenorrhea).[120,132] In light of this possibility, melatonin should be used with caution in developing children. In addition, exacerbation of seizure disorder during melatonin treatment in three neurologically disabled patients has been reported.[133]

Melatonin inactivation occurs in the liver by the P450-dependent microsomal mixed-function oxidase enzyme system. Thus, medication affecting this pathway could influence the metabolism of melatonin. In addition, data exist suggesting that melatonin may inhibit the CYP1A2 and CYP2C9 isoenzymes, theoretically affecting medications metabolized through these pathways (including theophylline, caffeine, clozapine, haloperidol, tacrine, nonsteroidal anti-inflammatory drugs, phenytoin, warfarin, and zafirlukast). Since production of melatonin depends on serotonin as a precursor and on increased noradrenergic innervation of the pineal gland at nighttime, psychotropic medications that affect serotonin or norepinephrine levels may affect the production of melatonin.[118]

LECITHIN

Lecithin has been examined for its possible role in the treatment of many neurological disorders, including mania, memory impairment, tardive dyskinesia, Gilles de la Tourette syndrome, Friedreich's ataxia, levodopa-induced dyskinesia, Huntington's disease, Alzheimer's disease, spastic spinocerebellar degeneration, and myasthenic syndromes.[134] Discovered by French scientist Maurice Gobley in 1805, lecithin is a naturally occurring phospholipid that acts as an emulsifier and is often used as an emulsification agent in processed foods. It is found in several foods, including egg yolks, soybeans, nuts, and whole grains, as well as in organ meats. Dietary lecithin intake varies, but, generally, it ranges from 1 to 5 g/d.[134] It has been theorized that low-fat and low-cholesterol diets may lower the amount of lecithin consumed, thus creating a deficit.[135]

Commercially available lecithin is a complex mixture of phosphatidyl esters, mainly phosphatidylcholine, phosphatidylethanolamine, phosphatidylserine, and phosphatidylinositol.[134] Phosphatidylcholine is an important structural component of cellular membranes. Choline is the precursor of the neurotransmitter acetylcholine. Underactivity of central cholinergic mechanisms has been hypothesized as an underlying feature in a number of neuropsychiatric disorders, including mania.[136,137] Neuroimaging studies have demonstrated altered membrane phospholipid metabolism in the frontal lobes and basal ganglia of patients with bipolar disorder; Cecil and colleagues[138] have reported lowered choline levels within the orbital frontal gray matter in adolescents and young adults with bipolar disorder, manic phase, found on MRS. The effect of lecithin taken orally has been noted to be considerably greater and more prolonged than that of ingestion of an equivalent amount of choline chloride.[139] In addition to its role in increasing acetylcholine, exposure to lecithin has been noted to cause changes in neurotransmitter receptor availability in cell membranes.[140]

In 1979 Cohen and colleagues[141] reported an open trial they conducted at a private psychiatric hospital in which eight newly admitted adults with manic-depressive illness, manic phase, were treated with lithium and/or neuroleptics plus either Lethicon (51%–55% pure lecithin) or Phospholipon 100 (>90% pure lecithin). Subjects received a dose of 15 g/d of lecithin in the first week and 30 g/d of lecithin in the second week. Manic subjects were found to be intolerant of 15 g/d of lecithin in the 50% pure form but were reported to be tolerant of as much as 30 g/d in the 90% pure form. All subjects who received Phospholipon 100 improved rapidly, and three of four showed some worsening following its withdrawal. Three years later, Cohen and colleagues[140] reported another study in which they looked at augmentation with lecithin in a double-blind, placebo-controlled trial of six adult psychiatric inpatients with DSM-III diagnosis of bipolar disorder, manic phase (except one patient with schizoaffective disorder). All patients had been on a stable medication regimen for 1 month before the study and remained on that regimen throughout the course of the study. Patients were given either 10 mg three times daily of >90% pure lecithin or placebo. Lecithin resulted in significant improvement compared with placebo and was noted to have a clear therapeutic effect in five of six patients studied. Lecithin did not lead to the appearance of depressive symptoms in any of the patients studied.

While there have been no similar trials in children and adolescents, in 1981 Schreier[142] reported the case of a 13-year-old manic girl who did not respond to neuroleptics or lithium but appeared to respond to 15 to 23 g/d of 90% pure lecithin monotherapy with a remission lasting at least 13 months.

Because lecithin is not considered an essential nutrient, no RDA has been set. Doses of 1 to 45 g/d of lecithin have been used for various conditions.[134] Commercially available lecithin is usually derived from soy and is available in capsule, liquid, and granule form. Most supplements sold in health food stores have been shown to contain only low levels of pure lecithin.[136]

As it is a dietary supplement, lecithin has not undergone the rigorous safety testing required for prescription drugs, though generally lecithin has been regarded as safe for most adults, except in those highly allergic to soy. High intakes of lecithin (>25 g/d) or choline have been reported to cause acute gastrointestinal distress, sweating, salivation, and anorexia.[134]

Caution must be used with lecithin, as it is possible that some patients may become depressed with increased cholinergic activity. Concerns regarding the development of supersensitivity of dopamine receptors and disturbance of the cholinergic-dopaminergic-serotonergic balance with prolonged, repeated intakes of large amounts of lecithin have also been raised.[134,136] Drug interactions with lecithin have not been well documented.

ACUPUNCTURE

One of the oldest medical procedures in the world, acupuncture has long been used for disorders including depression, anxiety, stress, and insomnia in China, Japan, and Korea.[143] Acupuncture is a family of procedures involving the stimulation of anatomical points on the body through a variety of styles and techniques. Common styles include traditional Chinese, Japanese, Korean, Vietnamese, and French acupuncture, as well as specialized forms such as hand, auricular, and scalp acupuncture. Common techniques include the insertion of ultrafine needles as well as the use of manual pressure, electrical stimulation, magnets, low-power lasers, heat, and ultrasound to stimulate acupoints.[144] Each school of acupuncture (eg, Chinese, Japanese, Korean, Indian) has its own approach to diagnosis and allocation of acupoints.[145] Acupuncture gained popularity in the United States in 1971, when New York Times reporter James Reston wrote about his experience with acupuncture to ease his postsurgical pain; it is now one of the most popular complementary therapies in the West.[143]

Acupuncture is based on the Traditional Chinese Medicine (TCM) concept that disease results from the disruption in the flow of energy, Qi (pronounced *chee*), along a series of points that connect bodily organs, *meridians*. Disease is thought to result when there is disharmony or imbalance in the body's energy system. By using acupuncture at certain points on the body that connect with meridians, Qi can be unblocked, thus restoring flow and balance. There are at least 2000 acupuncture points on the body.[143,145,146]

The exact mechanism of action of acupuncture is unknown, though its effect has been proposed to be due to the stimulation of afferent nerve fibers that transmit impulses to various parts of the central nervous system and induce release of neurotransmitters and peptides, including serotonin, norepinephrine, dopamine, substance P, β-endorphin, enkephalin, and dynorphins.[143,145] Additional proposed mechanisms of action include effects on the autonomic nervous system, the immune system, cytokines, and hormones.[144]

In their recent (2008) book chapter discussing acupuncture for the treatment of psychiatric disorders, Yeung and colleagues[147] refer to 3 reports on adults that address the use of acupuncture to treat bipolar disorder, though they noted that two were case reports that were published in Chinese journals and were not available in English.[148,149] The third report evaluated TCM acupuncture with manual stimulation (SPEC) against an active nonspecific acupuncture control (NSPEC) and against medication alone in 26 bipolar patients with depression refractory to treatment. Although augmentation of medication with acupuncture (SPEC and NSPEC) yielded significant improvement over medication alone in the primary outcome measures, including the Inventory of Depressive Symptomatology and the Global Assessment of Functioning, there were no significant differences among the acupuncture groups.[150]

A limited literature exists on the role of acupuncture in the treatment of adult depression. Because of the heterogeneity of acupuncture treatments, conducting randomized trials is difficult. Wang and colleagues[143] conducted a meta-analysis of 8 randomized clinical trials that compared acupuncture with sham acupuncture in adults with depression. Although this meta-analysis supported acupuncture as an effective treatment that could significantly reduce the severity of major depression and depressive neurosis in adults, they suggested that the results be read with caution due to the high heterogeneity of the studies and many limitations. Also in 2008, Samuels and colleagues[145] published a review that summarized clinical trials addressing acupuncture treatment of depression, anxiety, schizophrenia, and substance abuse and concluded that due to poor design and limited number of studies, there is insufficient evidence that acupuncture is effective for the treatment of depression. This agreed with a previous report by Leo and Ligot[151] in which they reviewed available randomized controlled trials dealing with acupuncture in treating depression. Further evaluation of the role of acupuncture in treating depression, therefore, is warranted.

There are no child and adolescent studies evaluating the use of acupuncture for the treatment of bipolar disorder or depression, although in our clinical experience, some parents have turned to acupuncture for this indication. In response to concerns that children and adolescents may not tolerate acupuncture due to fear of needles, Kemper and colleagues[152] published a retrospective study in which they spoke with 47 children and adolescents (or their parents) who received acupuncture after referral from the Pain Treatment Service. Most families found acupuncture to be a positive, pleasant, and relaxing experience (67% compared with 13% who found it negative/unpleasant/scary and 20% who found it other/neutral/strange); although some patients began with anxiety about the needles, many developed more positive perceptions over the course of treatment.

Acupuncture appears to be safe when provided by qualified acupuncturists. In 2001, Ernst and Adrian[153] published a systematic review of nine studies that evaluated the safety of nearly a quarter of a million acupuncture treatments. They found the most common adverse events to be needle pain (range, 0.2%–59% across studies), tiredness (2.3%–41%), bleeding (0.03%–38%), feeling faint (0.02%–7%), and nausea (0.01%–0.2%). Serious side effects were rare but included two cases of pneumothorax and two cases of needle fracture requiring surgical removal of the fragment (0.001% for both). Few of the studies in their review commented on loss to follow-up; thus long-term complications, such as nerve injury, may have been underestimated. In a subsequent prospective investigation of adverse effects of acupuncture in 97,733 patients (more than 760,000 acupuncture sessions) administered by 7050 German physicians with at least 140 hours of formal acupuncture training, a total of five potentially serious adverse effects were noted in six patients: pneumothorax in two patients (both recovered), exacerbation of depression, acute hypertensive crisis, vasovagal reaction, and acute asthma attack with angina and hypertension.[154]

Complications of acupuncture treatment can arise from inadequate sterilization of needles and improper delivery of treatments.[143] In the United States, acupuncturists should be certified by the National Certification Commission for Acupuncture and Oriental Medicine (NCCAOM) or the American Board of Medical Acupuncture (ABMA). The US Food and Drug Administration (FDA) regulates acupuncture needles for use by licensed practitioners.

Local contraindications to acupuncture include active infection or malignancy at insertion sites.[155] No drug interactions have been reported. Some insurance carriers will cover acupuncture.

ADDITIONAL INTERVENTIONS TO CONSIDER

There has been special interest in the role of exercise, massage, diet, and nutrients to address mood symptoms.[156] Although there are limited data in adult patients and minimal (if any) data in pediatric bipolar patients supporting the use of these interventions, given the low risk associated with their use, they warrant consideration for use as complementary/augmentation treatments.

Exercise has not been extensively studied in pediatric bipolar disorder, though improvements in cardiorespiratory fitness have been reported to have positive effects on depression, anxiety, mood status, and self-esteem in children and adolescents.[157] Although there are data supporting exercise as an effective intervention for depression,[158] other reports are less conclusive, largely due to the limitations of the available studies.[159] Bipolar patients have been reported to be more likely to engage in poor exercise habits and suboptimal eating behaviors compared with individuals without serious mental illness[160] and should be encouraged to pay attention to this aspect of their health. In 2005, Dunn and colleagues[161] published data of their DOSE trial in which 80 adults diagnosed with mild to moderate depression were randomized into one of five groups: total weekly energy expenditure of 7 kcal/kg/wk (low dose) for 3 days or 5 days a week, total weekly energy expenditure of 17.5 kcal/kg/wk (consensus public health recommended dose) for 3 days or 5 days a week, or placebo (3 d/wk of stretching flexibility exercise for 15 to 20 minutes per session) to determine not only whether or not exercise was effective for treatment of depression but also whether energy expenditure or frequency of exercise had an impact on the efficacy. They found that exercise at the public health dose (17.5 kcal/kg/wk) was significantly more effective than low dose and placebo, which both showed nonsignificant improvements in symptoms. There was no difference between exercising 3 d/wk versus 5 d/wk in improvement of depressive symptoms, suggesting that energy expenditure was the determining factor in the reduction of depressive symptoms.

While there are some data supporting the possible use of relaxation and massage to benefit depression and anxiety symptoms in children and adolescents,[162–165] two recent reviews of available randomized controlled trials did not support a significantly positive effect of massage therapy on pediatric depression.[166] Similar to exercise, however, given the low risk associated with massage therapy, it warrants consideration to target symptoms such as anxiety and tension that often occur in patients with bipolar disorder.

The role of vitamins and minerals in healthy mood has also been evaluated, although available data, especially in the pediatric population, are limited. In 2007, Kaplan and colleagues[167] reviewed available data, both correlational (eg, deficiency of a specific nutrient has been found in patients with depression) and investigational (eg, taking a specific nutritional supplement has been shown to improve depressive symptoms), for vitamins, including B, D, and E, and minerals, including calcium, iron, chromium, magnesium, zinc, and selenium (Vitamin C has also been linked to mood disorders).[168] B vitamins of particular interest included vitamins B_9 (folate), B_6 (pyridoxine), and B_1 (thiamine), all of which had some data to support their role in treatment of depression, as well as B_{12} (cobalamin), the repletion of which has been reported to treat vitamin-induced depressive and manic symptoms.[169] They also described evidence linking folate deficiency with poor response to treatment with traditional antidepressants.

Deficiencies of several minerals, including calcium, chromium, iron, magnesium, selenium, and zinc, have also been evaluated for their potential roles in affective symptoms in adults: calcium in depression,[167] chromium to treat rapid-cycling bipolar disorder (depressive episode),[170] magnesium augmentation in the treatment of mania,[171,172] and zinc to address depressive symptoms.[173] In addition, the amino acids tryptophan (precursor of serotonin),[174] tyrosine (converted to dopamine and norepinephrine), phenylalanine (precursor of tyrosine),[175] and methionine (combined with ATP to produce SAMe) have been reported to be helpful in treating mood disorders in adults.[173]

Table 1
Summary of complementary and alternative treatments for pediatric bipolar disorder and depression

Treatment	Child Studies for PBD	Proposed Mechanisms of Action	Most Common Side Effects	Precautions	Common Natural Sources
Acupuncture	None available	Unblocks the flow of *Qi*; stimulates afferent Group III nerve fibers that induce release of serotonin, norepinephrine, substance P, dopamine, β-endorphin, enkephalin, and dynorphins	Needle pain, tiredness, bleeding, feeling faint, and nausea	Acupuncturists should be certified by NCCAOM or ABMA	N/A
Inositol	Three neurochemical spectroscopic studies; no clinical trials	Serves as a precursor for, as well as a product of, the PI cycle, which is the second messenger system for neurotransmitter receptors including cholinergic, alpha 1 noradrenergic, serotonergic, and dopaminergic receptors	Mild increases in glucose, flatus, nausea, sleepiness and insomnia, dizziness, and headache	May induce mania	Beans, grains, nuts, and many fruits (especially cantaloupe and melons)
Lecithin	Case report of 13-year-old girl with mania who responded to 15–23 mg of 90% pure lecithin monotherapy	Increases acetylcholine, causes changes in neurotransmitter receptor availability in cell membranes	Gastrointestinal symptoms, sweating, salivation, and anorexia	May cause depression	Egg yolks, soybeans, nuts, whole grains, organ meats
Melatonin	Case report of 9-year-old boy with bipolar disorder responsive to melatonin 9–12 mg/d	Stabilizes possible circadian rhythm abnormalities	Drowsiness, headache, dizziness, and nausea	Withdrawal could induce circadian rhythm disorder; pharmacological doses could result in delayed puberty	Produced by the pineal gland

	Evidence	Mechanism	Side effects	Cautions	Source
Omega-3 fatty acid	Two positive studies: 1 open-label trial and 1 RCT	Increased cell membrane fluidity (affecting neurotransmitter receptors and ion channels), inflammatory mediator, inhibition of signal transduction	Mild gastrointestinal disturbance (loose stool), minimized by taking with food; "fishy" taste or fishy burps	Generally found to be safe	Oily fish, including salmon, herring, mackerel, and tuna; flaxseed oil; grass-fed beef; some eggs
SAMe	Case reports of 2 children and 1 adolescent with major depression responsive to SAMe 400–1800 mg/d	Possible metabolic or receptor effects on monoamine neurotransmission (eg, norepinephrine, dopamine, and serotonin) or on neuronal membrane structure and function in the brain	Gastrointestinal side effects, headache, dizziness, dry mouth, nausea, cold or flu-like symptoms, restlessness, and moderate increase in anxiety	May induce mania. May also affect homocysteine, prolactin, and thyroid hormone levels. Theoretically, may potentiate the activity and/or toxicities of MAOIs, tricyclic antidepressants, or SSRIs	Produced in mammals from the essential amino acid L-methionine and ATP; production requires vitamin B_{12} and folate
St. John's wort	Three positive open-label studies of St. John's wort 300–900 mg/d in pediatric depression	Modulation of neurotransmitter levels including serotonin, norepinephrine, and dopamine; induction of neurogenesis	Dry mouth, gastro intestinal symptoms, dizziness/confusion, tiredness/sedation, photosensitivity, urinary frequency, anorgasmia, and swelling	May induce mania, inducer of CYP450 system (especially 3A4), combinations with SSRIs, MAOIs, and other antidepressants may result in serotonin syndrome	Hypericum perforatum, a 5-petal perennial flowering plant

Abbreviations: ABMA, American Board of Medical Acupuncture; CYP450, Cytochrome P450; MAOIs, Monoamine oxidase inhibitors; N/A, not applicable; NCCAOM, National Certification Commission for Acupuncture and Oriental Medicine; PBD, Pediatric bipolar disorder; PI, Phosphatidylinositol; RCT, Randomized controlled trial; SAMe, S-Adenosyl-L-Methionine; SSRIs, Selective serotonin reuptake inhibitors.

In 2004, Kaplan and colleagues[176] published an open-label case series of 11 children and adolescents aged 8 to 15 years diagnosed with anxiety and mood or behavioral disorder who were given a supplement called E. M. Power Plus, which consisted of 36 minerals, vitamins, amino acids, and antioxidants in quantities that are higher than a person's usual level of daily dietary intake (eight capsules taken four times a day with food). The nine patients who completed the study demonstrated significant improvement on seven of the eight Child Behavior Checklist scales, the Youth Outcome Questionnaire, and the YMRS. Although more data are necessary regarding safety and efficacy before recommending this product, this study did provide evidence of the possible role of nutrients in stabilizing mood in children and adolescents. Despite the limited pediatric data for the role of vitamins, minerals, and amino acids in treating mood disorders, given the likely benefits and low risk associated with a balanced diet and proper nutrition, attention to nutritional intake should be considered to be a part of the treatment regimen.

SUMMARY

The high levels of morbidity and functional impairment caused by pediatric bipolar disorder often lead to a need for aggressive interventions. In light of moderate efficacy, difficult side effect profiles, unclear long-term effects, and a relatively high dropout/noncompliance rate associated with conventional mood stabilizing medications, parents and clinicians are forced to weigh benefits versus risks when considering treatments. With the perceived high risk associated with conventional treatments as well as the allure of using "natural remedies," there has been growing interest in complementary and alternative treatments. There are very limited data, however, regarding the safety and efficacy of complementary and alternative treatments in children and adolescents with bipolar disorder. It is important to note that the FDA regulates supplements as foods rather than drugs. As a result, safety and efficacy studies are not required before marketing of the supplement (but they will be pulled from the shelves if found to be unsafe postmarketing). Although historically there has also been concern about the content and purity of the products, in 2007, the FDA established regulations that set stringent standards on the quality and manufacturing of dietary supplements.[131]

This article covered select complementary and alternative treatments that have been considered for use in pediatric bipolar disorder and/or depression. Although several of the treatments have been shown to be safe and well tolerated as short-term treatment, long-term data are lacking. In light of limited data, as with conventional treatments of pediatric bipolar disorder, parents and clinicians should weigh risks and benefits when considering the use of complementary and alternative treatments. With the low risk associated with interventions such as exercise, balanced diet, massage, acupuncture, and omega-3 fatty acids (1–3 g/d), these interventions seem reasonable to use as augmentation despite limited (if any) data to support their efficacy in the treatment of pediatric bipolar disorder. On the other hand, interventions such as melatonin, inositol, and lecithin/choline require more evidence to support their use.

Dose ranges of the treatments can be extrapolated from a limited number of child studies and case reports, as most of the treatments do not have clear recommended doses in the pediatric patient population. As with conventional treatments, mechanisms of antidepressant or antimanic action in complementary treatments have been theorized but remain to be fully elucidated (**Table 1**). Given that drug interactions and long-term effects are not completely known for many of the treatments, use with conventional medications should be monitored closely. Across the board, more research is necessary and warranted regarding the long-term safety and efficacy of available complementary and alternative treatments for the management of pediatric bipolar disorder.

FURTHER READINGS

National Center for complementary and alternative Medicine. Available at: http://nccam.nih.gov/health.

American Academy of Pediatrics, Section on Complementary and Integrative Medicine. Available at: http://www.aap.org/sections/chim/.

Natural Medicines Comprehensive Database. Available at: www.NaturalDatabase.com.

REFERENCES

1. Biederman J, Mick E, Bostic J, et al. The naturalistic course of pharmacologic treatment of children with maniclike symptoms: a systematic chart review. J Clin Psychiatry 1998;59(11):628–37, quiz 638.
2. Kowatch RA, Suppes T, Carmody TJ, et al. Effect size of lithium, divalproex sodium, and carbamazepine in children and adolescents with bipolar disorder. J Am Acad Child Adolesc Psychiatry 2000;39(6):713–20.
3. Geller B, Cooper T, Zmermn B, et al. Lithium for prepubertal depressed children with family history predictors of future bipolarity: a double-blind, placebo-controlled study. J Affect Disord 1998;51(2):165–75.
4. Wagner KD. Management of bipolar disorder in children and adolescents. Psychopharmacol Bull 2002;36(4):151–9.
5. Frazier JA, Biederman J, Tohen M, et al. A prospective open-label treatment trial of olanzapine monotherapy in children and adolescents with bipolar disorder. J Child Adolesc Psychopharmacol 2001;11(3):239–50.
6. Frazier JA, Meyer MC, Biederman J, et al. Risperidone treatment for juvenile bipolar disorder: a retrospective chart review. J Am Acad Child Adolesc Psychiatry 1999;38(8):960–5.
7. Delbello MP, Schwiers ML, Rosenberg HL, et al. A double-blind, randomized, placebo-controlled study of quetiapine as adjunctive treatment for adolescent mania. J Am Acad Child Adolesc Psychiatry 2002;41(10):1216–23.
8. Biederman J. Comparative efficacy of atypical antipsychotics for pediatric bipolar disorder. In 158th Annual Meeting of the American Psychiatric Association. Atlanta (GA): American Psychiatric Association; May 21–26, 2005.
9. Findling RL, McNamara NK, Gracious BL, et al. Combination lithium and divalproex sodium in pediatric bipolarity. J Am Acad Child Adolesc Psychiatry 2003;42(8):895–901.
10. Findling RL, McNamara NK, Stansbrey R, et al. Combination lithium and divalproex sodium in pediatric bipolar symptom re-stabilization. J Am Acad Child Adolesc Psychiatry 2006;45(2):142–8.
11. Findling RL, McNamara NK, Youngstrom EA, et al. Double-blind 18-month trial of lithium versus divalproex maintenance treatment in pediatric bipolar disorder. J Am Acad Child Adolesc Psychiatry 2005;44(5):409–17.
12. Kowatch RA, Fristad M, Birmaher B, et al. Treatment guidelines for children and adolescents with bipolar disorder. J Am Acad Child Adolesc Psychiatry 2005; 44(3):213–35.
13. Hibbeln JR. Fish consumption and major depression. Lancet 1998;351(9110):1213.

14. Kris-Etherton PM, Taylor DS, Yu-Poth S, et al. Polyunsaturated fatty acids in the food chain in the United States. Am J Clin Nutr 2000;71:179S–88S.
15. Simopoulos AP. Evolutionary aspects of omega-3 fatty acids in the food supply. Prostaglandins Leukot Essent Fatty Acids 1999;60(6):421–9.
16. Tanskanen A, Hibbeln JR, Tuomilehto J, et al. Fish consumption and depressive symptoms in the general population in Finland. Psychiatr Serv 2001;52:529–31.
17. Noaghiul S, Hibbeln JR. Cross-national comparisons of seafood consumption and rates of bipolar disorders. Am J Psychiatry 2003;160(12):2222–7.
18. Peet M, Murphy B, Shay J, et al. Depletion of omega-3 fatty acid levels in red blood cell membranes of depressive patients. Biol Psychiatry 1998;43(5):315–9.
19. Edwards R, Peet M, Shay J, et al. Omega-3 polyunsaturated fatty acid levels in the diet and in red blood cell membranes of depressed patients. J Affect Disord 1998;48(2–3):149–55.
20. Maes M, Smith R, Christophe A, et al. Fatty acid composition in major depression: decreased omega 3 fractions in cholesteryl esters and increased C20: 4 omega 6/C20:5 omega 3 ratio in cholesteryl esters and phospholipids. J Affect Disord 1996; 38(1):35–46.
21. Hansen JB, Grimsgaard S, Nilsen H, et al. Effects of highly purified eicosapentaenoic acid and docosahexaenoic acid on fatty acid absorption, incorporation into serum phospholipids and postprandial triglyceridemia. Lipids 1998;33(2): 131–8.
22. Sato M, Katsuki Y, Fukuhara K, et al. Effects of highly purified ethyl all-cis-5,8,11,14,17-icosapentaenoate (EPA-E) on rabbit platelets. Biol Pharm Bull 1993;16(4):362–7.
23. Terano T, Hirai A, Hamazaki T, et al. Effect of oral administration of highly purified eicosapentaenoic acid on platelet function, blood viscosity and red cell deformability in healthy human subjects. Atherosclerosis 1983;46(3):321–31.
24. Nobukata H, Ishikawa T, Obata M, et al. Long-term administration of highly purified eicosapentaenoic acid ethyl ester prevents diabetes and abnormalities of blood coagulation in male WBN/Kob rats. Metamedicine 2000;49(7):912–9.
25. von Schacky C, Weber PC. Metabolism and effects on platelet function of the purified eicosapentaenoic and docosahexaenoic acids in humans. J Clin Invest 1985;76(6):2446–50.
26. von Schacky C, Angerer P, Kothny W, et al. The effect of dietary omega-3 fatty acids on coronary atherosclerosis. A randomized, double-blind, placebo-controlled trial. Ann Intern Med 1999;130(7):554–62.
27. Harper CR, Jacobson TA. The fats of life: the role of omega-3 fatty acids in the prevention of coronary heart disease. Arch Intern Med 2001;161(18):2185–92.
28. Stoll A, Severus E, Freeman M, et al. Omega 3 fatty acids in bipolar disorder. Arch Gen Psychiatry 1999;56:407–12.
29. Peet M, Laugharne J, Rangarajan N, et al. Depleted red cell membrane essential fatty acids in drug-treated schizophrenic patients. J Psychiatr Res 1995;29(3): 227–32.
30. Peet M, Brind J, Ramchand CN, et al. Two double-blind placebo-controlled pilot studies of eicosapentaenoic acid in the treatment of schizophrenia. Schizophr Res 2001;49(3):243–51.
31. Horrobin DF, Glen AI, Vaddadi K. The membrane hypothesis of schizophrenia. Schizophr Res 1994;13(3):195–207.
32. Horrobin DF. The membrane phospholipid hypothesis as a biochemical basis for the neurodevelopmental concept of schizophrenia. Schizophr Res 1998;30(3): 193–208.

33. Horrobin DF, Bennett CN. Depression and bipolar disorder: relationships to impaired fatty acid and phospholipid metabolism and to diabetes, cardiovascular disease, immunological abnormalities, cancer, ageing and osteoporosis. Possible candidate genes. Prostaglandins Leukot Essent Fatty Acids 1999; 60(4):217–34.

34. Horrobin DF, Bennett CN. The membrane phospholipid concept of schizophrenia. In: Hafner H, Gattaz WF, Janzarik W, editors. Search for the causes of schizophrenia. Berlin; New York: Springer Verlag; 1999. p. 1–17.

35. Adams PB, Lawson S, Sanigorski A, et al. Arachidonic acid to eicosapentaenoic acid ratio in blood correlates positively with clinical symptoms of depression. Lipids 1996;31(Suppl):S157–61.

36. Mahadik SP, Mukherjee S, Correnti EE, et al. Plasma membrane phospholipid and cholesterol distribution of skin fibroblasts from drug-naive patients at the onset of psychosis. Schizophr Res 1994;13(3):239–47.

37. Yao JK, Leonard S, Reddy RD. Membrane phospholipid abnormalities in post-mortem brains from schizophrenic patients. Schizophr Res 2000;42(1):7–17.

38. Prisco D, Filippini M, Francalanci I, et al. Effect of n-3 polyunsaturated fatty acid intake on phospholipid fatty acid composition in plasma and erythrocytes. Am J Clin Nutr 1996;63(6):925–32.

39. Kupka R, Nolen L, Altshuler L, et al. The Stanley Foundation Bipolar Network. 2. Preliminary summary of demographics, course of illness and response to novel treatments. Br J Psychiatry Suppl 2001;41:s177–83.

40. Post RM, Leverich GS, Nolen WA, et al. A re-evaluation of the role of antidepressants in the treatment of bipolar depression: data from the Stanley Foundation Bipolar Network. Bipolar Disord 2003;5(6):396–406.

41. Frangou S, Lewis M, McCrone P. Efficacy of ethyl-eicosapentaenoic acid in bipolar depression: randomised double-blind placebo-controlled study. Br J Psychiatry 2006;188:46–50.

42. Peet M, Horrobin DF. A dose-ranging study of the effects of ethyl-eicosapentaenoate in patients with ongoing depression despite apparently adequate treatment with standard drugs. Arch Gen Psychiatry 2002;59(10):913–9.

43. Wozniak J, Biederman J, Mick E, et al. Omega-3 fatty acid monotherapy for pediatric bipolar disorder: a prospective open-label trial. Eur Neuropsychopharmacol 2007;17(6–7):440–7.

44. Willatts P. Long chain polyunsaturated fatty acids improve cognitive development. J Fam Health Care 2002;12(6 Suppl):5.

45. Moore CMB, Janis L, Kukes Thellea J, et al. Effects of *myo*-inositol ingestion on human brain *myo*-inositol levels: a proton magnetic resonance spectroscopic imaging study. Biol Psychiatry 1999;45:1197–202.

46. Moore GJB, Joseph M, Parrish Julieclaire K, et al. Temporal dissociation between lithium-induced changes in frontal lobe *myo*-inositol and clinical response in manic-depressive illness. Am J Psychiatry 1999;156(12):1902–8.

47. Clements RS, Darnell B. *Myo*-inositol content of common foods: development of a high-*myo*-inositol diet. Am J Clin Nutr 1980;33:1954–67.

48. Belmaker RH, Levine J. Inositol in the treatment of psychiatric disorders. In: Mischoulon D, Rosenbaum JF, editors. Natural medications for psychiatry: considering the alternatives. Philadelphia: Lippincott Williams & Wilkins; 2008. p. 111.

49. Baraban JM, Worley PF, Snyder SH. Second messenger systems and psychoactive drug action: focus on the phosphoinositide system and lithium. Am J Psychiatry 1989;146(10):1251–60.

50. Barkai AID, David L, Gross Howard A, et al. Reduced *myo*-inositol levels in cerebrospinal fluid from patients with affective disorder. Biol Psychiatry 1978;13(1): 65–72.

51. Levine JKL, Rapoport A, Zimmerman J, et al. CSF inositol does not predict antidepressant response to inositol. J Neural Transm 1996;103:1457–62.

52. Atack JR, Levine J, Belmaker RH. Cerebrospinal fluid inositol monophosphatase: elevated activity in depression and neuroleptic-treated schizophrenia. Biol Psychiatry 1998;44(6):433–7.

53. Evins EA, Demopulos C, Yovel I, et al. Inositol augmentation of lithium or valproate for bipolar depression. Bipolar Disord 2006;8:168–74.

54. Shimon H, Agam G, Belmaker RH, et al. Reduced frontal cortex inositol levels in postmortem brain of suicide victims and patients with bipolar disorder. Am J Psychiatry 1997;154(8):1148–50.

55. Silverstone PHW, Ren H, O'Donnell Tina, et al. Chronic treatment with both lithium and sodium valproate may normalize phosphoinositol cycle activity in bipolar patients. Hum Psychopharmacol 2002;17:321–7.

56. Berridge MJD, Peter C, Hanley Michael R. Neural and developmental actions of lithium: a unifying hypothesis. Cellule 1989;59:411–9.

57. Einat HK, Karbovski H, Korik J, et al. Inositol reduces depressive-like behaviors in two different animal models of depression. Psychopharmacology 1999;144: 158–62.

58. Levine J. Controlled trials of inositol in psychiatry. Eur Neuropsychopharmacol 1997;7(2):147–55.

59. Belmaker RH, Yuly B, Agam Galila, et al. How does lithium work on manic depression? Clinical and psychological correlates of the inositol theory. Annu Rev Med 1996;47:47–56.

60. Agranoff BWF, Stephen K. Inositol, lithium, and the brain. Psychopharmacol Bull 2001;35(3):5–18.

61. Silverstone PHM, Brent M, Kim Hyeonjin. Bipolar disorder and *myo*-inositol: a review of the magnetic resonance spectroscopy findings. Bipolar Disord 2005;7:1–10.

62. Wolfson M, Bersudsky Y, Hertz E, et al. A model of inositol compartmentation in astrocytes based upon efflux kinetics and slow inositol depletion after uptake inhibition. Neurochem Res 2000;25(7):977–82.

63. Wolfson M, Bersudsky Y, Zinger E, et al. Chronic treatment of human astrocytoma cells with lithium, carbamazepine or valproic acid decreases inositol uptake at high inositol concentrations but increases it at low inositol concentrations. Brain Res 2000;855(1):158–61.

64. Wolfson M, Einat H, Bersudsky Y, et al. Nordidemnin potently inhibits inositol uptake in cultured astrocytes and dose-dependently augments lithium's proconvulsant effect in vivo. J Neurosci Res 2000;60(1):116–21.

65. Kaya NR, Resmi H, Ozerdem A, et al. Increased inositol-monophosphatase activity by lithium treatment in bipolar patients. Prog Neuropsychopharmacol Biol Psychiatry 2004;28(3):521–7.

66. Davanzo PT, Albert M, Yue Kenneth, et al. Decreased anterior cingulate *myo*-inositol/creatine spectroscopy resonance with lithium treatment in children with bipolar disorder. Neuropsychopharmacology 2001;24(4):359–69.

67. Silverstone PH, Hanstock CC, Fabian J, et al. Chronic lithium does not alter human *myo*-inositol or phosphomonoester concentrations as measured by 1H and 31P MRS. Biol Psychiatry 1996;40(4):235–46.

68. Davanzo P, Kenneth Y, Thomas M Albert, et al. Proton magnetic resonance spectroscopy of bipolar disorder versus intermittent explosive disorder in children and adolescents. Am J Psychiatry 2003;160(8):1442–52.

69. Patel NC, DelBello P, Cecil KM, et al. Lithium treatment effects on *myo*-inositol in adolescents with bipolar depression. Biol Psychiatry 2006;60:998–1004.

70. Friedman S, Dager S, Parow A, et al. Lithium and valproic acid treatment effects on brain chemistry in bipolar disorder. Biol Psychiatry 2004;56(5): 340–8.

71. Frey R, Metzler D, Fischer P, et al. *Myo*-inositol in depressive and healthy subjects determined by frontal H-magnetic resonance spectroscopy at 1.5 tesla. J Psychiatr Res 1998;32:411–20.

72. Levine J, Yoram B, Gonzalves Mirtha, et al. Double-blind, controlled trial of inositol treatment of depression. Am J Psychiatry 1995;152(5):792–4.

73. Levine J, Yoram B, Kofman Ora. Follow-up and relapse analysis of an inositol study of depression. Isr J Psychiatry Relat Sci 1995;32(1):14–21.

74. Levine J, Alex M, Susnosky Michael, et al. Combination of inositol and serotonin reuptake inhibitors in the treatment of depression. Biol Psychiatry 1999;45: 270–3.

75. Nemets B, Mishory A, Levine J, et al. Inositol addition does not improve depression in SSRI treatment failures. J Neural Transm 1999;106:795–8.

76. Chengappa KR, Joseph L, Gershon Samuel, et al. Inositol as an add-on treatment for bipolar depression. Bipolar Disord 2000;2(1):47–55.

77. Nierenberg AA, Ostacher MJ, Calabrese JR, et al. Treatment-resistant bipolar depression: a STEP-BD equipoise randomized effectiveness trial of antidepressant augmentation with lamotrigine, inositol, or risperidone. Am J Psychiatry 2006;163(2):210–6.

78. Levine J, Rapaport A, Lev L, et al. Inositol treatment raises CSF inositol levels. Brain Res 1993;627:168–70.

79. Findling RL, McNamara NK, O'Riordan MA, et al. An open-label pilot study of St. John's wort in juvenile depression. J Am Acad Child Adolesc Psychiatry 2003; 42(8):908–14.

80. Butterweck V. Mechanism of action of St John's wort in depression. CNS Drugs 2003;17(8):539–62.

81. Fegert JM, Kolch M, Zito JM, et al. Antidepressant use in children and adolescents in Germany. J Child Adolesc Psychopharmacol 2006;16(1–2):197–206.

82. Nierenberg AA, Lund HG, Mischoulon D. St. John's wort: a critical evaluation of the evidence for antidepressant effects. In: Mischoulon D, Rosenbaum JF, editors. Natural medications for psychiatry: considering the alternatives. Philadelphia: Lippincott Williams & Wilkins; 2008. p. 27–9.

83. Muller WE, Singer A, Wonnemann M, et al. Hyperforin represents the neurotransmitter reuptake inhibiting constituent of hypericum extract. Pharmacopsychiatry 1998;31(1):16–21.

84. Singer A, Wonnemann M, Muller WE. Hyperforin, a major antidepressant constituent of St. John's wort, inhibits serotonin uptake by elevating free intracellular Na. J Pharmacol Exp Ther 1999;290(1363):1–11.

85. Hammerness P, Ethan B, Ulbricht Catherine, et al. St. John's wort: a systematic review of adverse effects and drug interactions for the consultation psychiatrist. Psychosomatics 2003;44(4):271–82.

86. Bennett DA, Phun L, Pold JF, et al. Neuropharmacology of St. John's wort (hypericum). Ann Pharmacother 1998;32:1201–8.

87. Linde K, Knupel K. Large-scale observational studies of hypericum extracts in patients with depressive disorders - a systematic review. Phytomedicine 2005; 12(1–2):148–57.

88. Linde K, Mulrow CD, Berner M, et al. St. John's wort for depression. Cochrane Database Syst Rev 2005;18(2):1–70.

89. Simeon J, Nixon MK, Milin Robert, et al. Open-label pilot study of St. John's wort in adolescent depression. J Child Adolesc Psychopharmacol 2005;15(2):293–301.

90. Hubner W-D, Tilman K. Experience with St. John's wort (hypericum perforatum) in children under 12 years with symptoms of depression and psychovegetative disturbances. Phytother Res 2001;15:367–70.

91. Wurglics M, Westerhoff K, Kaunzinger A, et al. Comparison of German St. John's wort products according to hyperforin and total hypericin content. J Am Pharm Assoc (Wash) 2001;41(4):560–6.

92. Knuppel LL, Linde K. Adverse effects of St. John's wort: a systematic review. J Clin Psychiatry 2004;65(11):1470–9.

93. Brockmoller J, Reum T, Bauer S, et al. Hypericin and pseudohypericin: pharmacokinetics and effects on photosensitivity in humans. Pharmacopsychiatry 1997; 30(2):94–101.

94. Fahmi M, Huang C, Schweitzer I. A case of mania induced by hypericum. World J Biol Psychiatry 2002;3(1):58–9.

95. Nierenberg AA, Tal B, Matthews John, et al. Mania associated with St. John's wort. Biol Psychiatry 1999;46:1707–8.

96. Hauben M. The association of St. John's wort with elevated thyroid-stimulating hormone. Pharmacotherapy 2002;22(5):673–5.

97. Ferko NL, Mitchell AH. Evaluation of the association between St. John's wort and elevated thyroid-stimulating hormone. Pharmacotherapy 2001;21(12):1574–8.

98. Karalapillai DC, Bellomo R. Convulsions associated with an overdose of St. John's wort. Med J Aust 2007;186(4):213–4.

99. Whitten DL, Myers SP, Hawrelak JA, et al. The effect of St John's wort extracts on CYP3A: a systematic review of prospective clinical trials. Br J Clin Pharmacol 2006;62(5):512–26.

100. Zhou SF, Lai X. An update on clinical drug interactions with the herbal antidepressant St. John's wort. Curr Drug Metab 2008;9(5):394–409.

101. Markowitz JSD, Jennifer L, DeVane C, et al. Effect of St John's wort on drug metabolism by induction of cytochrome p450 3a4 enzyme. J Am Med Assoc 2003;290(11):1500–4.

102. Alpert JE, Papakostas GI, Mischoulon D. One-carbon metabolism and the treatment of depression: roles of S-Adenosyl-L-Methionine and folate. In: Mischoulon D, Rosenbaum JF, editors. Natural medications for psychiatry: considering the alternatives. Philadelphia: Lippincott Williams & Wilkins; 2008. p. 69.

103. Mischoulon DF, Fava M. Role of S-adenosyl-L-methionine in the treatment of depression: a review of the evidence. Am J Clin Nutr 2002;76:1158S–61S.

104. Saletu B, Peter A, di Padova C, et al. Gerda maria, electrophysiological neuroimaging of the central effects of S-adenosyl-L-methionine by mapping of electroencephalograms and event-related potentials and low-resolution brain electromagnetic tomography. Am J Clin Nutr 2002;76:1162S–71S.

105. Baldessarini R. Neuropharmacology of S-adenosyl-L-methionine. Am J Med 1987;83(5A):95–103.

106. Bottiglieri T, Godfrey P, Flynn T, et al. Cerebrospinal fluid S-adenosylmethionine in depression and dementia: effects of treatment with parental and oral S-adenosylmethionine. J Neurol Neurosurg Psychiatr 1990;53:1096–8.

107. Bell KM, Potkin SG, Carreon D, et al. S-adenosylmethionine blood levels in major depression: changes with drug treatment. Acta Neurol Scand 1994;154:15–8.
108. Williams A-I, Christine G, Jui Danny, et al. S-Adenosylmethionine (SAMe) as treatment for depression: a systematic review. Clin Invest Med 2005;28(3):132–9.
109. Hardy M, Coulter I, Morton SC, et al. S-adenosyl-L-methionine for treatment of depression, osteoarthritis, and liver disease. Complimentary and Alternative Medicine, 2002.
110. Schaller J, John T, Bazzan Anthony J. SAMe use in children and adolescents. Eur Child Adolesc Psychiatry 2004;13:332–4.
111. Goren JL, Stoll AL, Damico KE, et al. Bioavailability and lack of toxicity of S-Adenosyl-L-Methionine (SAMe) in humans. Pharmacotherapy 2004;24(11): 1501–7.
112. Alpert JE, George P, Mischoulon David, et al. S-Adenosyl-L-Methionine (SAMe) as an adjunct for resistant major depressive disorder. J Clin Psychopharmacol 2004;24(6):661–4.
113. Carney MW, Chary TK, Bottiglieri T, et al. The switch mechanism and the bipolar/unipolar dichotomy. Br J Psychiatry 1989;154:48–51.
114. Iruela LM, Minguez L, Merino J, et al. Toxic interaction of S-adenosylmethionine and clomipramine. Am J Psychiatry 1993;150(3):522.
115. Thomas CS, Bottiglieri T, Edeh J, et al. The influence of S-adenosylmethionine (SAM) on prolactin in depressed patients. Int Clin Psychopharmacol 1987; 2(2):97–102.
116. Fava MR, Jerrold F, MacLaughlin Robert, et al. Neuroendocrine effects of S-Adenosyl-L-Methionine, a novel putative antidepressant. J Psychiatr Res 1990;24(2):177–84.
117. Zhdanova IV. Melatonin as a hypnotic: pro. Sleep Med Rev 2005;9(1):51–65.
118. Zhdanova IV, Friedman L. Therapeutic potential of melatonin in sleep and circadian disorders. In: Mischoulon D, Rosenbaum JF, editors. Natural medications for psychiatry: considering the alternatives. Philadelphia: Lippincott Williams & Wilkins; 2008. p. 144.
119. Waldhauser F, Weiszenbacher G, Frisch H, et al. Fall in nocturnal serum melatonin during prepuberty and pubescence. Lancet 1984;1(8373):362–5.
120. Commentz JC, Uhlig H, Henke A, et al. Melatonin and 6-hydroxymelatonin sulfate excretion is inversely correlated with gonadal development in children. Horm Res 1997;47(3):97–101.
121. Leibenluft E, Feldman- NS, Turner EH, et al. Effects of exogenous melatonin administration and withdrawal in five patients with rapid-cycling bipolar disorder. J Clin Psychiatry 1997;58:383–8.
122. Lewy AJ, Nurnberger JI Jr, Wehr TA, et al. Supersensitivity to light: possible trait marker for manic-depressive illness. Am J Psychiatry 1985;142(6):725–7.
123. Nurnberger JI Jr, Wade B, Tamarkin Lawrence, et al. Supersensitivity to melatonin suppression by light in young people at high risk for affective disorder. Neuropsychopharmacology 1988;1(3):217–23.
124. Nathan PJ, Burrows GD, Norman TR. Melatonin sensitivity to dim white light in affective disorders. Neuropsychopharmacology 1999;21:408–13.
125. Lam RW, Alan L B, Berga Sarah L, et al. Melatonin suppression in bipolar and unipolar mood disorders. Psychiatry Res 1990;33:129–34.
126. Whalley LJ, Tony P, Shering Anne, et al. Melatonin response to bright light in recovered, drug-free, bipolar patients. Psychiatry Res 1991;38:13–9.
127. Bersani G, Alessandra G. Melatonin add-on in manic patients with treatment resistant insomnia. Prog Neuropsychopharmacol Biol Psychiatry 2000;24:185–91.

128. Robertson JM, Tanguay PE. Case study: the use of melatonin in a boy with refractory bipolar disorder. J Am Acad Child Adolesc Psychiatry 1997;36(6):822–5.
129. Buscemi N, Vandermeer B, Hooton N, et al. The efficacy and safety of exogenous melatonin for primary sleep disorders. A meta-analysis. J Gen Intern Med 2005;20(12):1151–8.
130. Buscemi N, et al. Efficacy and safety of exogenous melatonin for secondary sleep disorders and sleep disorders accompanying sleep restriction: meta-analysis. BMJ 2006;332(7538):385–93.
131. Available at: www.naturaldatabase.com. Accessed October 21, 2008.
132. Cavallo A. Melatonin and human puberty: current perspectives. J Pineal Res 2007;15(3):115–21.
133. Sheldon SH. Pro-convulsant effects of oral melatonin in neurologically disabled children. Lancet 1998;351:1254.
134. Wood JL, Allison RG. Effects of consumption of choline and lecithin on neurobiological and cardiovascular systems. Fed Proc 1982;41(14):3015–21.
135. Cooper A, Odle Teresa. Gale encyclopedia of alternative medicine. Detroit, MI: The Gale Group Inc.; 2005.
136. Rosenberg GSD, Kenneth L. The use of cholinergic precursors in neuropsychiatric diseases. Am J Clin Nutr 1982;36:709–20.
137. Janowsky DS, John M D, El-Yousef Khaled M, et al. A cholinergic-adrenergic hypothesis of mania and depression. Lancet 1972;2(7778):632–5.
138. Cecil KM, DelBello MP, Morey R, et al. Frontal lobe differences in bipolar disorder as determined by proton MR spectroscopy. Bipolar Disord 2002;4:357–65.
139. Wurtman RL, H Madelyn J, Growdon John H. Lecithin consumption rises serum-free choline levels. Lancet 1977;2:68–9.
140. Cohen BM, L Joseph F, Altesman Richard I. Lecithin in the treatment of mania: double-blind, placebo-controlled trials. Am J Psychiatry 1982;139(9):1162–4.
141. Cohen BM, Miller AL, Lipinski JF, et al. Lecithin in mania: a preliminary report. Am J Psychiatry 1980;137(2):242–3.
142. Schreier HA. Mania responsive to lecithin in a 13-year-old girl. Am J Psychiatry 1981;139(1):108–10.
143. Wang H, Hong Q, Wang Bai-song, et al. Is acupuncture beneficial in depression? A meta-analysis of 8 randomized controlled trials. J Affect Disord 2008;111:1–10.
144. Ahn AC. Acupuncture Up To Date Online 16.2, 2008 May. Accessed October 11, 2008.
145. Samuels N, Cornelius G, Singer Shepherd Roee, et al. Acupuncture for psychiatric illness: a literature review. Behav Med 2008;34:55–62.
146. Medicine, N.C.f.C.a.A. Available at: http://nccam.nih.gov/health/acupuncture/. Accessed October 9, 2008.
147. Yeung A, Schnyer RN, Yantao Ma, et al. Acupuncture for the treatment of psychiatric disorders. In: Mischoulon D, Rosenbaum JF, editors. Natural medications for psychiatry: considering the alternatives. Philadelphia: Lippincott Williams and Wilkins; 2008. p. 291.
148. Hu J. Acupuncture treatment of manic psychosis. J Tradit Chin Med 1996;16(3):238–40.
149. Ding D. Personal experience in acupuncture treatment of mental diseases. J Tradit Chin Med 2001;21(4):277–81.
150. Suppes T, Bersntein I, Dennehy E, et al. The safety, acceptability, and effectiveness of acupuncture as adjunctive treatment for bipolar disorder, in review.
151. Leo RJ, Ligot JS Jr. A systematic review of randomized controlled trials of acupuncture in the treatment of depression. J Affect Disord 2007;97:13–22.

152. Kemper KJ, Rebecca S, Silver-Highfield Ellen, et al. On pins and needles? Pediatric pain patients' experience with acupuncture. Pediatrics 2000;105(4):941–7.
153. Ernst EW, Adrian R. Prospective studies of the safety of acupuncture: a systematic review. Am J Med 2001;110:481–5.
154. Melchart D, Weidenhammer W, Streng A, et al. Prospective investigation of adverse effects of acupuncture in 97,733 patients. Arch Intern Med 2004;164: 104–5.
155. Guidelines on basic training and safety in acupuncture. Geneva: World Health Organization; 1999. p.1–31.
156. Kemper KJ, Scott S. Complementary and alternative medicine therapies to promote healthy moods. Pediatr Clin North Am 2007;54:901–26.
157. Ortega FB, Ruiz JR, Castillo MJ, et al. Physical fitness in childhood and adolescence: a powerful marker of health. Int J Obes (Lond) 2008;32(1):1–11.
158. Stathopoulou G, Powers MB, Berry AC, et al. Exercise interventions for mental health: a quantitative and qualitative review. Clin Psychol (New York) 2006;13: 179–93.
159. Lawlor DA, Hopker SW. The effectiveness of exercise as an intervention in the management of depression: systematic review and meta-regression analysis of randomised controlled trials. BMJ 2001;322(7289):763–7.
160. Kilbourne AM, Rofey DL, McCarthy JF, et al. Nutrition and exercise behavior among patients with bipolar disorder. Bipolar Disord 2007;9(5):443–52.
161. Dunn AL, Trivedi MH, Kampert JB, et al. Exercise treatment for depression: efficacy and dose response. Am J Prev Med 2005;28(1):1–8.
162. Jones NA, Field T. Massage and music therapies attenuate frontal EEG asymmetry in depressed adolescents. Adolescence 1999;34(135):529–34.
163. Field T, Morrow C, Valdeon C, et al. Massage reduces anxiety in child and adolescent psychiatric patients. J Am Acad Child Adolesc Psychiatry 1992; 31(1):125–31.
164. Khilnani S, Tiffany F, Hernandez-Reif Maria, et al. Massage therapy improves mood and behavior of students with attention-deficit/hyperactivity disorder. Adolescence 2003;38(152):623–38.
165. von Knorring AL, Soderberg A, Austin L, et al. Massage decreases aggression in preschool children: a long-term study. Acta Paediatr 2008;97(9):1265–9.
166. Coelho BS, Moyer CA. Randomized control trials of pediatric massage: a review. eCAM 2008;4:23–34.
167. Kaplan BJ, Crawford SG, Field CJ, et al. Vitamins, minerals, and mood. Psychol Bull 2007;133(5):747–60.
168. Naylor GJ, Smith AH. Vanadium: a possible aetiological factor in manic-depressive illness. Psychol Med 1981;11(2):249–56.
169. Goggans FC. A case of mania secondary to vitamin B12 deficiency. Am J Psychiatry 1984;141(2):300–1.
170. Amann BL, Mergl R, Vieta E, et al. A 2-year open-label pilot study of adjunctive chromium in patients with treatment-resistant rapid-cycling bipolar disorder. J Clin Psychopharmacol 2007;27(1):104–6.
171. Nechifor M. Interactions between magnesium and psychotropic drugs. Magnes Res 2008;21(2):97–100.
172. Heiden A, Frey R, Presslich O, et al. Treatment of severe mania with intravenous magnesium sulphate as a supplementary therapy. Psychiatry Res 1999;89: 239–46.
173. Lakhan SE, Vieira KF. Nutritional therapies for mental disorders. Nutr J 2008; 7(2).

174. Chouinard Gea. Tryptophan in the treatment of depression and mania. Recent Adv Biol Psychiatry 1983;10:46–66.
175. Sabelli HC, Fawcett J, Gusovsky F, et al. Clinical studies on the phenylethylamine hypothesis of affective disorder: urine and blood phenylacetic acid and phenylalanine dietary supplements. J Clin Psychiatry 1986;47(2):66–70.
176. Kaplan BJ, Fisher JE, Crawford SG, et al. Case report: improved mood and behavior during treatment with a mineral-vitamin supplement: an open-label case series of children. J Child Adolesc Psychopharmacol 2004;14(1):115–22.

Raising a Bipolar Child: A Family Perspective

Susan Resko, MM

KEYWORDS

• Childhood • Bipolar • Families

This article is intended to provide parents perspective on bipolar disorder in children and adolescents as is gathered from the experience of countless parents who participate in the activities of the organization known as the Child & Adolescent Bipolar Foundation (CABF; www.bpkids.org).

THE ROCKY ROAD TO THE PSYCHIATRIST'S OFFICE

By the time parents cross the threshold of a child psychiatrist's office with concerns about their child's behavior, they have traveled a long, twisted, and rocky road. While pregnant, a mother hopes and prays that her child will be born healthy; many worst-case scenarios may run through her mind about conditions, diseases, and deformities that might afflict her unborn child. Unless there is a strong family history of a *diagnosed* mental illness, seldom does a mother include bipolar disorder in her list of fears for her unborn child. It is hard for our society to fathom that a child's brain, just like any other organ of the body, is susceptible to illness. Although each decade brings new understanding about the diagnosis and treatment of mental illness, the general public still perceives that environment—parenting styles, socioeconomic conditions, and a supportive community—are the *sole* determinants of a child's behavior. We just cannot seem to grasp the concept that a child's behavior can be affected by an illness of the brain.

Perception is reality; our society first looks to the influences in a child's life to find blame for a child's baffling behavior. At ground zero is the parent. Just as *refrigerator mothers* were blamed for their autistic child's withdrawn and out-of-touch behavior several decades ago, we still blame mothers for a bipolar child's rages. *What is going on at home?* is often the first question parents receive from teachers, clinicians, and family members. Even the most well-adjusted mother soon feels like a *bad mom* and the subject of intense scrutiny rivaling that for a presidential candidate or an A-list celebrity.

Funding for this chapter was provided by the generous donations to the Child and Adolescent Bipolar Foundation. CABF neither seeks nor accepts support from the pharmaceutical industry. Child and Adolescent Bipolar Foundation, 1000 Skokie Boulevard, Suite 570, Wilmette, IL 60091, USA
E-mail address: sresko@bpkids.org

Child Adolesc Psychiatric Clin N Am 18 (2009) 515–521
doi:10.1016/j.chc.2008.12.001
1056-4993/08/$ – see front matter © 2009 Elsevier Inc. All rights reserved.

childpsych.theclinics.com

Parents also question what they could be doing wrong. They go to bookstores and libraries to find the answer in the latest parenting books. Yet today's *Dr. Phil*-type instant solutions to problems do not even scratch the surface of the complex challenges parents of children with bipolar disorder face.

Parents spend countless hours hovering outside classrooms, often unable to leave the school building due to their child's intense separation anxiety, or because they fear they may need to retrieve the child early. There is a revolving door outside school administrator's offices for parents of a bipolar child. Many parents report that their child has been kicked out of one if not several schools.

I find it almost comically ironic that Ryan was rejected even from residential treatment center.

—A CABF mom

Parents struggle, often in isolation, for years before they seek the advice of a child psychiatrist. For a parent, it is akin to a colonoscopy or oral surgery—deny, delay, and defer. They will seek the advice of any professional other than one who prescribes psychiatric medications; *I'm NOT putting MY child on psychotropics* is a common thought.

The media does not help to alleviate parents' angst. Almost without exception when the media reports on the use of psychiatric medications in children, it is prefaced with the words *powerful* or *mind-altering*. Very rarely do we see those adjectives used when describing the same medications for adult use or when toxic cancer-fighting medications are prescribed to children.

Further, recent headlines regarding pharmaceutical industry funding to psychiatric physicians, researchers, and advocacy groups have focused on the possibility of conflicts of interest—either real or perceived. When this controversy involves children, it is enough to give even the most well-informed parent pause.

Therefore, it is with much trepidation that a parent brings a child to a psychiatrist. The length of time between experiencing the first nagging thoughts that their child might have serious issues to the time they schedule an appointment varies from person to person, but the feelings they experience on the road to the psychiatrist's door are very similar.

FIRST STEPS

Parents with concerns about their child's extreme behaviors should consider the following steps:

- If the child is not safe, including if they are psychotic, suicidal, or menacing others: take him or her to the emergency room or call 911 for an ambulance (stress that the child needs medical care and an ambulance should be sent). If they are alone, they should also call a friend or relative to help immediately.
- Ensure the safety of the family. Find safe havens for siblings. Remove all firearms from the home (this is a matter of life and death, not a political statement). Lock up sharps (knives, razors, whatever). Lock up all prescription and over-the-counter medications. Childproof the home, no matter what the physical age of your child.
- Start a mood chart for your child. Make daily notes of the child's mood, behavior, sleep patterns, events, and medications. Include statements by the child that seem odd or concerning. Share notes with treatment professionals.

- Compile a brief family history on both sides. Include family members who have abused alcohol or drugs. Include family members who have been diagnosed with mood disorders, bipolar disorder, or other psychiatric diagnoses. Remember that even if a family member was not diagnosed, it may be a critical link if that person was hospitalized, attempted or completed suicide, or has a history of numerous marriages, employment instability, fighting, or reckless behavior.
- Keep a notebook or file of records of each doctor visit and results of laboratory tests. This notebook will be a good place to keep a list of all medications the child has trialed, the dates, the doses, and the effects. Mood charts and family history data can also be stored in this notebook.
- Join the CABF and connect with other parents who understand and can offer support.
- Parents are advised to take care of themselves! Remember the flight attendant's safety talk on the airplane: Put on your oxygen mask first so that you are in a position to put your children's masks on. Reduce stress, address your own mental health issues, and exercise.[1]
- Brothers and sisters are *always* affected when a sibling has bipolar disorder, and it is vital to tend to them too. They have gotten less of their parents' time and attention because their ill sibling has required so much, and they probably endured an unpredictable and sometimes threatening home environment. They may be sad, resentful, or angry, or they may hide their trauma and try to be the perfect child. They may develop anxiety, depression, eating disorders, self-injurious behaviors, or hostility toward their ill sibling or parents. Parents and psychiatrists must carefully assess how the "well" children are faring, even if they seem on the surface to be functioning well.

COMING OUT OF THE CLOSET

Once parents accept the fact that their child needs treatment, the journey is only just beginning. Many parents feel shame and stigma about their child's baffling behavior or the mere fact that their child has a psychiatric illness. We live in a society where blame is still affixed to psychiatric illness; parents of children with bipolar disorder are not big fans of Freud. It is very hard for parents to come out of the closet about their child's illness with friends, family, and school. When stigma triumphs over forthrightness, recovery and stability will be harder to reach.

> *Don't tell anyone that Johnny is really at a Residential Treatment Center; I've told everyone he's at boarding school.*
> —*A CABF member*

Some parents think they are doing their children a favor by keeping the illness private; they do not want their child to be labeled. Just as we kept epilepsy secret a generation ago, so do parents of children with severe psychiatric illness feel the need to protect their children by staying private. This shame and secrecy exacerbate the burden of parenting a child with bipolar disorder. Only through education and public awareness will parents feel safe to share the information with the people in their children's life. In doing so, they will find the enormous weight of secrecy lifted.

WELL-MEANING FRIENDS

While some parents never feel secure enough to come out of the closet, others gingerly take baby steps to share their problems with friends. Often, however, they receive meaningless advice such as "Your child just needs more love/discipline/

structure," or they endure admonishments for reaching for a medicinal quick fix from those who do not "believe in" psychotropic medications.

Many friends just do not "get it." They try to empathize in ways that make matters worse.

Katie never really connected with kids in her homeroom; I wouldn't worry so much about your son's lack of friends in homeroom.
—Advice from the mother of a daughter playing varsity hockey at an elite private east coast college to a mother whose son was facing residential treatment for severe depression.

It is difficult to imagine the enormity of the situation these families face unless you have walked in their shoes. They find themselves isolating themselves even further, because it hurts to hear the chatter of other moms in the carpool line as they discuss the current season's sports tryouts, play practice, or childhood milestones.

I just can't bear volunteering over at school and listening to the other moms talk. They whine and complain about the smallest issues. I wish Evan had the problems their children face.
—A mother of a suicide survivor

A SAFE HARBOR

Parents of children with bipolar disorder search unremittingly for understanding and compassion. Often, they turn to the Internet for answers and a place they can connect with other parents who walk in their shoes while in the privacy of their own homes. The CABF is a national not-for-profit organization dedicated to improving the lives of families, children, and teens living with bipolar disorder, depression, and related conditions. CABF offers resources, connection, and hope to families and teens who are struggling with mood disorders, often in isolation. CABF combats stigma by bringing mental illness into the light of public discourse through advocacy and education.

CABF supports thousands of families through its parent-to-parent network—Internet-based support programs designed to connect parents.

I understand; I've been there. Let me tell you what worked for my child.
—A CABF forum posting

CABF's online format utilizes message board forums, listservs, and digital chats and is available 24/7, requires no travel, speeds learning, and offers privacy. Most importantly, parents with ill, unstable children find it virtually impossible to leave the home to attend traditional, in-person support groups.

The model that CABF has used for the past decade works. Online delivery of support and resources is a cost-effective and highly accessible means of delivering needed services. According to a study conducted by Mary Fristad, PhD at The Ohio State University, CABF's online support programs help to end isolation, help parents recognize and obtain good treatment for their children, provide faster diagnosis from onset of symptoms to treatment, provide hope, and may improve outcomes for children.[2]

BRACE YOURSELF

Many parents complain that their child received multiple diagnoses before they landed on bipolar disorder. Parents want answers for their children, and they want to know the name of the demon they are facing. I recommend that you prepare any patient's parents to brace themselves for several changes in diagnoses, treatment plans, and courses of action. Although we have made great strides in understanding psychiatric illness in children, we still have much to learn. I tell parents that until there is a biological marker that can help aid clinicians in making more accurate diagnoses, it is par for the course for a child to have an alphabet soup of disorders. Just because clinicians may disagree on a child's diagnosis, it does not necessarily mean that one is right and another is wrong. Developing brains, immature emotional systems, and lack of biological markers make psychiatric diagnosis especially tricky in children. I tell parents to focus on outcomes and on providing accurate feedback to clinicians.

Bipolar disorder often involves comorbid disorders. In some children, proper treatment for bipolar disorder clears up the symptoms thought to indicate another diagnosis. In other children, bipolar disorder may explain only part of a more complicated case that includes neurologic, developmental, and other components. An accurate diagnosis of a child or teen presenting with severely troubled behavior is perhaps the most problematic issue facing families.[1]

After a decade of visiting the best experts around the country and countless medication trials, we still don't know if Will has Bipolar Disorder II or Major Depression.
—*A CABF dad*

THE GREAT DEBATE

There is little debate that bipolar disorder can emerge in childhood among well-informed physicians; the study results are definitive. Some ill children meet the textbook definition of bipolar disorder. Others with severe mood dysregulation might not meet the textbook definition, because they do not have distinct episodes of a certain duration or have few clear periods of wellness between episodes. They might have rapid and severe cycling between moods, or they might present in a mixed state that produces chronic irritability. Experts have not yet reached consensus as to whether children with chronic irritability and clear mood swings, but without elation, should be classified as having bipolar disorder.[1]

We have much ground to gain in finding consensus about how to accurately diagnose bipolar disorder in children, and about its manifestations, prevalence rates, and courses of treatment. Popular culture has won the battle over libraries in educating American parents. One could argue that bipolar disorder in children has become the diagnosis *du jour*. Many well-intentioned clinicians rail against the diagnosis because of the increased focus and attention it has received.

No matter where you position yourself in the great debate, we cannot forget that these children are seriously ill and deserve treatment.

A BITTER PILL

Common outcomes of pediatric bipolar disorder are school refusal, suspension, and dropping out; impulsive acts of aggression; self-injury; substance abuse; and suicide attempts and completions. Teens with symptoms of untreated bipolar disorder are arrested and incarcerated in alarming numbers. Suicide is the third leading cause of death among teens. Children as young as 6 years have attempted to hang, shoot, stab, or overdose themselves.[1]

The best treatment for pediatric bipolar disorder includes medication, therapy, lifestyle changes, and educational accommodations. Although you are primarily responsible for the first part, you can make an enormous difference in the outcome of your patients' well-being by spending a few minutes discussing the other treatments with your patients and their families at each visit. Refer your parents to resources, such as CABF's Web site, that can help significantly.

It is important for parents to realize that the worst outcome for a child with bipolar disorder is death, either by suicide, risk-taking behavior, or a cry for help gone horribly wrong. Events such as being open with friends and family about the illness, a move to an alternative school, hospitalization, residential treatment, incarceration, or even custody relinquishment are NOT the worst possible outcomes. After a decade of sharing stories with parents of children with bipolar disorder, I view many of these events as opportunities for children to gain a higher level of wellness. It is far from easy to view these events as *gifts,* but once a diagnosis is made, parents should be told that many of these events are not the exception, but the rule, and can actually speed their child's path along the road to wellness. The events that so many parents most fear can actually be the turning point in their children's lives.

This vantage point does not come easily, however, and it is sometimes only through years of struggle that parents realize that a more structured environment will improve their child's health. Many parents abhor the idea of making a change that will be perceived as less than "normal." For some parents, there is a defining moment that makes it obvious that further intervention is required; for others that realization never comes. However, just as parents of children with cancer are educated that with treatment often comes hair loss, nausea, and so on, so must parents of children with bipolar disorder be educated about the pain and discomfort their children's treatment might include. In this case, it is the emotional pain of making the tough decisions about a more restrictive environment.

Conversely, many parents recognize that changes in their child's environment are necessary, but they do not have the resources to access treatment. CABF's website at www.bpkids.org is replete with information including the following:

- Educational rights and how to effectively work with the school district to access treatment
- State-by-state directory of treatment professionals, state resources, advocates, and schools
- Professionally supervised parent-to-parent support
- Moderated real-time chats with treatment experts
- A section for teens, including a weekly audio podcast
- A library with journal articles, books, tips, and guides.

I knew for several years that my daughter needed residential treatment, but we could not afford it. After speaking with another CABF mom, I learned that there was an excellent RTC [residential treatment center] the cost of which my insurance plan covered 90% with no time limit! My daughter is getting the care she needs, my family is healing and we look forward to a healthier, happier child to return home.

—A CABF mom

Childhood is a window of opportunity in which parents have the chance to provide treatment that may profoundly benefit their children's development and save their children's lives. *Now* is the time to help establish as firm a foundation as possible for your patients to reach adulthood and be able to make sound independent judgments.[1]

OTHER RECENT REFERENCES HELPFUL FOR FAMILIES

Child & Adolescent Bipolar Foundation. Available at: www.bpkids.org.
American Academy of Child and Adolescent Psychiatry. Available at: www.aacap.org.
Bazelon Center for Mental Health Law. Available at: www.bazelon.org.

McDonnell MA, Wozniak J. Is your child bipolar? The definitive resource on how to identify, treat, and thrive with a bipolar child. New York: Bantam; 2008.

National Association of Therapeutic Schools and Programs (NATSAP). Available at: www.natsap.org.

National Institute of Mental Health (NIMH). Available at: www.nimh.nih.gov.

Pavuluri M. What works for bipolar kids: help and hope for parents. New York: Guilford Press; 2008.

Wrightslaw: special education law, education law, and advocacy for children with disabilities. Available at: www.wrightslaw.com.

REFERENCES

1. About pediatric bipolar disorder. Wilmette (IL): Child & Adolescent Bipolar Foundation; 2008. Available at: www.bpkids.org.
2. Bipolar disorder in childhood and early adolescence. In: Geller B, Del Bello MP, editors. New York: Guilford Press; 2003.

Index

Note: Page numbers of article titles are in **boldface** type.

A

Abuse, substance, bipolar disorder and, 284–285

Acupuncture, in bipolar disorder management, 499–500

S-Adenosyl-L-methionine, in bipolar disorder management, 493–495

ADHD. See *Attention-deficit hyperactivity disorder (ADHD).*

Adolescent(s), SUDs in, genes and, 301–302

Affect regulation
    basics of, 406–409
    brain regions implicated in, 408
    in bipolar disorder, **405–420**
        depression, 411
        described, 411–414
        euphoria, 410–411
        future research in, 414–415
        irritability, 410
    in typical development, 409–410
    sleep in, importance of, 324

Age, suicidality in bipolar disorder related to, 341

Anxiety disorders, bipolar disorder with, 302–307

Aripiprazole, for bipolar mania, 459

Artaeus of Cappadocia, in bipolar disorder, 258

Attention-deficit hyperactivity disorder (ADHD), bipolar disorder with, 293–295

B

Beck's Children's Depression Inventory, 265

Bedtime worry, sleep disturbance due to, 331–332

Behavioral problems, bipolar disorder and, 284–285

Biological factors, suicidality in bipolar disorder related to, 343

Bipolar controversy, birth of, 262–267

Bipolar depression, treatment of, 461–462

Bipolar disorder, **273–289**
    adults with, sleep disturbance in, current options and practices, 326–327
    affect regulation in, **405–420.** See also *Affect regulation, in bipolar disorder.*
    assessment of, **353–390**
        checklists in, 363–365, 376–377
        clinician ratings in, 376
        course specifiers in, 356–357
        cross-informant issues in, 372
        crossing treatment threshold in, 372–373
        developmental history in, 375
        diagnoses in, 355–356

Child Adolesc Psychiatric Clin N Am 18 (2009) 523–531

doi:10.1016/S1056-4993(09)00011-X

childpsych.theclinics.com

1056-4993/09/$ – see front matter © 2009 Elsevier Inc. All rights reserved.

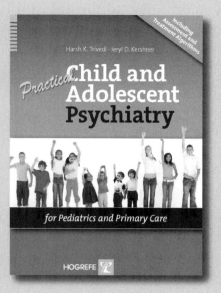
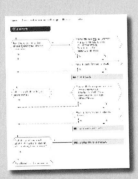
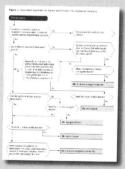
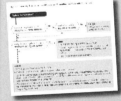
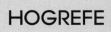